The Living Cleanse

Detoxification and Cleansing Using Living Foods and Safe Natural Strategies

By Case Adams, Naturopath

The Living Cleanse: Detoxification and Cleansing Using Living Foods and Safe
    Natural Strategies
Copyright © 2011, 2014 Casey Adams
LOGICAL BOOKS
Wilmington, Delaware
http://www.logicalbooks.org
All rights reserved.
Printed in USA
Front cover image © Dmitry

Publishers Cataloging in Publication Data
Adams, Casey
The Living Cleanse: Detoxification and Cleansing Using Living Foods
    and Safe Natural Strategies
First Edition
1. Medicine. 2. Health.
Bibliography and References; Index

ISBN-13: 978-1-936251-47-6

Other Books by the Author:

ARTHRITIS – THE BOTANICAL SOLUTION: Nature's Answer to Rheumatoid Arthritis, Osteoarthritis, Gout and Other Forms of Arthritis

ASTHMA SOLVED NATURALLY: The Surprising Underlying Causes and Hundreds of Natural Strategies to Beat Asthma

BREATHING TO HEAL: The Science of Healthy Respiration

ELECTROMAGNETIC HEALTH: Making Sense of the Research and Practical Solutions for Electromagnetic Fields (EMF) and Radio Frequencies (RF)

HAY FEVER AND ALLERGIES: Discovering the Real Culprits and Natural Solutions for Reversing Allergic Rhinitis

HEALTHY SUN: Healing with Sunshine and the Myths about Skin Cancer

HEARTBURN SOLVED: How to Reverse Acid Reflux and GERD Naturally

LIVING IMMUNITY: Supercharging Our Body's Defenses with Probiotics and Other Natural Strategies

NATURAL SLEEP SOLUTIONS FOR INSOMNIA: The Science of Sleep, Dreaming, and Nature's Sleep Remedies

NATURAL SOLUTIONS FOR FOOD ALLERGIES AND FOOD INTOLERANCES: Scientifically Proven Remedies for Food Sensitivities

ORAL PROBIOTICS: The Newest Way to Prevent Infection, Boost the Immune System and Fight Disease

PROBIOTICS: Protection Against Infection

PURE WATER: The Science of Water, Waves, Water Pollution, Water Treatment, Water Therapy and Water Ecology

THE ANCESTORS DIET: Living and Cultured Foods to Extend Life, Prevent Disease and Lose Weight

THE CONSCIOUS ANATOMY: Healing the Real You

THE SCIENCE OF LEAKY GUT SYNDROME: Intestinal Permeability and Digestive Health

TOTAL HARMONIC: The Healing Power of Nature's Elements

Table of Contents

Introduction

There are some intense cleansing programs offered out there. And they probably do provide detoxification, too. But this doesn't mean they make that much difference. That's because most cleansing programs are short lived. In other words, they are not sustained, while our the toxins in our environment continue to bombard us.

It is not as if we stop absorbing the toxins around us after the cleanse is over. Our bodies will continue to absorb toxins, and will continue to accumulate those toxins after the cleanse. This will produce an even greater risk of those accumulated toxins damaging our tissues.

Yes, we could maintain a regular cleansing program on a periodical basis. And this is probably good too. But in between those cleanses, toxins will still burden us, and damage our tissues. And the periodic cleansing will not reverse the damage done between the cleanses.

On a practical basis, most cleanses are not done periodically anyway. They might be done once or twice at the most. This infrequency might even do more harm than good; as we become lulled into a false sense of security.

Let's review some of the reasons most cleansing/detox programs are not sustained:

Most cleansing and detoxification systems are too complicated. They require an intense knowledge of nutritional components, herbs and recipes. The reason many of these cleansing plans are so complicated is because their developers are trying to create a proprietary system. Proprietary means that the program must have some complexity. Complexity produces uniqueness, which can in turn be patented and/or trademarked.

Most cleansing and detox systems require too much discipline. They require routines that are difficult to apply to our normal waking lives. Some of these routines require regimented times of action that may or may not apply to our daily obligations. They may also take a significant amount of time for preparation. In addition, many of these programs remove the possibility of going out to eat, simply because they involve programs that disallow eating foods that most other people eat.

Many cleansing and detox systems are too expensive. They require us to buy certain supplements and herbal combinations, often at riduculous prices. This is applicable to many of the colon cleanse herbal remedies. Some even cost hundreds of dollars for the same herbs that can be picked up at the health food bulk bin for a couple of bucks—or grown in our garden for pennies. Some cleansing protocols are put forth by those selling these formulations. Their websites and books often serve as advertising methods.

Most cleansing and detoxification protocols are unsafe. They push the body's detoxification systems too quickly, resulting in acidosis. Acidosis can cause dizziness, fainting and a number of other conditions.

Furthermore, many cleansing and detoxification systems produce a significant amount of toxin breakdown, followed by a re-accumulation of toxins.

This requires that we undergo one of these cleanses every month or two—an expensive and complicated process for most.

The program laid out in this text is not complicated. It does not require extreme discipline. And it certainly is not expensive. It can be applied to most lifestyles, and its ingredients are easily obtained.

Furthermore, significant research has indicated the protocols in this book are safe, gradual and sustainable. Why? Because they incorporate a wisdom of natural and living foods that has been utilized for thousands of years.

This protocol also allows for significant uniqueness. Every person is different, and thus a cleansing protocol must incorporate the differences between people with regard to their age, health status and lifestyle.

Many cleansing and detoxification programs are, quite simply, dangerous for some people. We each have a different build up of toxins. We each have a unique degree of immunosuppression. Each of us has a unique physiology, with a particular degree of immunity and tolerance.

For example, some of the cleansing programs out there might apply to a person in their twenties or thirties, but could not be safely applied by a person in their seventies. A person in their seventies might have a build up of toxins and a degree of immunosuppression that would produce a significantly adverse reaction should they use the detox program a younger person could. Their bloodstreams and lymphatic systems would be flooded with toxins, producing a level of acidosis that could harm the liver, the heart, the kidneys and/or other parts of the body.

How do we solve this problem? Do we have one detoxification program for a child, another for a adolescent, another for a young adult, another for a middle-aged person and another for an elderly person? That would render more complications, as well as create further issues, as some young people can be as immunosuppressed as an elderly person.

The answer is to provide what we are calling a living cleansing and detoxification program. This means simple guidelines on diet, nutrition and herbalism that can be easily applied to our lives to gradually and safely cleanse our bodies from our build up of toxins. Because these guidelines are incorporated into our lifestyles rather then require an extreme event, they allow for sustainability. We can continue to apply the program when applicable and available. When there are availability issues, other measures can be applied as appropriate to our lifestyle and application.

This is the only safe way to conduct detoxification. Otherwise, we face an outpouring of toxicity during a cleanse. This can result in an unexpected medical emergency as the body must deal with an immediate toxin burden.

Certainly, the reader with any health issues or on any medications should discuss any cleansing strategies with their health professional prior to implementation.

Chapter One

The Need to Detox

Elizabeth

Liz is an active 30-something with two small children and a happy marriage. Most of the time, she appears healthy and active. She jogs during the weekends, and takes the kids to the park during the weekdays after work. She isn't overweight, and has clear complexion.

Liz works with the phone company. She sits in a cubical in an older office building with a 1952 ventilation system, dealing with customers and their particular account issues. She says she enjoys her work because she gets to problem-solve. She works out each person's problems, and gets good feedback from her customers.

While she admits that her work is stressful, Liz has good relationships with her coworkers, and often goes out for after-work activities while her husband watches the kids. Liz enjoys fried foods and potato chips. While some of her friends are envious that she can keep the weight down, this has come with quite a bit of effort. Liz has participated in quite a few diet plans over the years. These have ranged from low-carb diets to prepared food diets. While she has kept her weight below the obese mark, and she is nowhere near as overweight as most of her friends, her current BMI classifies her as 'overweight' nonetheless.

On most days home from work, Liz often has a sneezing attack. Her eyes well up and her skin tends to itch. She used to think that it was hay fever until the symptoms began appearing year-round. She is also increasingly finding that her sneezing and watery eyes are coming on after going to friends' houses, or after a meal in a restaurant or other public activity.

Tom

Tom works for a local coal mining company. Everyday he takes an elevator about a mile underneath the earth's surface. The bottom of the mine is packed with mining equipment, conveyors and other equipment that spews exhaust and coal particulate. While ventilation systems are in place, the ventilation is negligible.

Not surprisingly, Tom has lung issues. He suffers from COPD, and has periodic coughing fits. His coughing bouts are worse at night, especially during the weekdays. During the weekends, he feels better and can sleep a little better. Sleep is one of Tom's biggest issues, because when he is tired at work he can more easily make a mistake at his job running the conveyors.

Tom enjoys his sports. His participation in sports usually consists of watching football or baseball while drinking 3-4 beers during the game, along with a burger or pizza. When he's lucky, his wife will make a pot roast or other meal for him to eat at his TV tray, where he won't miss a play.

Tony

Tony is retired at 72, and enjoys fishing. He and his wife bought a house on the lake a few years back, allowing Tony to fish nearly every day. Tony says it's the best thing for his health, because he gets to breathe fresh air every day and hang out in the sun.

The one drawback is an electric utility power plant, which also built near the lake. Luckily they are way on the other side of the lake, so Tony barely notices it. Nonetheless, the oil-burning plant spews mercury, arsenic and other toxins out around the clock. Luckily for Tony and his wife, they live upwind of the plant, so they don't smell the smoke billowing out of the stacks.

This doesn't prevent the plant from discharging its waste water into the lake. The power plant pulls water out of the lake to cool the engines, and empties the warmed waste water back into the lake.

The lake is well-stocked with fish, and Tony and his wife like their fish fried. Every day, Tony lands at least two or three spawned salmon or carp, giving them lunch meat and dinner meat.

While they've never tested the fish for pesticides, the state fish and game has posted warnings not to swim in the lake due to periodic mercury pollutants being found in the water.

Tony is grateful to be able to walk out on the lake every day, but he is fighting melanoma. While he wears a heat and long-sleeved shirt and puts on sunscreen when he goes outside, last year Tony was diagnosed with melanoma on his hip and groin—areas never exposed to the sun.

So Tony is currently undergoing chemotherapy, after completing six months of radiation treatment. His melanoma seems to be heading into remission, but his doctor says this has been going too slowly, so he warns of a possible malignancy.

Are We Toxic?

Tony, Elizabeth and Tom are. How do we know this? For Tony and Tom it is quite obvious. Tom is exposed to a constant barrage of pollutants from his mining job, while Tony is exposed to mercury, lead and other contaminants from the fish he eats out of the lake. Liz's toxicity, on the other hand, doesn't appear to be that obvious. However, the major suspect is the ventilation system at her work. Older HVAC systems are notorious for their old and mold-ridden ducting systems. Cleaning older duct systems can be more expensive than replacing them.

Yet beneath the obvious forms of toxicity, these three are also dealing with a multitude of toxins from the foods they eat, the clothes they wear, the personal hygiene items they use, the houses they live in and the furnishings they use every day.

The evidence for this is overwhelming. Thousands of studies over the past few decades have alerted us to the fact that the toxins in our environment are making us sick in one way or another.

So what about us? Are we toxic too? How can we tell if the reason I'm feeling a little out of sorts is because of a toxicity, versus just feeling ill for some other reason?

This is a difficult question, because just about every disease either can be associated with toxicity or may be directly caused by toxicity.

Instead of listing practically every disease imaginable, here we will simply list a few symptoms that may indicate a toxic condition. Note that these symptoms are not exclusive to toxicity. There may be a specific weakness, inflammation or infection that may be a more direct cause, regardless of whether toxicity is a contributing factor. The chart below summarizes a number of signs and symptoms that indicate possible toxicity:

Symptom
Abdominal aching
Abdominal cramping
Airway constriction
Anxiety
Blood pressure change
Change in voice quality
Chronic fatigue
Constipation
Coughing
Depression
Diarrhea
Difficulty concentrating
Dizziness
Drooling
Ear infections
Eye fatigue
Fainting
Fever or warmth (flushing)
Forgetfulness
Frequent colds or flus
General fatigue
Headaches
Hives
Inability to swallow
Irritable bowels
Itchy mouth
Itchy throat
Joint pain

Muscle fatigue
Lightheadedness
Low back pain
Nausea
Panic attacks
Rapid pulse
Redness
Runny nose
Shock
Skin eruptions
Skin Itchiness
Skin rash
Sore Throat
Stinging eyes
Stinging urine
Swelling
Swollen tongue
Toothache
Ulcers
Vomiting
Watery eyes
Weak pulse
Wheezing

As we will show, nearly any type of pain or inflammation may be related to, caused by, or worsened by toxicity. This is especially true for cramping pain or immediate bouts of inflammation. As we'll discuss, the body quickly and immediately responds to toxins with inflammation.

So what is inflammation and how can we lessen our bouts of inflammation? This calls for an understanding of the immune system, and how the immune system works to remove toxins from our body.

Before we focus there, let's review the potential toxins that we are faced with on a daily basis in modern living.

What is a Toxin?

The biochemicals natural to our environment undergo constant recycling. A single biochemical may be eaten by one organism, excreted by another, inhaled by yet another and become the skin of yet another organism. At the same time, an intricate chemical balance is kept through these changes, making biochemical a vital source for nutrition. In other words, the earth's natural biochemical recycling maintains its nutritional nature on a consistent basis. While one organism's waste may be another's food, that food/waste still maintains its nutritional content.

What we have then, is a living biochemical system.

However, should we interfere with any one part of nature's recycling, we can interrupt the balance of the rest of the cycle, often causing reverberations on an exponential basis. This is precisely what humans have unfortunately arrived at after two hundred years of industrial technological development.

An example is the delicate chemical pathway of nitrogen. Animals and humans consume nitrogen from the atmosphere and through nutrition—by breathing, eating plants, root nitrogen fixing, and so on. When an organism dies, *ammonifying bacteria* decompose the body and release ammonia into the soil. *Nitrosifying bacteria* oxidize the ammonia, converting it to nitrites, and *nitrifying bacteria* then oxidize the nitrites to soil nitrogen and ammonia ions. Plants utilize these to form amino acids and proteins. Nitrogen is also released into the air with *dentrifying* bacteria. As plant protein is eaten by animals and humans in plant food, these nitrogen amino acids become part of the proteins that make up our bodies. When our bodies die, the cycle begins again.

Throughout the nitrogen cycle, there is a precise balance of nitrogen in the atmosphere, the soils, and within each organism: Just enough to serve the combined purpose of all involved. Every species then gets a balanced dose of nitrogen, from the soil microbes and earthworms all the way up to humans.

Enter chemical fertilizer. The beneficial addition of nitrogen chemical fertilizers into the soil has increased crop production for agribusiness-based farms. While adding something already available in nature seems innocent enough, the dumping of pure nitrogen without the balance of nutrients provided by living organisms produces an imbalance throughout the nitrogen cycle.

Without the complex of nutrients produced by nature's nitrogen-fixing process, the soil begins to erode and thin. The heavy load of unused nitrogen leaches through the soil, settling into the ground water. This nitrogen leaching creates a build-up of dangerous nitrates within the ground water. Nitrate build up has been poisoning ground water in agricultural areas throughout the world. In areas of heavy fertilizer use, undrinkable ground water is reaching increasingly deeper wells. Nitrate levels above about 50 parts per million can make a person sick. Higher levels have been known to be fatal.

In addition, nitrogen-fertilizer-rich soils choke rivers and oceans with extra nitrogen, causing abnormal blooms of algae, cutting off oxygen supplies and leading to dead ocean zones with high toxicity levels.

The use of nitrogen fertilizers illustrates how the precise rhythms of nature—the use and recycling of natural biochemistry—can so easily be disrupted. Now why couldn't we simply have supplied the nitrogen produced by compost, as degraded by soil organisms and earthworms?

Our Synthetic World

Over the past century, humankind has opened a Pandora's box of chemical manipulation. The brilliant marketing efforts of chemical manufacturers of the twentieth century convinced us that synthetic chemicals made life easier, more productive and healthier. Not only did they get this wrong, but we all bought in to it.

And now we are paying the price.

As this grand synthetic experiment has unfolded, we have discovered that many of these chemicals are not only toxic. They now risk humankind's future existence. After only a few decades of massive synthetic chemical manufacturing, we are beginning to suffer the horrific price synthetic chemicals come with: We are faced with increasing epidemics of cancer, asthma, nerve degenerative diseases and so many others.

Much of our drinking supplies are now laced with mercury, arsenic, DDT, PCB, nitrates, HTMs, plasticizers, pharmaceuticals and hundreds of other dangerous toxins. Much of the non-organic food we eat is now to full of various pesticide residues. We are gradually discovering that agribusiness' use of chemical fertilizers and pesticides is slowly poisoning our bodies. The toxins are building up in our cells—mutating DNA and suffocating our immune systems.

Most of the furnishings we purchase now are filled with formaldehydes, synthetic materials and preservatives. Most office buildings and many houses still contain hazards like asbestos and other components that cause toxicity. Our entire environment is laced with synthetic chemistry. If the human race stopped chemical production today, we still would have done so much damage over the past fifty years that it will take centuries for the earth's detoxification systems to purify herself.

Today we are building mountains of synthetic chemistry loading up our dumps, landfills, lakes, rivers, and oceans with toxic brews. These mountains are decomposing very slowly—outgassing and breaking down into potent poisons. *Time Magazine* reported on June 25, 2007 that Americans generated 1,643 pounds of trash per person in 2005. A mere 32% of it was recycled.

Much of this waste is plastic. The problem with plastic is reflective of its benefit—it lasts far longer than do natural materials. While a plastic bag might not tear and rip as fast as a paper bag as we walk from the grocery store, a plastic bag will have as much as a 500-year half-life—depending upon its material. That is a long time. Whet happens to the bag while nature works to biodegrade it? It clogs our soils and waters. For this reason our lands, waters, and bodies are steadily becoming laced with polymers and plasticizers.

Plastics are made through reactions between monomers (small molecules) and plasticizers to create longer-chain molecules. Monomers are typically hydrocarbons such as petroleum. Combining ethane monomers and plasticizers forms polyethylene. Combining styrene monomers and plasticizers renders polystyrene. Combining vinyl chloride monomers and plasticizers results in polyvinyl chloride, or PVC. Combining propylene monomers and plasticizers gives us polypropylene. As these plastic combinations are broken down, guess what gets released into the environment?

Nature produces its own types of natural polymers such as rubber from rubber trees. But this isn't enough for our hungry appetite for luxury. In an attempt to improve upon nature, the 1855 lab of Alexander Parkes mixed pyroxylin from cellulose with alcohol and camphor to form the first type of plastic.

This clear, hard plastic was 'improved' by Dr. Leo Baekeland decades later with a polymer process using phenol and formaldehyde in early 1900s. "Bakelite" became a wildly successful product as it effectively replaced shellac and rubber as a general sheathing material. Because it was heat-resistant and moisture-proof, it quickly became the insulator of choice for engines, appliances, and electronics. Dr. Baekeland eventually sold his General Bakelite Company to Union Carbide in 1939 and retired a very wealthy man to Florida. His life was made easy through the 'miracle' of chemistry.

Nylon was an invention of DuPont researchers in the late 1930s. It was made initially with benzene from coal. The introduction of polypropylene as a synthetic rubber followed shortly thereafter. Polypropylene was an accidental discovery by a couple of researchers vying to convert natural gas for Phillips Petroleum.

The American industrial complex gearing up for World War II focused its attention on this synthetic version due to a shortage of natural rubber. Thanks to synthetic rubber, each soldier was able to wear 32 pounds of rubber in clothing and equipment. A tank needed about a ton. America's military might was as likely due to its synthetic rubber as were its bombs. Again, chemistry was seemingly making our lives easier.

The synthetic polymer revolution surged after the Second World War. The plastic revolution raged, as both consumers and manufacturers bonded to replace anything natural with synthetic polymers.

A polychlorinated biphenyl is a grouping of chlorine atoms bonded together with biphenyl. Biphenyl is a molecule composed of two phenyl rings. It is an aromatic hydrocarbon occurring naturally in coal and petroleum. When synthetically combined with chlorine—another naturally occurring element—the result is highly toxic. PCB was banned in the early 1970s when biologists studied a population of dead seabirds and found they died of a toxic dose of PCBs. For more than forty years, PCBs have been used in paints, pesticides, paper, adhesives, flame-retardants, surgical implants, lubricating oil and electrical equipment.

Referred innocently as "phenols" for many years, the PCB ban followed suspicion of toxicity for over a decade. Massive PCB contamination in the Hudson River was found caused by local electrical manufacturing plants. Some two hundred miles of the river was eventually designated a toxic *superfund site*. This woke us up to PCB toxicity. PCBs break down slowly and bioaccumulate in living organisms.

When PCBs get into our waterways, they build up in the smallest organisms and work their way up the food chain, eventually reaching humans.

Today the ban on PCBs does not include many applications considered "closed," such as capacitors and vacuum pump fluids. This means there are still considerable PCBs in our buildings and electrical equipment. PCB poisoning can cause immediate liver damage. Symptoms can include fever, rashes, nausea, and more.

One might argue that that combining earth-borne commodities like hydrocarbons cannot be so unnatural. After all, hydrocarbons are produced by the earth as part of her own recycling process. However, the process of converting nature's hydrocarbon monomers into polymers of our design requires various catalysts—*plasticizers*—to complete.

Plasticizers are used in plastic production to give the long polymer chain its flexibility. Without plasticizers inserted between the polymer chains, plastics would have no flexibility. Without plasticizers, polymers are clear, hard substances: rock-like. The gradations of flex added to polymer chains give the resulting plastic its particular usefulness. A plasticizer adds strength to this flexibility, making the new material difficult to tear or break.

Most plasticizers are *phthalates*. Phthalates are derived from phthalic acid, an aromatic ringed carbon molecule also referred to as dicarboxylic acid. Originally synthesized in 1836 through the oxidation of naphthalene tetrachloride, phthalic acid can also be synthesized from hydrocarbons and sulfuric acid with a mercury catalyst.

Common phthalates are di(2-ethylhexyl) phthalate (DEHP), dibutyl phthalate (DBP), and bisphenyl A (BPA), among others.

Biphenyl A, for example, is used in many types of containers, including baby bottles. BPA can easily leach into food or formula when the bottle is exposed to heat or sunlight. A 2000 Centers of Disease Control study found 75% of those tested had phthalates in their urine, and subsequent studies have found some 95% of the U.S. population has detectable levels of biphenyl A within body fluids. Biphenyls are considered endocrine system disruptors. Long-term effects as their residues build up in our cells, organs and tissue systems are largely unknown.

More recently, researchers from the University of Michigan (Meeker and Ferguson 2011) confirmed that common phthalate plasticizers DEHP, DBP and BPA all disrupt human thyroid hormones—linked to increasing the incidence of thyroid diseases. The research compared and analyzed the metabolites from urine and serum thyroid levels of 1,346 adults and 329 adolescents.

Higher DEHP, DBP, and BPA levels were found to be associated with lower levels of the thyroid hormone metabolites of T4, free T3, total T3 and thyroglobin. Higher DEHP levels were associated with higher TSH levels, while higher BPA levels were associated with lower T3 and TSH levels. This means that the more plasticizers in the bloodstream, the more deranged the hormone levels. The researchers found that lower T4 metabolite levels has the strongest association with higher phthalates. High DEHP levels were associated strongly with lower TSH levels, while BPA was associated with lower T4 and TSH levels.

The study, published in the scientific journal, *Environmental Health Perspectives,* is the first national human study confirming that BPA and other common plasticizers definitely disrupt hormones. Over the past decade, the chemical industry has been disputing the link between BPA and hormone disruption as coincidental. This large study confirmed previous research that led to the suspicion that these plasticizers, common among food packaging, water bottles, can linings and other consumer goods, disrupt hormone levels.

University of Michigan assistant professor and lead researcher, Dr. John Meeker, commented that the highest 20% of DEHP exposures had as high as 10% decreased thyroid hormones.

Most aromatic carbon rings like the phenyl ring or the benzyl ring used for these polymers have otherwise proven to be hazardous to our environment and well-being. Note there are a number of aromatic carbon rings produced in nature. These, however, do not affect hormone levels, turning males to females, as has been found among fish.

Today there are hundreds of different plasticizers used to produce plastics. Most are variations of aromatic carbons or similarly hazardous compounds. When plasticizers from plastic polymers break down in the environment, these aromatic carbons are released. Our backyards, landfills and oceans—our entire environment for that matter—are silently being inundated by these insidious compounds.

Benzene, for example, is a popular phenyl plasticizer. Benzene has been classified as a volatile organic compound and a carcinogen by the Natural Institutes of Health's National Toxicology Program. Benzene is among the top twenty most used industrial chemicals. It is used to make adhesives, paint, pharmaceuticals, printed materials, photographic chemicals, synthetic rubber, dyes, detergents, paint and even food processing equipment. As a result, benzene is found throughout our environment—notably in our air and water—and has been implicated in numerous types of cancers.

The problems of synthetic chemicals are pervasive. About 80,000 chemicals have been approved for commercialization over the past fifty years. The *Toxic Substances Control Act of 1976* was set up to evaluate chemicals being introduced. Yet only about 65,000 have been reviewed. However only a small percentage of these chemicals have been carefully analyzed for their environmental and health effects.

Meanwhile, more and more pharmaceuticals have been developed for the purpose of inhibiting inflammation, pain and nervous issues. These efforts are certainly commendable, and the intentions of some researchers may be valiant. Still, these efforts come with a considerable price.

The newest medical technologies, including pharmaceuticals, may well be creating as many problems as they might be resolving. Over the past few decades, our medical industry has become the leading cause of death and injury in the United States. Carolyn Dean, M.D., N.D., in her book *Death By Medicine* (2005), compiled the following statistics for 2005:

Medical Institutional Cause	Deaths
Hospital Adverse Reaction	106,000 deaths
Medical Error	98,000 deaths
Bedsores	115,000 deaths
Infection	88,000 deaths
Malnutrition	108,800 deaths
Outpatient Adverse Reaction	199,000 deaths
Unnecessary Procedures	37,136 deaths
Surgery-Related	32,000 deaths
Total Annual Deaths	**783,936 deaths**

Think about this. This accounting of deaths out-numbers U.S. cardiovascular disease death rates and cancer death rates. In 2002 for example, 450,637 people died of heart disease and about 476,009 died of cancer.

Furthermore, the *Journal of the American Medical Association* (Lazarou *et al.* 1998) reported that in 1994, 2,216,000 Americans were either hospitalized, permanently disabled, or died as a result of pharmaceuticals. *The Nutrition Institute of America* reports that over 20 million unnecessary antibiotic prescriptions are prescribed. Over seven million medical and surgical procedures a year are unnecessary. Over eight million people are hospitalized without need. Our medical institution is quite simply suffocating in its own mismanagement.

According to a nationwide poll conducted by Louis Harris and Associates released in 1997 by the National Patient Safety Foundation and the American Medical Association, an estimated 100 million Americans experienced a medical mistake: 42% of those randomly surveyed. Misdiagnosis and wrong treatments accounted for 40% of those mistakes. Medical medication errors accounted for 28% of these, and medical procedure errors accounted for 22% of these (NPSF 1997).

In a study of four Boston adult primary care practices involving 1202 outpatients, 27% (95% confidence) of responders experienced adverse drug events (Gandhi *et al.* 2003).

In a 2004 interview with Dr. Lucian Leape, an expert in patient safety and an author of a number of studies, reported that over the past ten years since the 1997 NPSF studies were performed, improvements in our medical system have been inadequate. Barriers to improvement cited physician denial, hospital environment, lack of leadership and little system review (Leape 2004).

The Environmental Working Group's *Human Toxome Project* has revealed some frightening statistics regarding the poisoning of our bodies by chemicals. In one study of nine adult participants, blood and urine contained 171 of the 214 toxic chemicals in the screen. These included industrial compounds and pollutants like alkylphenols, inorganic arsenic, organophosphates, phthalates, polychlorinated biphenyls (PCBs), volatile and semi-volatile organic compounds and chlorinated dioxins and furans.

In another study, the EWG found 287 of the 413 chemicals screened in the umbilical cord blood of ten mothers after giving birth. These included the chemical types mentioned above and more, including fifty different polychlorinated naphthalene compounds (EWG 2007).

By some accounts there are nearly nine hundred different pesticides being used in the United States. Of those, at least thirty-seven contain organophosphates—one of our more toxic chemical combinations. Organophosphates kill insects through nervous system disruption. These neurotoxins are also toxic to humans' nervous systems. The nerve gases Serin and VX are organophosphates, for example.

Organophosphates block cholinesterase—a key neuro-enzyme—from working properly within the body. With cholinesterase blocked, acetylcholine is not regulated. Unregulated acetylcholine causes an over-stimulation of nerve activity, resulting in nerve damage, paralysis, and muscle weakness.

Organophosphates are spreading through ground water, air and through dermal contact. They are exposing us through our breathing, skin contact, swimming, and consumption. Initial symptoms can include nausea, vomiting, shortness of breath, confusion, and muscle spasms. Some of the more common organophosphates include Malathion, Parathion, Diazinon, Phosmet, Clorpyrifos, Dursban and others.

The EPA actually banned Diazinon and Dursban in a phase-out beginning in March of 2001, to last through December 2003. Curiously, both Diazinon and Dursban are still in use today. Phased bans like this theoretically take several years to allow companies to run out their inventories. Also since these bans were aimed at consumer products, organophosphates are still used profusely in commercial agriculture—our food production.

In a 2003 study done by the Centers for Disease Control and Prevention, thousands of people were tested for 116 chemicals. Thirty-four of these were pesticides such as organophosphates, organochlorines, and carbamates. Nineteen of the thirty-four were found in either the blood or urine.

The use of pesticides on agricultural land, playgrounds, parks, home lawns, and gardens throughout the United States has growing by staggering proportions. In 1964, approximately 233 million pounds of pesticide active ingredients were used. By 1982, this amount tripled to 612 million pounds. In 1999, the U.S. Environmental Protection Agency reported that some five *billion* pounds of these chemicals were used per year throughout America's crops, forests, parks, and lawns.

One of the fastest growing of these pesticides has been imidacloprid, a neonicotinoid. Introduced by Bayer in 1994, imidacloprid is used against aphids and similar insects on over 140 different crops. Touted as a chemical with a fairly short half-life of thirty days in water and twenty-seven days in anaerobic soil, imidacloprid's half-life is about 997 days in aerobic soil. While it has a lower immediate toxicity compared with hazards like DDT, imidacloprid's use is now widespread. It is rated by the EPA and WHO as *"moderately toxic"* in small doses. Larger doses can disrupt liver and thyroid function. While this pesticide does well at killing off increasingly resistant pests, it also can decimate bee populations.

A world without bees, as described in Rachel Carson's classic *Silent Spring*, would insure a destiny of hunger and destitution in human society. In France for example, some 500,000 registered hives were lost in the mid-1990s. Imidacloprid was implicated, and was subsequently banned for many crops in that country. Massive bee destruction has occurred in other regions of Europe also appear connected to imidacloprid use. A 2006-2007 loss of hives throughout Europe and the U.S.—referred to as *colony collapse disorder*—is now increasingly being connected to imidacloprid, although it also appears that other chemicals as well as possibly unnatural electromagnetic radiation work together to weaken the bees' immunity to viruses and other diseases. Imidacloprid and other chemicals can weaken the bee's immune system just as they weaken the human immune system—depending of course on the level of exposure.

Chlorinated dioxins are also pervasive in today's environment. Significant sources include cigarettes, pesticides, coal-burning factories, diesel exhaust, and sewage sludge. Dioxins are also byproducts of the manufacturing of a number of products, including many resins, glues, plastics, and chlorine-treated products. Dioxins also bio-accumulate in fatty tissues and can take years to fully degrade. Dioxins are known endocrine disruptors. They have also been linked to liver toxicity and birth defects.

Thanks to the human industrial complex, there are now thousands of *volatile organic compounds* in our environment. A VOC is classified as such if it has a relatively high vapor pressure, allowing it to vaporize quickly and enter the atmosphere. Gasoline, paint thinners, cleaning solvents, ketones, and aldehydes are a few of the chemicals considered sources of VOCs. Methane-forming VOCs like benzene and toluene are also carcinogens. VOCs are often used as preservatives for pressed wood and other building materials. As a result, many buildings contain VOCs locked within its building materials. Once soaked in or inborn with the fabrication, VOCs are trapped within the material, causing them to outgas over time. This outgassing process is speeded up when the building is demolished or taken apart. As the building materials are broken up, VOCs can be released at toxic exposure levels.

VOCs will form ozone as they interact with sunlight and heat. VOC poisoning symptoms include nausea; headaches; eye irritation; inflammation of the nose and throat; liver damage; brain fog; and neurotoxic brain damage. Using cleaning or painting solvents indoors is a common cause of VOC poisoning.

In a study by Janssen *et al.* (2004) and *The Collaborative on Health and the Environment,* some two hundred diseases were found to be attributable to exposure to industrial chemicals. The diseases listed are some of the most prevalent diseases of our society—cancers, cardiovascular disease, autoimmune diseases and so on. The researchers found that over 120 diseases have been specifically linked by research to exposure to specific industrial chemicals. For another thirty-three diseases, the evidence for linking to specific chemicals was considered "good." For the rest of the diseases, research indicated a definite link but the evidence was considered "limited" (Lean 2004).

Synthetic versus Natural

The assumption of modern chemistry is there is no inherent difference between a chemical synthesized in a lab or manufacturing facility from one made in nature by living processes. This assumption has led humankind to haphazardly invent new synthetic chemical combinations with reckless abandon. Blinded by patents and profits, the industrial chemical complex has assumed there is no environmental cost.

Research has proven these assumptions wrong. Let's look at some interesting examples.

When palm and coconut oils are cooled, they become hardened. This makes them good thickening agents for cooking and good for frying. In an attempt to match nature, in 1902 German Wilhelm Normann patented the first hydrogenation process, which was eventually purchased by Proctor and Gamble, leading to Crisco® oil and eventually margarine. When nutritionists convinced us that *"all saturated fats are bad"* in the sixties and seventies, margarine sales took off. Processors also found that frying oil had a better shelf life and was cheaper if cottonseed oil and soybean oil were *partially hydrogenated.* Because these oils do not normally harden at room temperature as does palm, coconut and lard, hydrogenation allowed processors to use the less expensive oils for frying, spreading and cooking.

Hydrogenation means to *saturate* hydrogen onto all of the available bonds of the central molecule. Whereas a natural substance might have a double bond between carbon and other atoms, hydrogen gas can be bubbled through the substance—using a catalyst to spark the reaction—to attach more hydrogen to the molecule. To saturate carbon bonds with hydrogen, catalyst is added, and the oil undergoes the bubbling of hydrogen within a heated catalytic environment. This saturation synthetically changes the oil's melting point, giving it more versatility at a lower cost.

Let's review. Food scientists took real foods—oil extracted from soybeans or cottonseed—and synthetically converted it into what appeared to be the same molecular structure, but with a different melting point. Harmless, yes? Think again. After decades of use and millions of heart attacks and strokes later, health researchers began realizing that partially hydrogenated oils have damaging effects upon the cardiovascular system.

While the saturated or partially saturated molecule was the same formula, the synthetic process of hydrogenation created an unusual (transversed) molecular structure called a *trans-fat*. Trans-fat is now implicated in a various degenerative disorders, including atherosclerosis, dementia, liver disease, irritable bowel syndrome, and Alzheimer's disease among others. While the epidemic increase in cardiovascular disease has focused billions of dollars into research, the consumption of trans-fats was altogether overlooked. Why? Because researchers assumed that hydrogenated soybean oil was harmless because its molecularly-identical cousin—raw soybean oil—was harmless, and even healthy because it was a polyunsaturated oil.

The mechanism whereby trans-fats produce damage in the body—as we'll discuss later—is called lipid peroxidation. Because trans-fats are less stable than cis-fats, and because fats make up our cell membranes, trans-fats become more readily damaged, producing what is called lipid peroxides. Lipid peroxides damage blood vessel walls and other tissue systems, producing cardiovascular disease and other degenerative disorders.

So now researchers realize that the orientation—polarity and spin—of a molecule can have altogether different effects from the same molecule rotated in the orientation nature designed.

Nature normally orients healthy oil molecules—and many other nutrients—in *cis* formation: They are oriented so that the hydrogens are on the same side with the other molecular bonds. A *trans* configuration has hydrogens on the opposite side of the bonds.

This *cis* and *trans* orientation issue is also evident from the opposite perspective in the case of resveratrol. Resveratrol is a phytochemical constituent of more than seventy different plant species, including many fruits such as berries and grapes. Studies have shown natural resveratrol has many biological properties important to health. These include antioxidant, anti-bacterial, anti-viral, anti-fungal, liver-cleansing, mood-elevation, and amyloid-plaque-removal properties. Resveratrol also activates an enzyme-protein called sirtuin 1, which appears to promote DNA repair.

However, these effects are exclusive to the natural form: *trans*-resveratrol. Not surprisingly, pasteurization and other processing will convert the *trans*-resveratrol molecule to its less effective cousin, *cis*-resveratrol.

Another example of human meddling is vitamin E. While natural vitamin E is d-alpha-tocopherol, the synthetic version is dl-alpha-tocopherol. While d-alpha-tocopherol has one isomer, dl-alpha-tocopherol has eight. One of those eight is similar to the one natural isomer. The difference is that the natural version is more readily bioavailable than the dl-alpha version.

Illustrating this, in one study (Burton *et al.* 1998), subjects took either natural vitamin E or the synthetic vitamin E. Natural vitamin E levels in the bloodstream for all subjects were at least twice as high as levels of the synthetic versions. After twenty-three days, tissue levels were also significantly higher for the natural vitamin E group, compared to the synthetic vitamin E group. These tests illustrated that nature's form of vitamin E is more readily absorbed and utilized than the synthetic version.

Furthermore, Oregon State University researchers (Traber *et al.* 1998) found that humans excrete synthetic vitamin E three times faster than natural vitamin E. So not only does the human body not readily absorb the synthetic version, but it wants to rid the body of this version three times faster.

This ratio was confirmed in another test (Kiyose *et al.* 1997) showing that it took three times the quantity of synthetic vitamin E to reach the same levels achieved by natural vitamin E among seven women.

Vitamin C provides another example. Gas chromatography has revealed several structural differences between synthetic vitamin C (isolated ascorbic acid) and natural forms of vitamin C. While many people supplement with isolated ascorbic acid, nature provides a completely different structure. Not only is the molecule itself different, but natural vitamin C is naturally bonded—or *chelated*—to other natural compounds called biofactors. These include bioflavonoids, minerals, rutin, and other biochemicals produced by living organisms or nature's ecology. These are often referred to as *ascorbates*.

Synthetic vitamin D—referred to as vitamin D2 or ergocalciferol—is also molecularly different from naturally produced cholecalciferol. In a study published in 2012 from France's International Prevention Research Institute (Tripkovic *et al.*), scientists conducted a meta-analysis of studies that compared blood-levels of 25-hydroxyvitamin D resulting from the supplementation of either vitamin D2 or vitamin D3 among those over the age of 50. Among the 76 clinical studies between 1984 and 2011, vitamin D2 (ergocalciferol) did not increase blood levels of 25(OH)D (blood form of D) anywhere near as much as did vitamin D3 (cholecalciferol).

Yes, we can now conclude that vitamin D2 is not as therapeutic and new research finds it can even reduce our blood levels of the more therapeutic 25(OH)D3.

Synthetic forms of vitamin D3 don't match nature's form. The vitamin D produced by the sun is 25-Hydroxyvitamin D3-beta-sulphate. This is a water-soluble form of 25(OH)D3—sometimes referred to as vitamin D3-sulfate.

Yes, the form of vitamin D3 from supplements is not conjugated with sulfate as is nature's form. Does this make a difference? Yes, it certainly does. Other research has shown the sulfated form is sequestered into fat cells (for later use) significantly greater than supplemented forms will.

Illustrating nature's role further, in a recent study from Washington University's School of Medicine (Nicola *et al.* 2007), 168 healthy postmenopausal women were tested for supplemented calcium versus dietary (natural) sources of calcium. Women whose calcium intake was primarily from supplementation—even though their dosages were higher—had lower bone mineral density levels than the women whose calcium intake was primarily from dietary sources. Those taking supplements plus good dietary sources had the highest totals.

Naturally occurring nutrients are electromagnetically different than synthesized chemicals. The resulting quanta of spin, angular momentum and so on will vary between nature's version and a version synthesized in a lab or processed beyond nature's intended course.

Spectroscopy tests show that when two different ions with different atomic character are brought together, the resulting compound will display different spectra than either did independently. The combination's waveforms are not necessarily a composite of the two. It is a new waveform combination resulting from the resonating interference of the combining elements together with its natural catalysts and environment.

Most biological combinations require a catalyst (a facilitator) to complete. These catalysts may supply or borrow electrons in an oxidizing or reducing mechanism to assist in the combination. They will also supply the needed electromagnetic energy to speed up the reaction. Nature's catalysts provide specific changes in molecular structure—creating a unique *fingerprint* of sorts.

Synthetic catalysts will produce a different molecular combination, even if the original ions or compounds are the same as found in nature. Even if the combination may be similar to nature's version, often the molecular orientation—as with trans-fats—will be subtly different.

Because it is not cohesive—or stable—with the body's components, a synthetically combined compound throws off the balance between oxidizers and reducers in the body. This produces increased levels of oxidized or oxidative radicals, which will rob electrons or ions from the molecules that make up our tissues—notably our cell membranes, and the membranes that make up our mitochondria.

This later point—damage to the membranes of our mitochondria—is now implicated as the functional event that causes dementia, chronic fatigue and fibromyalgia. When the mitochondria within our brain cells is damaged by free radicals, these brain cells begin to shut down.

In chronic fatigue and fibromyalgia—often considered the same condition—damage to the membranes of mitochondria shuts down the energy production of muscle cells.

This is because mitochondria is where are energy is produced. The mitochondria house the Krebs cycle, which converts glucose and oxygen to heat and energy. As they become damaged and dysfunctional, we experience fatigue.

While our bodies are built to handle moderate levels of free radicals, our synthetic world is overloading our body with synthetics, which produce these oxidized or oxidative radicals within the body. This oxidizing potency of toxins leads to an overload of acids (H+), causing excessive acidosis, and the subsequent degeneration of our tissue systems.

And among those synthetic chemicals that do not readily metabolize (break down) within the body, many will build up among the body's fat cells. This is because many synthetic toxins are *lipohilic:* fat-loving, or fat-soluble.

This has the effect of the body storing up synthetic toxins within our fat cells, only to break down and pollute our bodies days, weeks or years later.

Natural versus Synthetic Medicines

Even with trillions of dollars of research, chemical manufacturers cannot seem to synthesize safe chemicals. As one chemical's toxicity is discovered, another one is launched in its place: Perhaps with different or delayed toxic effects. While there might be reductions in dilution or dosage to lower its toxic effects, practically every synthetic medication will either readily metabolize into toxins or accumulate within fat cells for later break down.

This was illustrated in a 1998 report published in the *Journal of the American Medical Association* (Lazarou *et al.* 1998). Approximately 2,300,000 people either end up being hospitalized, permanently disabled, or fatally injured as a result of pharmaceutical use in the United States alone every year. That is over 2.2 million people annually with *reported* injury from pharmaceuticals.

This study, done at the University of Toronto, also showed that approximately 106,000 people in the U.S. die each year from taking correctly prescribed pharmaceuticals approved by the FDA. This does not include the number of deaths resulting by overdose or by addiction to these same drugs. The U.S. FDA was sent 258,000 adverse drug events in 1999.

Harvard researcher and associate professor of medicine Dr. David Bates told the *Los Angeles Times* in 2001: *"...these numbers translate to 36 million adverse drug events per year"* (Rappoport 2006).

The plausibility of this number was confirmed in another study published in the *Journal of the American Medical Association* in 1995 (Bates *et al.*). This revealed that over a sixth month period, 12% of 4,031 adult hospital admissions had either a confirmed adverse drug event or a potentially adverse drug event. If we extrapolate this rate using the population of 300 million Americans, we would arrive at the same 36 million calculated in the study.

Now let's compare these numbers with the side-effects and fatalities due to nature's herbal medicines.

By comparison, the 2007 annual report of the American Association of Poison Control Centers reported a grand total of three deaths from natural remedies over the year. This included herbs, homeopathy, essential oils, minerals, vitamins and other supplements. Quite a difference from 106,000 deaths and 36 million adverse drug events among pharmaceuticals.

Oh but the reader thinks that more people take pharmaceuticals? Just consider research from the National Institutes of Health National Center for Complementary and Alternative Medicine. This revealed that 38% of adults and 12% of children in the U.S. use some form of alternative medicine. While not as many Americans are taking drugs as herbs, this number (approaching 100 million people) is significant enough for comparison. A 2007 report by Medco Health Solutions, Inc. calculated that about 51% of Americans take one or more pharmaceutical drugs—more than any other country on a per-person basis.

Pharmaceuticals are a recent development among humans. Many drugs have only been developed over the past decade or two, and nearly all drugs have been developed over the past few decades.

Drug tests typically test clinical population of maybe a thousand or two people, over a span of six weeks to a couple-three months. Rarely do drug tests extend much longer, as this would be too expensive for drug companies.

Now millions of people are taking pharmaceuticals—some of them for many years. This means that we are undertaking a grand experiment on humanity. We are effectively testing the long-range effects of synthetic pharmaceutical use among our own kind. And what have the results of this grand experiment been so far? We can see the results from the side effect and fatality statistics discussed earlier: It's been a disaster of epidemic proportions, with over a hundred thousand people dying every year from pharmaceuticals. Not to mention the tens of millions of people getting sick from pharmaceuticals each year: *And this is only in the United States.*

Let's now compare this with a little history of herbal medicine use.

For thousands of years, traditional doctors and scientists have been documenting the clinical use of particular herbal medicines to treat particular ailments. One of the earliest advanced records of herbal medicine is the *Pen Ts'ao,* written some 4,500 years ago by a Chinese herbalist. The *Pen Ts'ao* recorded 366 different plant medicines and their specific uses.

Meanwhile some Ayurvedic medicine texts appear to be older, documenting herbal medicine use over 5,000 years ago.

These two medicines predate the use of herbal medicines by many other ancient civilizations. These include the Egyptians, the Greeks, the Romans, the Polynesians, the New Zealand Maoris, the Aboriginals, the North American Indians, the Indonesians, the Mayans, the various African tribes, the Northern Europeans and the tribes among the ancient British Isles. This means that literally billions of people have been using herbal medicine for thousands of years.

Over the centuries, traditional yet clinically established treatises on herbal medicine have accumulated from these societies and traditions—all confirming tremendous healing results and a record of safety among botanicals.

Today we can use these treatises to make herbal formulations and herbal teas that render various health benefits. And these have been proven by thousands of modern clinical studies, all showing an almost virtual lack of serious side effects.

All of these ancient cultures and traditions together assemble a grand study—complete with blindedness among billions of participants of different cultures, most unknown to the other cultures that were also testing most of the same herbs. Each culture developed and used various botanical medicines, many unaware that other cultures were using some of the same botanicals or botanical families, yet experiencing the same results. These different cultures all found the same families of herbs with primarily the same curative properties.

It is only over the past century or two that humankind's quest for ownership and profits drove humans to isolate and attempt to synthetically reproduce the constituents of these natural medicines. The primary fact that modern societies have given patent rights to those who develop an isolated synthetic chemical has promoted an increasing concept of molecular ownership. This policy of molecular ownership is frankly, a crime against humanity. And the damage to our environment and our bodies is the evidence for such a crime.

Yet isn't it interesting that some 50-60% of chemical pharmaceuticals are founded upon one or more naturally occurring biochemicals, many from herbal medicines. Some sources iterate that at least 30% of currently prescribed medicines are actually synthetic analogues of herbal medicine constituents.

There are other critical differences between herbs and pharmaceuticals. Pharmaceuticals are isolated constituents with typically has one mechanism of action—usually to inhibit a particular metabolic process in the body. In contrast, most botanicals have multiple—some even hundreds—of pharmacological constituents.

For example, according to the research of James Duke, PhD of the *U.S. Department of Agriculture* and Norman Farnsworth, PhD, a research professor at the University of Illinois, ginger has at least 477 active constituents (Schulick 1996). Compared to single-constituent pharmaceuticals, this fact is simply astonishing. While nature produces multiple active biochemicals that act in a healing manner upon our bodies, she also produces multiple biochemicals that that buffer and balance the active ones and each other.

Furthermore, many of these hundreds of active compounds in a medicinal herb will be bonded (chelated) biofactors nutrients that nourish our bodies!

Now should we isolate one of ginger's active ingredients—say gingerol—from those chelated nutrients and balancing actives, we will undoubtedly find that while it might have some medicinal action by itself, it may very well cause side effects due to the lack of balancing agents in nature's ginger. We'll illustrate this effect in a moment as we discuss aspirin and the herbs willow bark and meadowsweet.

One reason ginger has had such success among traditional medicines is because it suppresses the expression of both cyclooxygenase-1 and cyclooxygenase-2, two enzymes that stimulate inflammation. Ginger also slows leukotriene production through the blocking of the 5-lipooxygenase enzyme (Grzanna *et al.* 2005).

Unlike the parade of side effect-ridden COX-inhibiting non-steroidal anti-inflammatory drugs (NSAIDs) introduced by the pharmaceutical industry over the past century, ginger provides a level of safety and a myriad of nutritional benefits. We might add that these COX-2 pharmaceuticals—some of which have been pulled from the market for serious cardiovascular problems such as Bextra—have required billions of dollars of commercial research by the pharmaceutical industry and vast amounts of taxpayer investment in government oversight. If even a small amount of this wasted effort was diverted to the development of the availability of natural ginger, we could have saved the planet and our population billions of dollars of resources, and millions of tons of toxic pollution.

Illustrating this later point, on March 10, 2008, a report released by the *American Press National Investigation Team* that pharmaceutical drugs taken for pain, high cholesterol, asthma, epilepsy, infection, heart problems and mood disorders had contaminated the water supplies of over forty-one million Americans. In a finding that confirmed a 2002 report by the U.S. Geological Survey, pharmaceutical drugs are infecting the country's rivers and streams nationally. These drug residues slip through the filtration systems of municipalities, as they were not designed for treatment for these pollutants. The source of this pharmaceutical pollution appears to be primarily the flushing of medications down the toilet as those medications expire or are otherwise thrown out. This is of course compounded by the waste streams of pharmaceutical manufacturers.

One report recently stated, for example, that a quite large and well-known pharmaceutical manufacturer generates some 2,400,000 pounds of hazardous waste every year, which escapes into the surrounding countryside and its waters in Europe. The report also stated this same manufacturing facility caused genetic pollution among a variety of crops near its manufacturing facility.

Through 1996, the pharmaceutical industry had launched at least two hundred pharmaceuticals and spent over $70 billion aimed at reproducing the eicanosoidal-inhibitory effects ginger and other anti-inflammatory botanicals. Not only does ginger act thoroughly and without side effects, but it is also a tasty ingredient for various dishes, and grows profusely among natural environments. How much better can nature get?

Pharmaceutical eiconasoid manipulation using the various NSAID pharmaceuticals has been a disaster in almost every respect. Each has some negative side effects. Some such as aspirin and COX-2 inhibitors alter the stomach lining, causing ulcers. Some, like acetaminophen, damage or overburden the liver. Some have been linked to hypertension. Some have been linked to thin skin and bone weakness. Some have been known to weaken immunity.

Ginger does none of this. Rather than *cause* negative side effects, ginger and other botanicals in the same category—such as curcumin, feverfew, holy basil, oregano, rosemary and baikal skullcap—modulate eicanosoids, reduce fever and inflammation while having other healthy side effects. According to various sources, ginger also stimulates immune function; increases healthy appetite; reduces nausea; protects against ulcers; increases liver vitality and circulation; calms nerves; stimulates endocrine function; encourages bone healing; increases lung and gum health; and neutralizes oxidative radicals. Ginger is antiseptic, anesthetic, and antimetic—among so many other characteristics and affects. Laboratory studies have also shown ginger to be protective against cancer (Shukla and Singh 2007).

There are a number of other excellent botanical treatments for pain to consider before resorting to the array of increasingly toxic pharmaceutical painkillers. Botanicals such as *cayenne pepper, white willow tree bark* and *meadowsweet* are good examples.

The latter two botanicals contain a constituent called *salicin*. This of course is the natural version of the synthetic *acetyl-salicylic acid,* known by its expired patented trademark name of *aspirin.* Acetyl-salicylic acid and its nonacetylated *salicylic acid* come with a side effect of gastro-intestinal upset, sometimes leading to ulceration and stomach bleeding. Other documented side effects of aspirin include *Reye's Syndrome*, liver damage, nephritis, central nervous system issues such as tinnitus, dizziness, vertigo, and the risk of uncontrolled bleeding due to the thinning of the blood.

Far from being natural, today's aspirin is usually manufactured from phenol, which can be derived from coal or isolated from other components. The phenol is treated with sodium and then carbon dioxide under pressure, rendering salicylate. After acidification into salicylic acid, it is acetylated with acetic anhydride to yield the final product. The environment surrounding each of these reactions produces significant magnetic influence to yield the synthetic result. Though it successfully relieves pain, it also creates imbalances. We know that aspirin has been shown to disrupt the cyclooxygenation (COX) process, which oxygenates fatty acids utilizing an enzyme called cyclooxygenase. The inflammatory process that produces prostaglandins and prostanoids such as thromboxane—which inhibits the inflammatory immune response of the body—is thus blocked. When the body's immune system senses an invader, this cascading inflammatory process helps rid the body of the invader is interrupted.

This means the fever the body produces is part of its detoxification process to rid the body of a foreign agent. Yes, the headache—a signal indicating a metabolic problem exists—may be squelched by inhibiting part of this inflammatory process. The problem is, without a correction of the *cause* of this inflammation, the problem will continue. The headache will come back or the joint pain will remain.

Pain is, after all, a signal for us to make a correction to remove the cause.

Aspirin's disruptive mechanisms are illustrated in its effective depletion of a number of nutrients from the body. These include iron, potassium, folic acid, and vitamin C. According to Kauffman (2000), death rates among populations of aspirin users are significantly higher than non-aspirin populations. Conservative estimates state 7,600 deaths and 76,000 hospitalizations occur within the U.S. from NSAIDS like aspirin (including others, such as Motrin®, Aleve® and Celebrex®).

On the other hand, white willow bark and meadowsweet—by nature's design—contain salicin buffered by a variety of constituents to balance these side effects. Their molecular arrangements are synergistically oriented with a balance of constituents, which buffer and ameliorate any negative effects. To the contrary, these herbs actually stimulate a healthy stomach lining! Quite the opposite effect of isolated, synthetic salicin.

Willow and meadowsweet also contain constituents that help the body detoxify of those invaders or conditions that may be causing the headache. In this way, these herbs, if used correctly, can help the body turn around the condition that originally caused the headache, joint pain or whatever.

Other pain-relieving herbs have similar effects. Cayenne is another example. Cayenne contains the alkaloid *capsaicin*—known to reduce the amount of *substance* P in nerves, thereby reducing pain transmission.

Cayenne also has tremendous antioxidant and antimicrobial effects as well, however. These effects help the body correct the condition that caused the pain in the first place. *Capiscium frutescens,* as it is known in botanical terms, contains not only capsaicin but also various carotenoids, flavonoids, volatile oils and vitamins A and C. These constituents work together to not only detoxify and cleanse the liver, bloodstream and lymphatic system, but they stimulate the immune system while rendering useful nutrients!

Back to meadowsweet, or *Filipendula ulmaria*. This herb actually has three types of salicylates: opiraein, salicin and gaultherine. These three act conjunctively to reduce fever and reduce inflammation for such issues like headaches or rheumatism. Whole meadowsweet herb also contains mucilage and tannins, which buffer the salicylates' potential negative effects within the gastrointestinal system. The tannins in meadowsweet also have therapeutic effects upon the digestive tract. For this reason, meadowsweet has been used successfully in cases of digestive disorders, including diarrhea and colitis. Meadowsweet also has antiseptic diuretic action, making it useful for detoxifying excess uric acid. Meadowsweet also increases detoxification through sweating, all the while reducing fever through its salicylate action. Aspirin can't hold a candle to this kind of synergistic healing.

Cancer prevention provides another basis for comparison between synthetic chemicals and nature's biochemicals. As cancer researchers have probed for various anti-cancer prevention strategies, the overwhelming evidence points to natural foods—especially those from plant sources—as most assuredly chemo-protective. In other words, those chemicals produced within botanical living organisms prevent cancer. They prevent DNA mutation. They stimulate the immune system. They augment the process of detoxification. New anti-cancer biochemicals are continuously being found among nature's foods, herbs, and mushrooms.

Foods noted for anti-cancer benefits include *apples, asparagus, barley, basil, beans, beets, various berries, broccoli, Brussels sprouts, buckwheat, bulgur, cabbage, cantaloupe, carrots, cauliflower, celery, cherries, chili peppers, corn, fiber, flaxseed, garlic, grapefruit, grape juice, mangoes, milk, mushrooms, nuts, oats, olive oil, oranges, pears, peas, pectin, prunes, raisins, rhubarb, rice, saponins, soy, various spices, wheat,* and many others (Yeager 1998).

For example, research indicates the intake of selenium—a mineral contained in Brazil nuts, grains and other foods—appears to protect the cell from the mutation of the p53 gene (Fischer *et al.* 2007). The p53 gene is now referred to as the *tumor suppressor gene.*

We are hard pressed to find edible botanicals that do not contribute to the immune system in one way or another, in contrast to pharmaceuticals, where we are hard pressed to find safe synthetic medications.

On the other hand, as researchers have investigated the causes of cancer, overwhelmingly the biggest culprits appear to be synthetic chemicals amongst our pervasive chemical-laced environment. Air and water pollution, synthetic building materials, cleaning agents, chemical food additives, and many others have been implicated as absolute carcinogens. Unnatural elements are carcinogens because they render free radicals that inflict, disrupt, and damage cells and tissues throughout the body, including the vital cells of artery walls, the stomach, the intestines, the heart, the liver and the brain—creating a basis for genetic mutation while switching off the protective p53 gene.

It is evident that plant-based natural biomolecules are for the most part chemoprotective, while synthetic substances are mostly carcinogenic.

What does this tell us about the difference between the two types of chemistry—synthetic versus natural? While natural biochemicals are produced within living organisms within a living natural ecosystem, synthetic chemicals are created in sealed laboratories and factories using extraordinary heat and unnatural catalysts. While natural biochemicals work harmonically within nature's balance, synthetic chemicals have produced a myriad of natural disasters, from toxic soup waterways to poisoned air.

Chapter Two

Toxins and Their Sources

We've talked about a wide range of toxins already. Let's now get a little more specific about toxin sources and some strategies to avoid them. Listing every toxin and its sources would fill many volumes. Instead, we will clarify the major toxin categories and discuss why they are toxic, together with a few strategies to avoid them.

Why Toxins are so Bad

A considerable amount of research has illustrated that selenium deficiencies are common among those who have muscle fatigue, thyroid issues, reproductive issues, lung disorders, immune disorders and cognitive issues. While many diets might be lacking in selenium, it should be noted that selenium deficiency is dramatically *more common* among those with these issues than the general population.

Significant research confirms that selenium deficiency relates directly to systemic inflammation:

Researchers from the University of Alabama's School of Public Health (Stone et al. 2010) reviewed the association between low levels of selenium and higher rates of AIDS, HIV infections and other immune diseases. They found that HIV-infected persons who have low selenium levels have a faster progression of their disease to AIDS, and higher rates of mortality.

Selenium is a key ingredient in the liver's production of glutathione peroxidase. Glutathione peroxidase neutralizes toxins and free radicals, especially those relating to lipid peroxides.

In one of the early studies that established this link, researchers from Stockholm's Karolinska Institute (Hasselmark *et al.* 1993) gave 24 intrinsic asthma patients either placebo or 100 micrograms of sodium selenite per day for two weeks. The selenium group had higher glutathione levels and activity, and their asthma significantly improved as compared with the placebo group.

Researchers from Slovakia's Institute of Preventive and Clinical Medicine (Jahnova *et al.* 2002) also gave 20 asthmatic adults either a placebo or 200 micrograms of selenium per day for six months, in addition to inhaled corticosteroids and beta-agonists. They found that the selenium blocked IFN-gamma adhesion molecules, reducing inflammation.

Researchers from Britain's Imperial College (Shaheen *et al.* 2007) tested 197 patients with 100 micrograms of a selenium-yeast formula or a placebo for 24 weeks. Quality of life increased among the selenium patients but in this study, there was little difference between the selenium group and the placebo (yeast only) group. It should be noted, however, that the patients were all taking regular steroid medication and this study only used 100 micrograms of a blend of selenium and yeast. So the selenium dosage was substantially (less than half) the dosage of the studies that showed reductions in inflammation symptoms and improvement in lung function.

The recommended daily allowance for selenium is 55 micrograms. The studies above illustrated that those with inflammation require more like 200 micrograms for a therapeutic effect.

The critical component in this mystery is glutathione peroxidase—an enzyme produced in the liver. Glutathione peroxidase is the leading enzyme responsible for the breakdown and removal of lipid hydroperoxides. Lipid hydroperoxides are oxidized fats that damage cell membranes. As they do this, they create pores in the cell. The resulting damage eventually kills most cells. Lipid hydroperoxides are one of the most damaging molecules within the body. They are responsible for many deadly metabolic diseases, including heart disease, artery disease, Alzheimer's disease and many others.

When lipid hydroperoxides accumulate in the body, they can also damage the cells of the airways, causing irritation and inflammation. The damage from lipid hydroperoxides stimulates an inflammatory response. Researchers have called the initial signal from the cell that initiates this inflammatory response *lipid peroxidation/LOOH-mediated stress signaling*. In other words, the cells are stressed by lipid peroxidation, and this initiates a distress signal to the immune system.

This distress signal stimulates the contraction of the smooth bronchial muscles while stimulating leukotriene activity—which delivers cytotoxic (cell-destroying) T-cells and eosinophils into the region. This stimulates the production of more mucous, which drowns the cilia and restricts breathing.

The production of more mucous is intended to clear out the damaged cells. In other words, much of the increased mucous that drowns the cilia and produces wheezing is caused by the influx of dead cell matter from lipid hydroperoxide damage.

By virtue of removing lipid hydroperoxides, glutathione peroxidase—not to be confused with glutathione reductase—regulates pro-inflammatory arachidonic acid metabolism. In other words, glutathione regulates the release and populations of those pro-inflammatory mediators, the leukotrienes. Leukotriene activity is directly associated with the damage created by lipid hydroperoxides. Thus, when lipid hydroperoxide levels are reduced by glutathione peroxidase, leukotriene density is reduced.

Selenium is required for glutathione peroxidase production. Should the body be overloaded with lipid hydroperoxides, more glutathione is required to clear out the damage. As more glutathione is produced, more selenium is utilized, which runs selenium levels down.

This issue was illustrated by research from Britain's South Manchester University Hospital (Hassan 2008). The researchers studied 13 aspirin-induced asthmatics and a healthy matched control group. They found that the asthmatics maintained higher levels of selenium in the bloodstream—especially among blood platelets. This high selenium content in the bloodstream correlated with higher glutathione peroxidase activity. The research illustrated how selenium is used up faster in by those with inflammation through this glutathione peroxidase process.

Lipid Peroxidation

As we touched on earlier, lipid peroxidation means that the lipids that make up the cell membrane are being robbed of electrons. This 'robbery' results in an unstable cell membrane. Let's take a closer look at the process of lipid peroxidation.

The first step takes place with the entry of a reactive oxygen species into the proximity of the cell. Reactive oxygen species are elements that require an electron—such as hydrogen (H+)—in order to become stable.

Fatty acids that make up the membranes of cells are the likely candidates for peroxidation. Remember, the name "lipid" refers to a fatty acid. Fatty acids include saturated fats, polyunsaturates, monounsaturates, and so on (see fatty acid discussions later on).

Several types of lipids make up the cell membrane. Fatty acids will combine with other molecules to make phospholipids, cholesterols and glycolipids. Saturates and polyunsaturates are typical, but there are several species of polyunsaturates. These range from long chain versions to short versions. They also include the cis- configuration and the trans- configuration. Cell membranes that utilize predominantly cis- versions with long chains are the most durable. Those cell membranes with trans- configurations can be highly unstable, and irregularly porous. This is one reason why trans fats are unhealthy. The other reason is that trans fats easily become peroxidized.

Cell membranes with more long chain fatty acids are more stable and are less subject to peroxidation. Shorter chains that provide more double bonds are less stable, because these are more easily broken. Also, monounsaturated fatty acids such as GLA are more stable.

Once the fatty acid is degraded by an oxygen species, it becomes a fatty acid radical. The fatty acid will usually become oxidized, making it a peroxyl-fatty acid radical. This radical will react with other fatty acids, forming a cyclic process involving radicals called cyclic peroxides.

This becomes a chain reaction that results in the cell membrane becoming completely destroyed and dysfunctional. This forces the cell to signal to the immune system that it is under attack and about to become malignant. The T-cell immune response will often initiate the cell's self-destruct switch: TNF—tumor necrosis factor. Alternatively, the cell may be directly destroyed by cytotoxic T-cells. The combined process stimulates inflammation. As these cells are killed or self-destruct, they are purged from the system—provoking increased mucous formation.

While this peroxidation and cell destruction is taking place, the immune system is not simply standing by. The body enters a state called *systemic inflammation*. As we discussed earlier, during systemic inflammation, the immune system launches an ongoing supply of eosinophils, neutrophils and mast cells, which release granulocytes that inflame the airways.

In other words, due to this ongoing peroxidation, the immune system is on a hair-trigger. Imagine a person at work who is stressed from being buried in work and a myriad of problems. You walk into their office and they immediately react: "And what do *you* want?" they ask.

If they were not overloaded with work, problems and deadlines, your coming into their office would probably be met without such a frantic response. But since they were overloaded, they reacted (hyper reacted is a better word) more defensively than needed, *because they thought you were going to add to their workload.*

In other words, inflammation is simply a defense measure by an immune system that is overwhelmed.

Typical associations with inflammation include artery damage and plaque build-up, obesity, diabetes, a sedentary lifestyle, and a diet high in saturated fats and/or fried foods. High blood pressure and fast or irregular heart rate, especially in persons over 40 years old, are also strong markers.

Along with these associations come higher levels of total cholesterol, low-density lipoprotein (LDL) and very low-density lipoprotein (VLDL) cholesterol, and total triglycerides are also key markers. The link between small LDL particle size and atherosclerosis is a key factor, and the oxidation of LDL particles is the match that lights the fuse. These involve hyperperoxides, as they readily form oxidative radicals. The cascade towards LDL oxidation also seems to be accelerated by lipooxygenases like 15-LOX-2 along with cyclooxygenases. The process as a whole is lipid peroxidation.

In addition to launching systemic inflammation due to widespread cell damage, the body also produces processes that attempt to halt the peroxidation cycle. One of these components is the glutathione peroxidase enzyme discussed earlier, formed by the body using selenium as a substrate. Depending upon the rate of lipid peroxidation, however, this could be like trying to blow out a forest fire. There is simply too much fire spreading too quickly.

Reactive Oxygen Species

Let's take a wider perspective on the problem. The initiation process of the lipid peroxidation is started by a reactive oxygen species. What is this?

This is also often called a free radical. A free radical is an unstable molecule or ion that forms during a chemical reaction. In other words, the molecule or ion needs another atom, ion or molecule to stabilize it. Once it is stable, it is not reactive.

While a free radical is unstable, it can damage any number of elements it meets. These include the cells, organs and tissues of the body.

Nature produces many, many free radicals. However, nature typically accompanies radicals with the molecules, atoms or ions that stabilize the radical. In the atmosphere, for example, radicals become stabilized by ozone and other elements. In plants, radicals become stabilized by antioxidants from nutrients derived from the sun, soil and oxygen. In the body, radicals are stabilized by antioxidizing enzymes, nutrients and other elements. These include glutathione peroxidase, as we discussed earlier.

Confirming this, the research from South Manchester University Hospital mentioned earlier concluded with a comment that the increased glutathione peroxidase activity related to radical oxidation: *"administration of aspirin to these patients increases the generation of immediate oxygen products..."*

Another anti-oxidation process within the body utilizes the *superoxide dismutase* (SOD) enzyme. The SOD enzyme is typically available within the cytoplasm of most cells. Here SOD is complexed by either copper and zinc, or manganese—similar to the way selenium is complexed with the glutathione peroxidase enzyme. Several types of SOD enzymes reside within the body—some in the mitochondria and some in the intercellular tissue fluids. SOD neutralizes superoxides before they can damage the inside and outside of the cell—assuming the body is healthy, with substantial amounts of SOD. The immune system produces superoxides as part of its strategy to attack microorganisms and toxins.

Another broad anti-oxidation process utilizes *catalase*. Here the body provides an enzyme bound by iron to neutralize peroxides to oxygen and water. It is a standard component of many metabolic reactions within the body.

Yet another enzyme utilized for radical reduction is *glutathione reductase*. This enzyme works with NADP in the cell to stabilize hydrogen peroxide oxidized radicals before they can damage the cell.

Notice that all of these antioxidizing enzymes require minerals. We have seen either selenium, copper, zinc, manganese or iron as necessary to keep these enzymes in good supply. Many other minerals and trace elements are used by other antioxidant and detoxifying enzyme processes. These minerals, and many of the enzymes themselves, are supplied by various foods and supplements, as we'll discuss further.

Another tool that the healthy body utilizes to stabilize radicals are the antioxidants supplied by plant foods. Plants produce antioxidants to protect their own cells from radical damage. Thus, their plant material contains a host of these oxidation stabilizers, which our bodies use to neutralize radicals.

C-reactive Protein

A plethora of research has shown that higher C-reactive protein levels are indicative of systemic inflammation occurring somewhere in the body. The diagnostic measurement of CRP for cardiovascular disease is now standard care. This is because cardiovascular disease is typically the result of inflammation within the artery walls. This is usually companied by a body-wide inflammation condition called systemic inflammation.

CRP is now seen among many other inflammatory diseases. For expel, researchers from the Texas Tech University Health Sciences Center (Arif *et al.*

2007) studied the relationships between C-reactive protein (CRP) and asthma among 8,020 adults over the age of twenty. They found that those in the highest quarter of CRP levels had a 60% greater risk of current asthma than those with lower CRP levels. Those with the highest quartile of CRP levels had more than double the incidence of asthmatic wheezing, and more than triple the incidence of nighttime coughing. In other words, as we discussed in *Asthma Solved Naturally*, asthma is another sign of systemic inflammation.

So what causes systemic inflammation? As we'll discuss in the next chapter, localized inflammation is often caused by physical injuries like broken bones or tissue damage. Systemic inflammation, however, is typically caused by the bombardment and overload of toxins or pathological microorganisms.

Systemic inflammation indicates that the immune system is overburdened. The extent or combination of the elements mentioned simply overwhelms the immune system. Typically, the immune system can resolve most of these problems when it is presented with a small amount or a few of them at a time. But when an avalanche of them becomes too great, the immune system goes on alert, resulting in systemic inflammation.

Systemic inflammation is the immune system's version of all-out war. The immune system begins to launch the nukes. These can include fever, vomiting, diarrhea, swelling and pain.

The rest of this chapter will more specifically discuss lifestyle choices that produce or worsen systemic inflammation within the body. In other words, these are all *contributing causes*. This means that just one of these factors may not in itself cause systemic inflammation. But any one of these, in addition to others, can overwhelm the immune system—producing systemic inflammation.

Systemic Inflammation Factors

While toxin overload is the primary condition, the following list summarizes conditions that collectively contribute to systemic inflammation:

1) **Toxemia:** An overload of toxins that produce radicals.
2) **Infections:** Infection with microorganisms that produce mutagenicity, toxins and radicals: viruses, bacteria, yeasts and parasites.
3) **Antioxidant enzyme deficiencies:** An undersupply of antioxidizing enzymes that stabilize radicals, including glutathione peroxidase, glutathione reductase, catalase and superoxide dismutase.
4) **Dietary antioxidant deficiencies:** An undersupply of antioxidants from our foods to help stabilize radicals.
5) **Barriers to detoxification:** Lifestyle or physiological factors that block our body's ability to rid waste products and toxins. Detoxification requires exercise, fresh air, sweating, sunshine and so on.
6) **Poor dietary choices:** A poor diet burdens the body with toxins, unstable fatty acids, refined sugars and overly processed foods.
7) **Immunosuppression:** A burdened or defective immune system.

Chemical Toxin Overload

Clinical research by Professor John G Ionescu, Ph.D. (2009) concluded that environmental pollution is clearly associated with the development of hypersensitivities. Dr. Ionescu's research indicated that environmental noxious agents, including many chemicals, contribute to the total immune burden, producing increased susceptibility for intolerances due to inflammation.

According to Dr. Ionescu, toxic inputs such as formaldehyde, smog, industrial waste, wood preservatives, microbial toxins, alcohol, pesticides, processed foods, nicotine, solvents and amalgam-heavy metals have been observed to be mediating toxins that produce the physical susceptibilities for toxin sensitization and subsequent inflammation.

This is also consistent with findings of other scientists—as discussed—that chemicals overload the immune system and cause inflammation.

Chemical toxins such as DDT, PBDEs, dioxin, formaldehyde, benzene, butane and chlorinated chemicals tend to accumulate within the body's tissues. This is because many of these are fat-soluble. Other compounds, such as phthalate plasticizers and parabens tend to clear the body faster because they are not fat soluble. Still, these can also cause toxicity issues if they are regularly presented to the body.

The compounding of these synthetics contributes to the body-wide status of systemic inflammation. As the immune system gears up to overdrive due to the overloading of multiple toxins, it becomes weaker and hypersensitive. This can cause a host of issues, including allergies, irritable bowel syndrome and many others.

This is a gigantic discussion, so here we will summarize the major categories and sources of toxic chemicals that add to our immune system burden:

Plasticizers and Parabens

Today, plasticizers and parabens are common amongst many of our medications, toys, foods packaged in plastic and other consumer items. Phthalates are also found in many household items. While phthalates have shorter half-lives than some toxins, they have been implicated in systemic inflammatory issues, hormone disruption, cancers and other conditions. Many cosmetics and antiperspirants contain parabens. They are thus readily absorbed into the skin where they can provoke inflammatory responses (Crinnion 2010).

Heavy Metals

Heavy metals are metal elements that exist naturally in trace quantities within our soils, waters and foods. However, extraordinary levels of heavy metals such as cadmium, lead and mercury are produced by humanity's industrial complex in the manufacturing of various consumer items.

We can cite many studies that have associated heavy metal exposure to immunosuppression. Mercury is one of these.

For example, in multicenter research from the Department of Medicine from the Lavoro Medical Center in Bari, Italy (Soleo *et al.* 2002), researchers studied the effects of low levels of inorganic mercury exposure on 117 workers. They compared these with 172 general population subjects. They found no difference in the white blood cell count between the two groups. However, the worker group exposed to mercury had increased levels of CD4+ and CD8+ cytokines, and CD4+ levels were particularly high. These indicated a state of systemic inflammation. In addition, significantly lower levels of interleukin (IL-8) occurred among the exposed workers—indicating immunosuppression.

This research concluded that even low levels of environmental exposure to mercury and other heavy metals (beyond the trace levels normally found in nature) suppresses the immune system and stimulates inflammation.

Cadmium is another heavy metal bombarding us. Among consumer products, cadmium is used in a number of metal coatings, batteries and colorings. Most cigarettes also contain cadmium.

Consumer Toxins

In conjunction with a mandate to lower toxin levels among the state's residents, in 2010 the Minnesota Department of Health compiled and released a list of the most toxic chemicals used in consumer products, building materials, pesticides, hair dyes, detergents, aerosols, cosmetics, furniture polish, herbicides, paints, cleaning solutions and many other common sources. The list also referenced research connecting the toxins to disease conditions.

The list contained 1,755 chemicals.

For each of these toxins, the liver and immune system must launch a variety of macrophages, T-cells and B-cells to break them apart and escort them out of the body. This means that each toxin represents an additional load the immune system must carry.

We might compare this to moving dirt. A small handful of dirt can be carried around easily, and dispersed without much effort. However, a truckload of dirt is another matter completely. What can we do with a truckload of dirt? If we dumped a truckload of dirt on our lawn, we'd have a hill of dirt that would bury the access to our front door and annihilate our lawn and/or garden.

This is a useful comparison because while our bodies can handle a small amount of toxins quite easily, modern society is increasingly dumping toxic 'dirt' into our atmosphere, water and foods, effectively inundating our bodies 'by the truckload.'

With this increased burden, the research shows that the body's defenses are lowered. The mucosal membrane is weakened. The immune system is on alert. Systemic inflammation becomes evident. In this immunosuppressed state, the body is more likely to succumb to a variety of disease conditions.

Water Pollutants

Our industrial society has been dumping massive amounts of synthetic chemistry into our waters for many decades, and we are paying the price. Water contamination comes from manufacturing, wastewater streams from houses, air pollution, ship and boat waste streams and pollutants, run-off from farms and the gutters and streets. All of these to one degree or another end up in our drinking water supplies.

While municipalities have extensive chlorination systems in place to clear microbiological content, removal systems for chemical pollutants are still in various stages of development. As a result, our drinking water supplies have numerous contaminants.

Even some of the cleaning agents used in some municipal water supplies are toxic. This includes trichloroethylene. Trichloroethylene is a chlorinated hydrocarbon used to separate oil from water. The solvent was popularized in the dry cleaning business, and is a common cleansing agent in many local water municipalities.

Pharmaceutical medicines in our water supplies make for a perfect example. In 2007, researchers from Finland's Abo Akademi University (Vieno *et al.*) released a study showing that pharmaceutical beta-blockers, antiepileptic drugs, lipid regulators, anti-inflammatory drugs and fluoroquinolone drugs were all found in river waters. The concentrations of these were well above drinking water limits. The researchers also found that water treatment only eliminated an average of 13% of the concentration of these pharmaceuticals. This means that 87% of these pharmaceutical medicines remained in the drinking water, ready to dose each and every person drinking that water with prescription medication.

Other pollutants that are commonly found in our drinking water supplies include PCBs, and other biphenol compounds, dioxin, chlorine metabolites, pesticides, herbicides, petroleum byproducts, nitrates, and many others.

Agricultural runoff is a huge source of drinking water contamination. In addition, nitrogen-rich fertilizers choke rivers and oceans with extra nitrogen, causing abnormal blooms of algae. These massive algal blooms cut off oxygen supplies and lead to the die-offs of many species of marine life. *Dead zones* have been reportedly growing in many of the world's waterways, as we will discuss shortly. The cause is the massive use of nitrogen-based synthetic fertilizers.

The use of pesticides on agricultural land, playgrounds, parks, home lawns, and gardens throughout the United States is staggering, and it is growing. In 1964, approximately 233 million pounds of pesticides were applied in the U.S. By 1982, this amount tripled to 612 million pounds. In 2006 and 2007, the U.S. Environmental Protection Agency reported that some five *billion* pounds of these chemicals were applied per year throughout America's crops, forests, parks, and lawns.

One of the more increasingly popular pesticides is imidacloprid, a neoni-cotinoid. Introduced by Bayer in 1994, imidacloprid is used against aphids and similar insects on over 140 different crops. Touted as a chemical with a fairly short half-life of thirty days in water and twenty-seven days in anaerobic soil, imidacloprid's half-life is about 997 days in aerobic soil. While it has a lower immediate toxicity compared with hazards like DDT, imidacloprid's use is now widespread. It is rated by the EPA and WHO as *"moderately toxic"* in small doses. Larger doses can disrupt liver and thyroid function. While this pesticide does well at killing off increasingly resistant pests, it has also been shown to decimate bee populations.

Cleaning agents are used with or rinsed by water. They will thus immedi-ately enter our greywater systems. According to the U.S. Poison Control Centers, about ten percent of all toxin exposure is caused by cleaning prod-ucts, with almost two-thirds involving children under six years old. While we might be shocked to find a child toying with a bottle of drain cleaner contain-ing sulfuric acid, hydrochloric acid and lye, we do not think twice about feed-ing this same product into our waterways. We wear gloves to protect our skin from the harmful affects of ammonia and bleach while we do our cleaning but assume they disappear once poured down the sink.

An example of this is 1,4-dioxane, a common ingredient in many sham-poos and other cleaning products. The California EPA documented that 1,4-dioxane is a carcinogen that can also damage kidneys, nerves and lungs. It biodegrades very slowly and is becoming a threat to drinking water supplies. This is but one of many.

In a 2002 U.S. Geological Survey report on stream water contaminants, 69% of stream samples revealed non-biodegradable detergents, and 66% of the samples contained disinfectant chemicals. Phosphates—central ingredi-ents in many commercial laundry soaps—have been banned for dumping in over eleven states in the U.S. because of their dangerous effects upon the environment. Yet many people still use these soaps without any consideration of their effects upon our waters.

Biphenyls are considered *xenoestrogens,* or endocrine system disruptors. Long-term effects as their residues build up in the tissues of aquatic species, and bio-accumulate up the ladder to our cells, organs and tissue systems. Research has found that biphenyls have produced sexual re-orientation of fish in some water supplies.

Our waters are filling up with plastic particles. As plastics break down into smaller particles, they are absorbed by filtering marine plants and aquat-ics and passed up the food chain. Research led by Captain Charles Moore of the *Algalita Marine Research Foundation* (2001; 2002; 2008) found an astound-ing six-to-one ratio of plastic particles-to-plankton in some areas. This means that for every pound of algae—the key nutrient for nearly all marine life—there are six pounds of plastic in the oceans. This also means that our marine life is eating plastic particles with their meals: and so are humans who eat fish.

Captain Moore was first alerted to the plastic problem in 1997 when he sailed through a region of the Pacific Ocean between Hawaii and California called the *North Pacific Gyre*. He came upon a large area of floating garbage, consisting primarily of plastic debris. The *Great Pacific Garbage Patch* is now documented from a number of studies, the earliest from a 1988 National Oceanic and Atmospheric Administration paper.

Requiring some 500 years to breakdown, plastics are known to disrupt hormones and accumulate hydrocarbons as mentioned earlier. It is estimated that about twenty percent of the plastic polluting our waters comes from discarded plastic pellets used to make plastic by manufacturers. These pellets are being swept or blown into the water from careless manufacturers and transport companies. The other eighty percent of the ocean's plastics is estimated to come from daily consumer use and the careless littering of waterways and runoffs.

These combined factors are increasingly problematic to a human population seeking to sustain life on the planet. Research by Slovenian researchers Tatjana Tisler and Jana Zagorc-Koncan (2003) has shown that we are drastically underestimating the effects of toxic industrial waste. Our typical method for toxicity research has been to study each individual chemical and its possible toxicity. What we are missing with this type of research is the combined effects of the thousands of chemicals we are putting into our waters. As these chemicals mix, they create a toxic soup of new chemical combinations. Some of these are combinations are exponentially more toxic than the individual chemicals.

Insect Endotoxins

Insect endotoxins—such as from dust mites—can be allergens as well as toxins. They can overload our immune system with toxicity and produce systemic inflammation. This overloaded immune system produces the allergy response.

Many other insects also produce endotoxins that one may become sensitized to. These include cockroaches, ladybugs, aphids and other household pests. We should be clear that insect endotoxins are practically everywhere. They are unavoidable. They are in our water, air, foods, carpets, seats, floors... literally everywhere.

Humans have been dealing with insect endotoxins since time immemorial. Furthermore, a strong immune system can easily tolerate these, simply because a natural immune system has the technology to break down and cleanse these toxins from the body.

However, an immune system that already is overloaded with toxins may have difficulty breaking these down and purging their metabolites from the body. In this case, there might be a need to reduce our exposure to dust mites and insect endotoxins.

While insects are ubiquitous, dust mites are especially insidious because they are so tiny and hardy. They live in beds, pillows, carpets, and other fabrics, and their favorite food is dead skin cells that slough off of our bodies and the bodies of our pets.

There are two prevalent household species: The American house dust mite (*Dermatophagoides farinae*) and the European house dust mite *(D. pteronyssinus)*. Storage mite species include the *Acarus spp.* and *Tyrophagus spp.* Dust mites feed on organic matter—and they love dead skin. The primary allergens these mites create are the skin moltings they shed as they grow, and their feces. Because of their propensity for eating skin, mites are usually not found in vents or ducts.

Many health experts have advised that dust mites like warm and humid places, so they suggest placing a dehumidifier in the house. University of Cambridge researchers (Hyndman *et al.* 2000) tested this theory. They investigated 76 households given a dehumidifier, a behavior program, or nothing for one year. Other trap measures were also instituted to reduce dust mites. Every three months they tested each house for humidity, temperature, dust mite counts, dust mite allergens, and several other environmental elements. Not surprisingly, they found the relative humidity in houses with dehumidifiers were significantly lower than houses without dehumidifiers. However, the houses with dehumidifiers had no fewer dust mites than did the other houses.

Confirming this, researchers from New Zealand's Wellington School of Medicine (Crane *et al.* 1998) studied lowering humidity levels in heat-exchanger systems (MVHE) units. They tested ten buildings in Wellington, NZ. Again, lowering the humidity in these buildings did not reduce concentrations of the *Der p1* dust mite allergen.

German researchers (Kroidl *et al.* 2007) found, in a study of 132 patients with bronchial asthma, over half were sensitized to either storage mites or house mites. Only three patients were allergic to storage mites and not household dust mites. Farm workers, bakers and forestry and paper mill workers had the most risk of storage mite allergies.

Researchers from Italy's G. D'Annunzio University (Riccioni *et al.* 2001) studied the seasonal nature of mite and pollen sensitivity among 165 allergic patients. They found that pollen bronchial symptoms increased with pollen seasons as expected. However, asthmatic symptoms among patients allergic to dust mites increased in the fall—seemingly as mites or their endotoxin populations also increase.

Researchers from the UK's Imperial College (Atkinson *et al.* 1999) studied the relationship between allergen exposure and subsequent asthma among infants. They collected and analyzed dust samples from 643 homes. They coupled this with surveying each house and studying each infant. They found that higher dust mite allergen content was seen among houses that were carpeted, had double-glazed windows and less ventilation. Houses sampled in the winter had more dust mites than those sampled in other parts of the year.

These conditions did not produce greater levels of cat allergens, however. Homes with more occupants had more dust mite and fewer cat allergens, regardless of cat ownership. Homes with smoking inhabitants had significantly fewer dust mites, but again had no difference in cat allergens.

Animal Dander

Animal dander is another toxin produced by the waste products of a living organism. A strong immune system should be well equipped to tolerate and manage these, but an overburdened immune system may not be.

Animal dander can come from any number of animals, including pets, farm animals, zoo animals and wild animals. This means that sources for animal dander include pet stores, zoos, vet clinics, farms, barns, and just about anywhere else that animals may occupy for extended periods.

The allergic or sensitive element of animal dander is not necessarily their hair, as one might think. It is typically the shedding of their skin as it flakes off their bodies. This can resemble dandruff, but may also be invisible to the naked eye. Dead skin or waste matter excreted by their skin is included in this. In other words, we are talking about the waste products of animals.

While we know now that greater levels of pet dander do not necessarily cause allergies, pet dander is one of the most prevalent allergy triggers. Illustrating this, researchers from Denmark's Roskilde County Hospital and Sweden's Sahlgrenska University Hospital (Plaschke *et al.* 1999) studied 1,859 adults to test atopic sensitization and asthma. They found that positive skin prick tests for allergens and allergen-specific IgEs included pets, grass pollens and mites. The greatest associations between allergies were made with cat and dog allergens.

Today, cat allergens (such as protein *Fel d1*) are found virtually everywhere. Scientists from New Zealand's Canterbury Respiratory Research Group and Christchurch Hospital (Martin *et al.* 1998) tested a variety of public places to understand exposure levels for the *Fel d1* cat allergen. They tested 203 floors, 64 beds and 24 seats in hotels, hospitals, rest homes, churches, schools, daycare centers, ski lodges, movie theaters, banks and airplanes. They found that 95% of the floors, 91% of the beds, and 100% of the seats maintained exposure levels of *Fel d1*. Furthermore, they found that theater seats and airplane seats contained the greatest levels, with more cat allergens than other public places, and most floors. Not surprisingly, cat allergen levels were greater on carpeted floors than on hard floors.

New Zealand has relatively high rates of asthma and allergies. About half of Kiwi households also have a cat, according to the research. To test the relationship between cat allergens and asthma, Wellington School of Medicine researchers (Patchett *et al.* 1997) tested the cat allergen (*Fel d1*) levels within schools and the clothing of children. They analyzed the clothing of 202 children and floors of 11 school classrooms. They found cat allergen practically everywhere, and (duh) highest on the clothing of children from homes that had cats. They also found a significant amount of cat allergen among the carpeted classes, significantly more than the floors without carpets.

While the researchers concluded that carpeting should be discouraged from schools and daycare centers, they could not correlate asthma frequency with increased cat allergens.

We are surrounded by microorganisms. Trillions upon trillions of bacteria, fungi, viruses, parasites, nanobacteria and extremophiles live within our clothes, cars, bathrooms, beds, floors, air, and all over our bodies. Just about everything we touch has millions of microbes living on it. Bacteria also live in and around just about every food. Our bodies are also densely populated with bacteria. There are more bacteria in our bodies than there are cells.

This situation has not changed for millions of years. Bacteria have been living amongst us and other creatures of our planet through the duration. Not only that, but for most of humankind's existence, we slept on earthen floors and straw beds. We farmed in our bare feet or in sandals made of rope. We crapped in holes in the ground and ate with our fingers. We drank out of the streams with our hands, and used twigs to brush our teeth.

How is it that over the past century we have become so fearful of bacteria? How is it that we now live in disinfectant-cleaned houses, and wash our hands with antibacterial soaps, and we still have a mortal fear of bacteria? How is it that despite these measures, we are still becoming infected?

Today, despite our various antibiotics, antivirals, disinfectants, mouthwashes and antiseptic cleaners, infectious diseases are on the rise. Rates of tuberculosis, influenza, shingles, mononucleosis, cytomegalovirus, malaria, HIV, AIDS and herpes are increasing worldwide. Estimates have calculated that 80% of the U.S. population may be infected with Herpes Simplex 1, while some 45 million are infected with the genital variety, HS2. More than half the world's population harbors *Helicobacter pylori* bacteria. About 1.5 million Americans are infected with sexually transmitted diseases gonorrhea, syphilis or chlamydia. Over 33 million people around the world were theoretically infected with HIV in 2005—a rise of 16% per year. In the U.S. alone, there are about 40,000 new cases of HIV documented every year. About one third of the world's population is infected with the tuberculosis bacterium. Every year about 6 million people die from TB according to the CDC. Millions more are infected with water-borne diseases throughout the world.

Microorganisms

Microorganisms and their endotoxins are collectively called *biological pollutants*. These microorganisms include bacteria, viruses, fungi and mold.

Bacteria can come from rotting food, plants, people and pets. Dander also can carry these creatures. Viruses can trigger inflammation initially, or once they infect the body's cells. Viruses damage DNA within the cells, and reproduce through the body via the DNA damage.

Microorganisms can grow on anything wet—especially mold. Almost any type of sitting water or dampness will grow mold, especially those in dark areas (as many fungi abhor sunlight).

Research has confirmed that infective microorganisms from viruses, bacteria and fungi can stimulate serious systemic inflammation. As we'll discuss later, microorganism infection requires a sharp living immune system—as we'll discuss in the next chapter. While a periodic super-cleanse might be helpful to clear microorganism toxins, a vibrant living immune system will consistently protect the body against infection. Let's talk about the possible microorganism infections we can face.

Bacteria were first discovered in 1673 by Dutch scientist Antony van Leeuwenhoek. Leeuwenhoek began writing letters to the Royal Society of London about the images he was seeing in his newly invented microscope. In 1674, Leeuwenhoek described his microscopic creatures as "wound serpent-wise and orderly arranged, after the manner of the copper or tin worms." He described "many very little living animalcules."

There are a variety of different

Types of Microbes

Fungi	Yeasts, molds and others; over 100,000 species; live in earth, air, water and damp, moist environments; can infect the body via food, water, air, and skin
Bacteria	Single-celled organisms; live in water, earth, air, on and inside other living organisms; can infect via food, water, air, and skin
Viruses	Non-living; genetic mutation triggers; exist in water, earth, air and skin; infect by altering cellular DNA, and spreading through ongoing cell division and mutation
Mycoplasmas	Ancient slow-moving bacteria; live primarily on earth and water; infect mostly via food, water and touch
Parasites	Tiny organisms that infect and live within another living organism. Includes worms, protozoa and amoeba
Thermophiles	Opportunistic bacteria that can live in very hot environments, such as deserts, boiling water or even in ovens
Psychophiles	Opportunistic bacteria that can live in the very cold, such as the artic or in freezers
Nanobacteria	Extremely small bacteria that typically have a hard calcium shell. Are thought to cause some diseases considered autoimmune.

Bacterial Infections

Today we are dealing with a multitude of infections from all of these types of microorganisms. Growing infectious diseases from this list include lyme disease (*Borrelia burgdorferi*), pneumonia, staphylococcus, streptococcus, salmonella, *E. coli*, cholera, listeria, salmonella, Shigella, dengue fever, yellow fever, tuberculosis, cryptosporidiosis, hepatitis, rabies and others. Many of these microorganisms are growing despite our antibiotic and antiviral medications. Some are growing because of unsafe sex, unclean water or changes in land use. Many are growing because of new opportunities arising from our destruction of nature. Many are becoming resistant to our antibiotics. These are often referred to as *superbugs*.

One of the more dangerous of these superbugs is methicillin-resistant *Staphylococcus aureus* (MRSA). MRSA rates are on the rise, and nearly every hospital—the crown jewels of our antimicrobial kingdom—is infected with MRSA. In a 2007 survey of 1200 U.S. hospitals, 46 of every 1,000 hospital inpatients are colonized or infected with MRSA, with 75% of those being infected. Among the general population, the incidence of MRSA has skyrocketed from 24 cases per 100,000 people in 2000 to 164 cases per 100,000 people in 2005 (Hota *et al.* 2007). This means that MRSA is infecting nearly seven times the number of people it did in 2000.

The virulence of *Staphylococcus aureus* was first realized in 1929 by Alexander Fleming, a microbiologist who cultured a combination of *Staphylococcus aureus* in the vicinity of a growing mold. He noticed that the penicillin mold would kill some bacteria and not others. Fleming soon realized that *Staphylococcus aureus* adapted quickly to the penicillin. It became resistant. Even to this day, *Staphylococcus aureus* is still one of the most antibiotic-resistant bacteria.

Staphylococcus aureus is also one of the most lethal bacteria known to man. It secretes three cell-killing toxins: alpha toxin, beta toxin and leukocidin. Together these poisons bind to and dissolve cell membranes, allowing cytoplasm and cell contents to leak out. This, of course, immediately kills the cell. The immune system also has difficulty attacking and removing *Staphylococcus aureus* because it secretes enzymes that neutralize the immune system's attack strategies. *Staphylococcus aureus* adapts very quickly, so the more we throw at it, the stronger it becomes.

Multiple pathogenic microorganisms can grow and prosper within the mouth, teeth and gums. These include *Streptococcus mutans, Streptococcus pyogenes, Porphyromonas gingivalis, Tannerella forsynthensis* and *Prevotella*. Additional microbes can grow within root canals. Root canals provide protected spaces for bacterial growth. Bacteria infecting root canals can include a variety of steptococci, staphylococci, and even dangerous spirochetes such as *Borrelia burgdorferi* among many others. Just about any bacteria that can infect the body internally can hibernate inside root canals. Because root canals are enclosed and the tissues around them die, the immune system cannot reach these areas to remove bacteria. As a result, a growing number of diseases are now being associated with root canal-harbored bacteria.

As these microbial populations grow, they not only can infect teeth and gums with gingivitis: They can also infect various other parts of the body. Infected gums have been implicated in a variety of fatal disorders, including heart disease, lung disease, liver disease, kidney disease, septic arthritis and others. A recent report from the Jos University Teaching Hospital in Nigeria (Adoga *et al.* 2009) reported that, "Most often the cause of cervical necrotizing fascitis is of dental origin." Necrotizing fascitis is a growing lethal infection of multiple bacteria that rapidly destroy tissues around the body, causing death very quickly.

Bacterial infections can cause an overload on the immune system because they produce endotoxins that form radicals in the body.

Lipopolysaccharides are common bacteria endotoxins. Lipopolysaccharides make up the cell membranes of gram negative bacteria, and they make up a significant part of their waste stream. Lipopolysaccharides also have shown in research to produce inflammation and immunosuppression.

A few diseases linked to microorganisms:

Disease	Some Suspected Microbes
Stroke and cardiovascular diseases	*Helicobacter. pylori* *Treponema pallidum* (syphilis) *Staphylococcus aureus* *Enterococci faecalis* *Streptococcus* spp. Herpes Simplex (I and II) *Pneumonococcal aerogenes* *Candida albicans* *Streptococcus mutans* *Escherichia coli* *Chlamydia pneumonia* *Porphyromonas gingivalis* *Tannerella forsynthensis* *Prevotella intermedia*
Gallstones	Eubacteria *Clostridium* spp.
Ulcers, ulcerative colitis and Crohn's	*Helicobacter pylori* *Clostridium* spp. *E. coli* *Mycobacterium pneumoniae*
Cancers	*Staphylococcus aureus* *Enterococci faecalis* *Streptococcus* spp. *Pneumonococcal aerogenes* *Streptococcus mutans*

	E. coli mammary tumor virus papilloma virus (HPV) *H. pylori* Heptitis B
Diabetes	Coxackle B virus Cytomegalovirus *Salmonella osteomyelitis* others suspected (see arthritis below)
Arthritis	*Bacteroides fragilis* *Borrelia burgdorferi* *Brucella melitensis* *Brucellae* spp. *Campylobacter jejuni* *Chlamydia trachomatis* *Clostridium difficile* *Corynebacterium striatum* *Cryptococcal pyarthrosis* *Gardnerella vaginalis* *Kingella kingae* *Listeria monocytogenes* *Moraxella canis* *Mycobacterium lepromatosis* *Mycobacterium marinum* *Mycobacterium terrae* *Mycoplasma arthritidis* *Mycoplasma hominis* *Mycoplasma leachii sp.* *Neisseria gonorrhoeae* *Ochrobactrum anthropi* *Pasteurella multocida* *Pneumocystis jiroveci* *Porphyromonas gingivalis* *Prevotella bivia* *Prevotella intermedia* *Prevotella loescheii* *Pseudomonas aeruginosa* *Pyoderma gangrenosum* *Roseomonas gilardii* *Salmonella entertidis* *Scedosporium prolificans* *Serratia fonticola* *Sphingomonas paucimobilis* *Staphylococcus aureus* *Staphylococcus lugdunensis*

	Streptococcus agalactiae
	Streptococcus equisimilis
	Streptococcus pneumoniae
	Streptococcus pyogenes
	Streptococcus uberis
	Tannerella forsynthensis
	Treponema pallidum
	Vibrio vulnificus
	Yersinia enterocolitica
Alzheimer's	*Chlamydia pneumoniae*
	Borna virus
	H. pylori
	Spirochetes
	Herpes simplex I
	picornavirus

Viral Infections

Viruses that infect the lower respiratory tract or digestive tract can produce significant inflammatory conditions. These include pneumonia, viral dysentery, influenza and so many others.

An example of a serious viruses is the respiratory syncytial virus (RSV). RSV is fairly common among premature children. As a result, doctors often give premature children anti-viral medications during infancy to help prevent an RSV infection. RSV has specifically been shown cause wheezing in children, and other conditions later on.

Another virus is the human metapneumovirus (hMPV). This virus also can infect the lower respiratory airways. In a study from Iran's Shiraz University of Medical Sciences (Moattari *et al.* 2010) of 120 children found that 17% of the children were infected with hMPV.

Researchers from the City University of New York (Dowd *et al.* 2009) explored the association of various viral infections among U.S. families of different socioeconomic means. Using the Third National Health and Nutrition Examination Survey (NHANES III), they found that infections of herpes simplex virus-1 (HSV-1), cytomegalovirus, hepatitis A and B related to higher levels of illness among U.S. children over the age of six. They also found that non-white children with lower family income, and parents with lower levels of education, had greater incidences of these infections.

Certainly, while infections relate to exposure, they relate more to a weakened or compromised immune system. As to family income and education, these also likely relate to a weakened and compromised immune system due to a lack of wholesome foods. Other research has shown that Americans of lower income status tend to consume more processed and inexpensive mass market foods containing more fried foods, additives and refined sugars.

Surprisingly, the human rhinovirus (HRV), which will cause the common cold in most people, can also infect the lower respiratory airways. Indeed, the association between HRV during infancy and a weakened immune system later in life is stronger with HRV than with other viruses (Jackson and Lemanske 2010).

This study confirms what other studies have indicated: An early serious viral lung infection seriously weakens the immune system. This results in a compromised ability to remove toxins later on.

Yeast, Molds and other Fungi

Yeast and mold are members of the fungi family. While many fungi such as mushrooms are protective to the immune system, an overburdened immune system can become sensitive to microorganism yeasts and molds. Yeasts can become infective and can directly overload the immune system. Mold and their airborne spores can also overload the immune system. This makes these fungi can contribute to an already-overloaded system.

Mold spores reproduce and float through both the outdoor and indoor air. Once they land, they can begin multiplying into larger cultures. While there are several species of mold, almost all require moisture to grow and populate. A concentration of spores riding the indoor air currents can cause various sensitivities, allergies, and sickness (Sahakian et al. 2008).

Mold spores also produce a number of substances called mycotoxins, which can create health concerns if inhaled. Homeowners and renters should be aware of this, and make sure the houses they live in have no water entry into the basement. Moist appliances like air conditioners, bathtubs, bathroom carpets, and air ducts can also grow mold.

For these reasons, we might want to frequently check the various corners and dark places in our houses and workplaces for moisture, because the fungal or bacterial populations growing on these surfaces will only get bigger with time—disbursing toxins into the air as they grow. Once found, the area should be dried, the mold or bacteria should be cleaned up (water with a few drops of rubbing alcohol, vinegar or chlorine will kill most mold or bacteria) thoroughly. If a mold growth is over several feet, a mold specialist may need to be called in to eliminate the mold.

This was confirmed by researchers from the National University of Singapore (Tham et al. 2007), who found that home dampness and indoor mold is linked to an increase in asthma and allergy symptoms among children. They studied 4,759 children from 120 daycare centers. After eliminating other possible effects, home humidity was significantly associated with increased rates of allergic rhinoconjunctivitis. As discussed earlier, allergic rhinoconjunctivitis is the inflammation of the conjunctiva and sinuses as a result of histamine release following an allergic immune response. As mold burdens the immune system, the body can respond with hypersensitivity.

Overgrowths of yeasts like *Candida albicans* can also contribute to or overload the immune system. While Candida is a typical resident of the immune system, when it is unchallenged by our probiotic system it can grow to incredible colony sizes. Like most other organisms, it is typically not the Candida organism that overloads the immune system: it is the endotoxins that these microscopic living beings produce.

Candida albicans can grow conjunctively with *Staphylococcus aureus,* resulting in the accelerated growth of both microorganisms. This can result in a tremendous burden for the immune and probiotic systems as they try to defend against the incursion of combined yeast and bacteria infections.

As the immune system becomes overloaded with microorganism endotoxins, it will often respond with an acute inflammatory response. This inflammatory response may be diagnosed variously, from fibromyalgia to COPD to cardiovascular disease.

The Superbugs

The use of antibiotics has soared over the past few decades. Today, over 3,000,000 pounds of pure antibiotics are taken by humans annually in the United States. This is complemented by the approximately 25,000,000 pounds of antibiotics given to animals each year.

Meanwhile, many of these antibiotics either are given in vain or are ineffectual. The example is respiratory infections, which are typically viral infections. The Centers for Disease Control states that, *"Almost half of patients with upper respiratory tract infections in the U.S. still receive antibiotics from their doctor."* This said, the CDC also warns that *"90% of upper respiratory infections, including children's ear infections, are viral, and antibiotics don't treat viral infection. More than 40% of about 50 million prescriptions for antibiotics each year in physicians' offices were inappropriate."*

Indeed, the growing use of antibiotics has also created a Pandora's Box of superbugs. As bacteria are repeatedly hit with the same antibiotic, they learn to adapt. Just as any living organism does (yes, bacteria are alive), bacteria learn to counter and resist repeatedly utilized antibiotics. As a result, many bacteria today are resistant to a variety of antibiotics. This is because bacteria tend to adjust to their surroundings. If they are attacked enough times with a certain challenge, they are likely to figure out how to avoid it and thrive despite it.

This has been the case for a number of other new antibiotic-resistant strains of bacteria. They have simply evolved to become stronger and more able to counteract these antibiotic measures.

This phenomenon has created *multi-drug resistant organisms.* Some of the more dangerous MDROs include species of *Enterococcus, Staphylococcus, Salmonella, Campylobacter, Escherichia coli,* and others. Superbugs such as MRSA are only the tip of the bacterial iceberg.

Another growing infectious bacterium is *Clostridium difficile.* This bacterium will infect the intestines of people of any age. Among children, this is one of the world's biggest killers—causing acute, watery diarrhea. It is also a growing infection among adults. Every year *C. difficile* infects tens of thousands of people in the U.S. according to the Mayo Clinic. Worse, *C. difficile* are increasingly becoming resistant to antibiotics and infections from clostridia are growing in incidence each year.

Pharmaceuticals

As we discussed in the last chapter, pharmaceuticals can harm the mucosal membranes, harm the liver and cause free radicals.

Practically any and every synthetic pharmaceutical can add to our body's total toxin burden. This is because the body must eventually break down any synthetic chemical in order to purge it from the body. The isolated or active chemical within the pharmaceutical may have its biological effect upon the body, but it must be broken down at some point. The body rarely if ever utilizes these chemicals as nutrients, in other words. They are foreigners to the body. Thus, enzymes such as glutathione must break down these chemical molecules into forms that can be excreted in urine, sweat, exhalation or stool.

This breakdown and disposal process requires work by the body's detoxification systems. This means that they further burden or stress a system that must remove many other toxins within the body, including other environmental toxins, microorganisms and their endotoxins, inflammatory mediators, broken-down cells and other toxins the body must get rid of. In other words, pharmaceuticals can contribute to, and even become another straw that breaks the camel's back.

Illustrating this, researchers from Britain's Imperial College (Shaheen *et al.* 2008) studied the association between acetaminophen use and asthma incidence among 1,028 asthmatics and healthy matched controls. They found that the weekly use of acetaminophen was significantly related to a diagnosis of asthma. The researchers concluded that: *"These data add to the increasing and consistent epidemiological evidence implicating frequent paracetamol [acetaminophen] use in asthma in diverse populations."*

Researchers from Norway's Oslo University Hospital (Bakkeheim *et al.* 2011) studied 1,016 mothers and their children from birth until six months old, and then followed up with the children at 10 years old. They found that acetaminophen use by the mother during the first trimester significantly increased incidence of allergic rhinitis at age ten. Furthermore, girls given acetaminophen had more than double the asthma incidence at age ten.

While these pharmaceuticals may be of concern specifically, we should look at any pharmaceutical as having the potential to increase the body's total toxic burden and raise the risk of systemic inflammation.

The Tryptophan Defect

As another example of the potential for pharmaceuticals to stimulate systemic inflammation is that some people have a defect in the availability of tryptophan, caused indirectly by the use of pharmaceuticals. Tryptophan is an amino acid critical for a number of processes in the body. If tryptophan is not properly metabolized, it can remain in the body at unhealthy high levels. This can be evidenced by extraordinary high levels of xanthurenic and knurenic acid in the urine.

One of the problems with high levels of tryptophan is that tryptophan is the precursor of serotonin. Thus, high tryptophan levels produce high levels of serotonin. And high serotonin levels can cause a variety of conditions, from fatigue and fibromyalgia to wheezing and lung disorders.

A link between tryptophan and inflammation is the indoleamine dioxygenase enzyme, or IDO. IDO regulates eosinophil inflammation, and tryptophan reduces IDO availability. This means that increased tryptophan presence in the blood has the effect of leaving eosinophils unregulated—which are directly involved in inflammation and pain, as we've discussed earlier.

There is reason to believe that oral steroids may increase the loss of vitamin B6 levels (Holt 1998). Vitamin B6 (pyridoxine) is required to metabolize and reduce tryptophan levels. Vitamin B6 also happens to diminish the effectiveness of steroid medications, because it inhibits steroid update into the nucleus and DNA (Gropper *et al.* 2008).

A number of pharmaceuticals have the effect of reducing levels of vitamin B6, which in turn increases tryptophan availability. This effectively produces continuous inflammation associated with high eosinophil levels by virtue of decreased levels of the IDO enzyme.

This effect was confirmed by researchers (Sur *et al.* 1993), who found that the medication theophylline significantly reduced pyridoxine (vitamin B6) levels within patients.

Another study (Collipp *et al.* 1975) found that asthmatic symptoms were significantly improved, together with a reduction of asthma medications, after B6 supplementation. This study followed 76 asthmatic children who were given 200 milligrams per day of pyridoxine (vitamin B6) for five months.

While this should not be interpreted as vitamin B6 as a panacea, its reduction is simply one sign that synthetic chemicals can interrupt the body's normal cleansing processes. Should we interrupt these processes, our body's ability to purify the body is blocked.

We can add to this discussion particular drugs and drug types that have been shown to be particularly toxic to particular organs, or toxic in general:

Drugs particularly hard on the liver:
- ➢ Acetaminophen
- ➢ Analgesics (pain-killers)
- ➢ Anesthetics (given during surgery)
- ➢ Antibiotics
- ➢ Anticoagulants
- ➢ Antihistamines
- ➢ Anti-inflammatory drugs
- ➢ Blood pressure drugs
- ➢ Chemotherapy drugs

- Cholesterol-lowering drugs
- Diabetes drugs
- Heart disease drugs
- Oral contraceptives
- Parkinson's drugs
- Tuberculosis drugs

Drugs that can stress or damage the kidneys:
- ACE inhibitors
- Acyoclovir
- Allopurinol
- Aminoglycosides
- Amphotericin
- Beta-blockers
- Captopril
- Cephalothin
- Chemotherapy drugs
- Chlorothiazide
- Chlopropamide
- Clofibrate
- Cyclosporine
- Diuretics
- Furosemide
- Isoproterenol
- Lithium
- Macanylamine
- Methotrexate
- Methysergide
- Morphine
- NSAIDs (acetaminophen, aspirin, ibuprofen)
- Penicillins
- Phenytoin
- Piperidine
- Probenecid
- Procaine
- Quinidine
- Sulfonamides
- Tolazoline

There are several conditions that will change the body's ability to metabolize drugs, and different factors that will increase or decrease the drug's effects. This can lead to serious outcomes. The factors include sex, age, race, weight, pregnancy, nursing, illness, alcohol consumption, food, multiple drugs, digestion variation, kidney damage, liver damage, nutritional deficiencies, supplements used, exposure to other toxins, exercise, stress and time of the day.

In particular, a number of drugs are metabolized differently in women than men. These include amitriptyline, benzodiazepines, beta-blockers, chlordiazepoxide, diflunisal, imipramine, methylprednisoline, oxazepam, piroxicam, prednisolone and trazodone.

Some drugs can lead to breast enlargement among men. These include AACE inhibitors, amitryptyline, cimetidine, digoxin, famotidine, ibuprofen, indomethacin, ketoconazole, ketoprofen, methyldopa, naproxen, spironolactone and terfenadine.

A number of drugs can cause intestinal issues and diarrhea. These include antibiotics, antidepressants, antihypertensive drugs, statins and heart drugs like digitalis, quinidine, hydralazine, beta-blockers, and ACE inhibitors.

The liver uses what is called the P-450 enzyme pathway to break down many drugs. However, the P-450 pathway can easily become overloaded by too many drugs, combined with other toxins. This can result in a few dire circumstances:

> The liver can be seriously damaged
> The drug's effects can be exaggerated, causing dangerous effects.
> The drugs can remain in the system longer, causing more side effects
> The unprocessed metabolites of these drugs can produce fatigue, chemical overload and immunosuppression.

Several drugs can block or overload the liver's P-450 pathway:

> Antirrhythmic drugs (disopyramide)
> Antihistamines (terfenadine, astemizole)
> Benzodiazepines
> Bromocriptine
> Caffeine
> Calcium channel blockers
> Statins
> Cimetidine
> Cisapride
> Macrolides
> Antifungals
> Phenytoin
> Tacrine
> Theophyllines
> Tricyclic antidepressants
> Warfarin

(Adapted from Mindell and Hopkins 1998)

51

Food Additives

This is a large topic, because so many processed foods are chock full of many different artificial additives. These include hundreds of artificial food colors, preservatives, stabilizers, flavorings and a variety of food processing aids. A number of these additives have been found to cause sensitivities in some people.

Illustrating the effects that food additives can have, Australian researchers (Dengate and Ruben 2002) studied 27 children with irritability, restlessness, inattention and sleep difficulties. The researchers saw many of these symptoms subside after putting the children on the Royal Prince Alfred Hospital Diet, which is absent of food additives, natural salicylates, amines and glutamates.

Using preservative challenges, the researchers were also able to determine that the preservatives significantly affected the children's behavior and physiology adversely.

Researchers from Britain's University of Southampton (Bateman *et al.* 2004) screened 1,873 three-year old children for hyperactivity and the consumption of artificial food colors and preservatives. They gave the children 20 mg daily of artificial colors and 45 mg daily of sodium benzoate, or a placebo mixture. The additive group showed significantly higher levels of hyperactivity than the group that did not consume the artificial colors and preservative.

While these studies are not proof that these food additives are allergens, we can say that with confidence that they can cause food intolerances, as hyperactivity is considered a reaction to eating these "foods."

Once an additive has caused intolerance symptoms such as those from the research above, there is always the possibility that the immune system may begin to become sensitive to some of the foods these additives are associated with. This likelihood increases should the immune system become continually exposed to the foods together with the additives over a considerable period of time.

Sulfites

Sulfites provide a classic case. The sulfite ion will aggressively preserve a food. Sulfites can also produce wheezing, tightness of the throat and other symptoms almost immediately after eating foods preserved with them. However, the effects of sulfites may not be as significant as often portrayed. It may well be that many sulfite-sensitivities seen among wine drinkers are actually the product of the alcohol rather than the sulfites.

Illustrating this, researchers from Australia's Centre for Asthma (Vally *et al.* 2007) tested eight wine-sensitive subjects with sulfite wine and non-sulfite wine. The researchers found that the wine sensitivities were unlikely caused by the sulfites in the wine.

Today, sulfites are used to preserve many wines, dehydrated potatoes and numerous dried fruits. Sulfites include potassium bisulfite, sulfur dioxide, potassium matabisulfite and others. Often labels do not disclose the use of sulfites, because the preservative may have been used early in the processing of the raw ingredients instead of added into the finished product. In addition, under current U.S. labeling laws, if an ingredient such as sulfite is less than 10 parts per million, there is no requirement for putting the ingredient on the panel.

Sulfite sensitivity may be the result of B12 deficiency. In a study presented to the American Academy of Allergy and Immunology, 18 sulfite-sensitive persons were given sublingual B12. The B12 effectively blocked adverse reactions to sulfites in 17 of the 18 (Werbach 1996).

Monosodium Glutamate

Monosodium glutamate also gets a lot of attention for producing sensitivity symptoms. This has also been echoed among a number of studies.

To better understand this, Harvard researchers (Geha *et al.* 2000) set out to study the effects of MSG sensitivities in a multi-center study. They found that of 130 human volunteers who thought they were sensitive to MSG, 38% physically responded to MSG with allergic symptoms. However, 13% also responded to a placebo (they thought contained MSG). Subsequent retesting continued to show inconsistent responses among some of those who thought they were MSG-sensitive.

This led the researchers to conclude that people who believe they are sensitive tend to react more strongly to MSG, but their responses were not always consistent. This of course may be the result of differing levels of tolerance and periods of sensitivity—again depending upon immunity.

This research still confirms that MSG can cause sensitivity responses. Possibly MSG may be overhyped somewhat, but like so many other food additives, there is no doubt that it is not a natural part of our food supply.

Microparticles

Some researchers have suggested that substances with microparticles can lead to increased intestinal permeability and food sensitivities (Korzenik 2005).

Microparticles are particles smaller than 100 μm, but larger than 0.1 μm. (Smaller molecules, in the nanometer range, are called nanoparticles.) Products that are produced with microparticles include toothpaste and mouthwashes. Food products that contain microparticles include powdered sugars and some refined flours.

We might better classify microparticles in the same category as overly processed foods. The bottom line is that the body can become sensitive to unnaturally-processed constituents should they be exposed to intestinal tissues and bloodstream—and not be recognized by the immune system.

Artificial Sweeteners

A number of artificial sweeteners should be considered toxic. One is aspartame. Aspartame is a chemical combination of the amino acids phenylalanine and aspartic acid, bonded by methyl ester—a wood alcohol. Once inside the body, the wood alcohol and formaldehyde are released.

Another artificial sweetener sucralose. This is sweet yet not readily absorbed according to manufacturers. Yet studies have found that 11-27% is absorbed, and 20-30% of that absorbed quantity can be metabolized by the body. This requires the liver and kidneys to break it down and excrete it.

While this is a huge topic in itself, other questionable sweeteners that may provide toxicity once within the body include saccharin, acesulfame potassium and cyclamates. Stevia, mannitol and xylitol are plant-derived sweeteners that are considered by most to be relatively safe and non-toxic.

Air Pollutants

Clean air contains about 78% nitrogen, 21% oxygen, .9% argon, .03% carbon dioxide and a host of other trace elements. Depending upon the location and source, outdoor air pollution can contain carbon monoxide, nitrogen dioxide, sulphur dioxide, excess carbon dioxide, ammonia, various particulates, chlorofluorocarbons (CFCs), radon daughters, and a variety of toxic metals and volatile organic compounds (VOCs).

There are several types of air pollution, and most of them can overload the body with toxins. The first is *air particle* pollution—when particulate size ranges from .1 micron to 10 microns. This type of pollution is from soot, typical of automobile exhaust, industrial smoke stack exhaust, fireplace smoke, and smoke from forest fires, barbeques and other combustion. Soot is also called *black carbon* pollution, because the excess carbon burn off from burning fossil fuels is the primary component.

Noxious gases are another type of pollution category. These include gasses such as carbon monoxide, chlorine gas, nitrogen oxide, sulphur dioxide and various other chemical gases and vapors. CFCs are a type of noxious gas.

While these two pollution types are distinct, they are often tough to differentiate. Many pollutants are actually vaporized liquids. Molecules become suspended in vapor, appearing like gases or liquid vapors. They are airborne elements derived from synthetic solid and liquid compounds.

We should also specify a difference between *indoor* and *outdoor* air pollution. There are a number of pollutants specifically pervading building ventilation systems and indoor facilities. To this, we can add outdoor pollution entering the house. Examples of indoor pollutants include formaldehyde emitted by foam, treated wood plastics, and chlorine gas emitted in indoor swimming pools.

According to a 2007 *American Lung Association State of the Air* report, 46% or about 136 million Americans live within a county having *"unhealthful"* levels of either ozone or particle-based outdoor pollution. Over 38 million Americans live in a county with *"unhealthful"* levels of both ozone and particle pollution. A third of Americans live in *"unhealthful"* ozone level counties.

Interestingly, this is substantially better than a 2006 report indicating that almost half of Americans live in ozone-rich areas. It is unlikely that the source of ozone pollution—carbon emissions—went down this much in a year. Most likely—just as the ozone hole has been fluctuating with atmospheric rhythms—there are complicated relationships between weather systems, temperature, pressure and so on.

Meanwhile, more than ninety-three million Americans—about one in three—live in areas seasonally high in short-term particle pollution and about one in five Americans lives in an area of high year-round particle pollution. Unlike the fluctuating ozone levels, the number of high particle pollution areas has steadily increased over the past few years.

Smog

Research has illustrated that increased exposure to the particulates within smog, as well as the toxic burden presented by mercury, arsenic, sulfur dioxide, nitrogen dioxide and others, can contribute to systemic inflammation.

Illustrating this, researchers from Australia's University of Queensland (Barnett *et al.* 2005) studied respiratory hospital admissions among children of different ages in five Australian cities and two New Zealand cities. They found that increased rates of hospital admissions for asthma correlated with increased levels of particulate matter smaller than 2.5 micrometer and less than 10 micrometer (PM10-2.5), along with increased nitrogen and sulfur levels. A 6% hike in asthma admissions for children between five and fourteen years old related to a five parts per billion increase in nitrogen levels.

Ozone

Smog is primarily made up of ozone. There are two forms of ozone: The ozone that naturally makes up part of the stratosphere, often referred to as the ozone hole; and the ozone within the lower atmosphere, or troposphere. This latter ozone is called tropospheric ozone or ozone pollution. This form of O_3 gas is caused not by a nature's interaction between radiation and the atmosphere, but through the reaction between fuel vapors from automobiles and sunlight. For this reason, smog levels tend to peak during hot weather.

Smog levels are also higher in warmer regions like Southern California and urban areas in the southern U.S., such as Atlanta. Other cities also experience greater smog levels during the summer months. Wherever higher concentrations of vehicles combine with warm sunshine, smog levels go up. The 'perfect storm' of almost constant sunshine, warm weather, and vehicle concentration makes Southern California one of the worst smog and ozone regions in the United States.

Ozone will oxidize on a cellular and internal tissue level when taken into the body. These tissues will be damaged in almost the same way other oxidized radicals damage tissues. Ozone is readily absorbed through the alveoli as a gas. From there it can enter the bloodstream and damage artery walls and tissues. Ozone is also a major lung tissue irritant, causing inflammation and epithelial cell damage. This can result in decreased lung capacity and/or decreased lung growth development among children.

Ozone is directly linked to the incidence and worsening of respiratory conditions such as asthma, bronchitis, and COPD. Recent research indicates that this mechanism is the oxidation of lung surface lipids that line the cells of the lung. These oxidized lipids stimulate inflammation as the body seeks to mitigate ozone's damaging effects. The oxidation stimulates scavenger macrophages, which bind to the oxidized lipids in an effort to reverse the damage (Postlethwait 2007).

This means that ozone will release unpaired oxygen radicals, which can damage cell membranes and tissues, as we discussed earlier.

Ozone has some redeeming qualities as well. Ozone therapy is gaining recognition among the alternative medical community. Ozone is used in hot tubs as a purification measure. It is also used as an industrial cleaning and sanitizing substance. Ozone is part of our natural mix of gases in our air as well. Typical levels are between 25 and 75 parts per billion.

However, dangerous ozone levels occur with higher levels of carbon monoxide levels, sulphur dioxide, and other pollutants. Like the canary in the coalmine, high ozone levels provide a good indicator of unhealthy air. When combined with other pollutants, ozone has a worsening detrimental effect upon the body.

The EPA's Air quality index rates 85 parts per billion of ozone as unhealthy for sensitive people, and over 105 ppb as unhealthy for anyone. As ozone levels rise, it can irritate the lungs and throat, increasing the potential for inflammatory throat and lung infections. As a result, indoor ozone generating machines—which have become popular over the last decade—are discouraged by both the EPA and the FDA if they emit levels higher than 50 parts per billion.

Ironically, higher ozone levels in the air reflect its cleansing action upon other pollutants. Ozone is part of the atmosphere's normalizing systems. The very same cleaning and antibacterial effect we have begun to utilize are part of the earth's detoxification mechanisms to clean and break down particulate pollution. This doesn't mean it is healthy to breathe in ozone at these levels, however.

Particulates

Particulate pollution can produce severe toxicity. PM(10-2.5) refers to a particle size from 2.5 micron to 10 micron, and PM(2.5) refers to particle sizes below 2.5 micron. 2.5 micron or less is a *fine particulate*, while less than .1 micron is *ultra-fine*. Ultra-fine particles may also be considered noxious gas pollutants, because their molecular size is small enough to pass through the alveoli into the bloodstream.

Particles above 10 micron in size are usually trapped by the cilia and mucous membranes in the nose, throat, or mouth. As mentioned earlier, these are usually disposed through the movement of mucous or broken down by immune cells.

Fine particulates are small enough to escape this labyrinth and get into our lungs, but they are usually too large to get directly into the bloodstream. These particles can become lodged in the tissues of the lungs and bronchi and slowly break down. As they break down, their toxins become absorbed and dumped into the bloodstream. This accumulation of toxins can quickly overburden the liver and bloodstream, producing an inflammatory airway response. In other words, the pollution of the air quickly becomes the pollution of our bloodstream and liver—producing systemic inflammation.

The chemical makeup of these toxins depends upon the source of the pollution. Particle pollution caused by automobile exhaust will have various fluorocarbons and nitrate particles, while coal fired power plants will emit large numbers of sulphur dioxide molecules.

Course particulate pollutants are typically caused by mining, construction, or demolition. Building demolition can rain fumes of various dangerous substances a mile or more from the demolition site.

The most blatant illustration of the demolition effect is the World Trade Center bombing of 2001. The collapse of the towers caused such a toxic fume that there are still thousands of people suffering from a slow poisoning of the lungs. Dangerous chemicals like asbestos, formaldehyde and many others were breathed by thousands of people.

This effect was not limited to rescuers and those who escaped from the twin towers. Many others who happened to be in the vicinity are now suffering. One of the more prevalent diseases has been *sarcoidosis*—a life-threatening inflammation of the lungs. As toxin deposits build up and damage the airways, scar tissue forms—making mild asthma seem like a walk in the park.

This scar tissue affects the elasticity and efficiency of the lungs, causing life-threatening lung collapse. A recent study released by nine doctors (Izbicki *et al.* 2007) who researched the delayed health effects at Ground Zero reported that firefighters and rescue workers were diagnosed with sarcoidosis at a rate of five times the incidence rate prior to 9/11.

An epidemic of respiratory disorders and lung cancer was also an unfortunate result of the Trade Center bombing. While we know asbestos is toxic to the lungs, it is still a popular building material. Many structural components of new buildings use asbestos as an ingredient. Because it is a cheap fire retardant material, buildings still go up using it. Asbestos has been linked to thyroid cancer and lung cancer in many studies, which caused a number of high profile lawsuits and residential building restrictions.

Another toxin released when buildings collapse or are demolished is benzene. Benzene has been identified as a carcinogen, and certain types of leukemia are associated with benzene exposure. Other toxins thought to be released by building collapse include mercury, lead, cadmium, dioxin, polycyclic aromatic hydrocarbons (PAHs) and polychlorinated biphenyls (PCBs). Many of these components are still used to build buildings. All of them were used in buildings a few decades ago, when many of our current skyscrapers were built.

Besides the more publicized cases of cancer and sarcoidosis, ailments associated with the WTC bombing include reactive-airways syndrome, asthma, chronic throat irritation, gastroesophageal reflux disease (GERD—also referred to as heartburn) and persistent sinusitis. Other cases thought to be associated with the WTC have included miner's lung and thyroid cancer. While many thought these disorders were temporary, new diagnoses have continually increased. This is because toxins can build up and reside in lung tissue cells, affecting future lung capacity for many years to come. Studies on firefighters involved in the rescue report an average loss of 300 milliliters of lung capacity (Senior 2003).

It is thus safe to say that exposure to these sorts of particulates may not be symptomatic for years after the exposure. This was certainly the case with those exposed to Agent Orange in Vietnam. Cases of prostate cancer, skin cancer, and chronic lymphocytic leukemia did not appear in some veterans for decades later (Beaulieu and Fessele 2003).

Particulate pollution or soot is the most dangerous form of outdoor pollution. Auto exhaust, aerosols, and chemicals from power plants and wood burning are the major sources. While the particles themselves are too small to be seen by the naked eye, they can be seen as a whole in the form of a haze in the sunlight. While the body's cilia hair and mucous membranes in the nose and throat might filter and catch some of these particles, many will make it into the lungs where they can trigger inflammation.

Like any living organism, the earth and its atmosphere have means to cleanse toxins out of the system. The atmosphere conducts a number of self-cleaning currents, which move and break down pollutants. One such mechanism is the hydroxyl radical (OH) molecule. The immediate effect of the hydroxyl radical is to form photo-oxidants like nitric acid, which undergoes a photolysis reaction with nitrous acids. These can be highly toxic.

Humanity's intrusions into nature's course can produce other types of toxins. We might consider, for example, Owens Lake, California. For thousands of years, this beautiful lake offered respite from the heat and inhospitality of the California desert region known as Death Valley. The size of Owens lake was nearly 28,500 hectares—a huge body of water fed by the Sierra mountains. In 1900, the mountain rivers feeding the lake were diverted into the Los Angeles basin to feed a growing legion of humanity.

Within ten years, Owns Lake, which was often compared to the Aral Sea, turned into a dustbowl. Now the silt covering the water basin is coated with arsenic. Arsenic is a natural element, and in this case, it is providing resistance and restructuring for the soil at the lake bottom. This arsenic is also blowing around the region with the winds, increasing cancer rates among local residents (Raloff 2001).

Carbon Monoxide

Carbon monoxide is a substantial indoor air toxin. Carbon monoxide is released by burning gas, kerosene, or wood. It can thus arise from the use of wood stoves, fireplaces, gas stoves, generators, automobiles, kitchen stoves, and furnaces. Low concentrations of carbon monoxide in the indoor environment might cause fatigue and even chest pain.

Higher concentrations may result in headaches, confusion, dizziness, nausea, vision impairment and fever. This is due to carboxyhemoglobin formation in the bloodstream, which takes place when carbon monoxide attaches to hemoglobin instead of oxygen. This will in effect starve the body of oxygen, and higher concentrations can easily lead to death.

Acceptable carbon monoxide levels in households are about .5 to 5 parts per million. Levels near a gas stove might be 5 to 15 ppm. An improperly vented or leaking stove might cause 30 ppm or more near the stove, which becomes hazardous. The U.S. National Ambient Air Quality Standard for maximum carbon monoxide levels outside is 35 ppm for one hour and 9 ppm for eight hours. Standards for indoor carbon monoxide have not been determined.

Making sure that every appliance is vented properly is task number one in avoiding carbon monoxide poisoning. The appliance should also be checked for leaks, and those leaks should be sealed prior to use. Central heating systems should be inspected for leaks as well. Idling the car in the garage is a no-no. Open fireplaces should be avoided indoors, and wood stove doors should be kept closed. We shouldn't solely rely upon the draft up the fireplace chimney for the escape of carbon monoxide.

Nitrogen oxide

Nitrogen oxide is a gas byproduct of most engines and practically any gas-run appliance. Gas stoves, water heaters, wood stoves, gas heaters and cars are probably the biggest emitters in the home. Homes without these appliances will have very low levels of NO_2 compared to outside. Homes with these appliances may have double the levels. Nitrogen oxide can be a significant toxin if significant levels are taken in.

Researchers from Birmingham Heartlands Hospital (Tunnicliffe *et al.* 1994) tested one hour exposure to nitrogen dioxide on ten mild asthmatics with dust mite sensitivities. Forced expiratory volume (FEV1) levels were tested with non-NO_2 air, air with 100 parts per billion of NO_2, and air containing 400 ppb of nitrogen dioxide. FEV1 levels were 27% lower between the non-NO_2 air and the 400 ppb of NO_2 air. The average FEV1 among the asthmatics was nearly three times lower in the 400 ppb NO_2 air than in the clear air. The 100 ppb NO_2 air content did not seem to make a significant difference in FEV1, however. This gives us a yardstick for determining un-healthy NO_2 levels.

Cooking and Heating

Research from the University at Albany (Kaplan 2010) has revealed that about half of the people around the world utilize biomass such as wood, agricultural residues or coal to cook by and heat their homes with.

These fuels are not completely consumed by their ignition. They leave toxic residues in the form of carbon monoxide, arsenic and others that can significantly increase the body's burden of toxins when breathed in. This in turn increases the risk of systemic inflammation, as the body works to break down and remove these toxins.

Volatile Organic Compounds (VOCs)

Researchers from the Texas Tech University Health Sciences Center (Arif and Shah 2007) studied the effects of volatile organic compounds (VOCs). They collected data on ten VOCs and 550 adults. Aromatic compounds and chlorinated hydrocarbons were specifically categorized. Exposure to aromatic compounds increased the incidence of asthma by 63%. In addition, exposure to aromatic compounds increased wheezing incidence from the previous year by 68%, and chlorinated hydrocarbon exposure increased wheezing incidence from the previous year by 50%.

Exposures to VOCs ranged from 0.03 micrograms per cubic meter for trichloroethene up to 14 microg/m3 for toluene. In other words, the higher the level of toxic inhalation, the higher the incidence of respiratory disorders. This is because VOCs present toxins that are quickly absorbed into the bloodstream through the airways. Once in the bloodstream, the body launches an inflammatory response to remove them.

The researchers also found that as a group, Mexican-Americans experience the highest exposure levels to benzene—averaging 2.38 micrograms per cubic meter—compared with whites—who averaged 1.15 microg/m3—and blacks—who averaged 1.07 microg/m3. This relates to exposure levels that are relative to the type of work being done. In other words, this study indicates that Mexican-Americans are likely doing more work involving the use of VOCs, which in turn expose them to greater levels of benzene.

Benzene, like toluene and other VOCs, is highly disruptive to cells and tissues because of its highly reactive aromatic hydrocarbon structure. It can thus damage practically every cell and tissue system in the body, releasing numerous radicals. Not surprisingly, benzene is also known to be significantly carcinogenic.

Benzene and other VOCs can be found in many paints, glues, solvents, rubbers and many other workplace materials. Industries that use aromatic hydrocarbon solvents must provide significant ventilation and protection to avoid poisoning their workers.

First-, Second- and Third-Hand Smoke

Tobacco smoke is also an important source of indoor pollution. The American Cancer Society estimated in 2004 that 160,000 Americans die each year from lung cancer caused by smoking. Lung cancer maintains between an eleven and fifteen percent chance of survival beyond five years. It should be noted that the highest rates of global lung cancer occur for both men and women in North America and Europe (Field *et al.* 2006). Of course, these are also countries where indoor smoking rates are the highest.

Recent research has indicated that not only is second-hand smoke dangerous to non-smokers, but it has more than twice the amount of tar, nicotine and other toxins than the smoker inhales. While the smoker will inhale the smoke through the filtering mechanism provided by the packed tobacco inside the cigarette paper—and many cigarettes also have additional filters to screen out toxins—the second-hand smoker will breathe all the smoke. Second-hand smoke contains five times the amount of carbon monoxide—the lethal gas that de-oxygenates the blood—than the smoker inhales.

Second-hand smoke also contains higher levels of ammonia and cadmium. Its nitrogen dioxide levels are fifty times higher than levels considered harmful, and the concentration of hydrogen cyanide approaches toxic levels. Constant exposure to second-hand smoke increases the risk of lung disease by 25%, and increases the risk of heart disease by 10%. Second-hand smoke exposure has also been irrefutably linked to emphysema, chronic bronchitis, asthma and other ailments.

Despite significant educational programs, second-hand and third-hand smoke poisoning is still prevalent in the United States. The Centers for Disease Control's National Health and Nutrition Examination Survey from 1999-2008 (CDC 2010) revealed that between 2007 and 2008, about 88 million American nonsmokers over the age of three were consistently exposed to secondhand smoke. The good news is that the detectible blood nicotine levels among nonsmokers have declined from 52% between 1999 and 2000 to 40% between 2007 and 2008. Still, 40% is simply not acceptable. It should be noted that rates were the highest among children living in households below federal poverty levels.

Researchers from Britain's University of Southampton School of Medicine (Edgecombe *et al.* 2010) found in a study of 22 adolescents with severe asthma, that two-thirds lived with a smoker.

Researchers from the Respiratory Diseases Department of France's Hospital of Haut-Lévèque in Bordeaux (Raherison *et al.* 2008) studied 7,798 children among six cities in France. This focused on asthma and allergies among families who smoked. They found that about 20% of children were exposed to tobacco via their mother's smoking. Furthermore, they found that children born of mothers who smoked during pregnancy had significantly greater incidence of asthma.

There is now research that shows that anti-smoking laws decrease disease rates. Researchers from the Harvard School of Public Health (Dove *et al.* 2011) studied the National Health and Nutrition Examination Survey (NHANES) data—a research program run by the U.S. Centers for Disease Control and Prevention's National Center for Health Statistics (NCHS). NCHS's directive has been a continuous survey method focused on specific diseases among representative samples throughout the United States. About 5,000 persons each year are included in the data, from different counties across the nation.

The Harvard researchers used the 1999-2006 NHANES data to correlate locations that had some semblance of required smoke-free public places with asthma incidence. They found that smoke-free laws significantly reduced the odds of asthmatic symptoms among nonsmoking children and adolescents. Smoke-free laws were also linked to reduced asthma episodes ("attacks"), persistent wheeze, chronic night coughing and asthma medication use.

Fragrances

Various scents and fragrances used in deodorizers, decorations, soaps, and furniture can be downright toxic. While a fragrance might smell like flowers or delicious foods, the typical commercial fragrance contains at least ninety-five percent synthetic chemicals. A single perfume may contain more than 500 different chemicals. Benzene derivatives, aldehydes, toluene, and petroleum-derived chemicals are just a few synthetics used in commercial fragrances. Toluene alone, for example, has been linked to respiratory disorders among previously healthy people.

For this reason, we should carefully consider any product with an ingredient called "fragrances." This includes laundry detergents, dishwashing and other soaps, shampoos and other types of hair products, disinfectants, shaving creams, fabric softeners, fragrant candles, air fresheners, and of course perfumes and colognes. Discernment also should also be given to the word "unscented," as this still may have some of the same synthetics, used instead as fragrance masking elements.

In one study (Anderson and Anderson 1997), mice were submitted to breathing with a commercial air freshener for one hour at different concentrations. A number of concentrations, including levels typically used by humans in everyday use, caused sensory and pulmonary irritation, decreased breathing velocity, and functional behavior abnormalities.

Another study, performed by the same researchers (Anderson and Anderson 1998) and published a year later, revealed that mice who were subjected to five commercial colognes or toilet water for an hour suffered various combinations of negative effects, including sensory irritation, pulmonary irritation, decreased airflow expiration, and neurotoxicity.

Skin Lotions

Many of the chemical ingredients in many sunscreens have been identified as carcinogenic. These include benzophenone-3, homosalate, 4-methyl-
benzylidene camphor, octylmethoxycinnamate, and octyl-dimethyl-PABA.
These five, alone or in some combination thereof, are contained in about
90% of today's commercial sunscreens. All five have showed increased cancer
cell proliferation both *in vitro* and *in vivo* in a study conducted at the Institute
of Pharmacology and Toxicology at the University of Zurich (Schlumpf *et al.*
2001). This study also showed negative estrogenic and endocrine effects
among mice from several of these chemicals.

A study done at the University of Manitoba in Winnipeg (Sarveiya *et al.*
2004) reported that all sunscreen ingredients tested—including octymethoxy-
cinnamate and oxybenzone—significantly penetrate the skin. The penetration
of common sunscreens was found to increase the penetration of even more
dangerous herbicides—a concern for agricultural workers and non-organic
gardeners (Pont *et al.* 2004). Furthermore, it has been established that some
organic sunscreens can cause photo-contact allergies (Maier and Korting
2005). Research from Australia's Skin and Cancer Foundation (Cook and
Freeman 2001) reported 21 cases of photo-allergic contact dermatitis caused
by oxybenzone, butyl methoxy dibenzoylmethane, methoxycinnamate or
benzophenone. The Cook and Freeman research has led to a conclusion that
these sunscreen ingredients are the leading cause of photo-allergic contact
dermatitis.

Contact dermatitis is actually quite rare amongst the general population.
A study at the National Institute of Dermatology in Colombia conducted a
study of eighty-two patients with clinical photo-allergic contact dermatitis.
Their testing showed that twenty-six of those patients—31.7%—were shown
to be positive for sensitivity to one or several of the sunscreen ingredients
(Rodriguez *et al.* 2006).

The widespread proliferation of these harmful sunscreen ingredients—an
occurrence increasing since the 1960s sunbathing era—is a significant factor
in the skin cancer epidemic. Their addition to the epidermis layer create an
environment of excessive oxidative radicals, as the sun in the presence of
oxygen further oxidizes these synthetic molecules without nature's balancing
biomolecules. At the bare minimum, these chemicals substantially increase
the toxic burden within skin cells. This burden minimizes the body's ability to
neutralize the oxidizing effects of the sun's radiation—intensifying the oxidizing factor. This intensification would essentially convert the sun's rays from
therapeutic to dangerous.

Prior and concurrent to the prevalent use of sunscreen, sun-worshipers
have ceremoniously applied various chemical- and oil-based sun lotions onto
the skin. This is done to intensify the sun's tanning effects: to obtain that rich,
brown tan to look more attractive. Many chemicals are/were in these products, including various hydrocarbons, which revert to oxidized radicals when

exposed to the sun. In addition to sun lotion, sunbathers also apply various other chemical-based lotions onto the skin to condition, hydrate or treat sunburn. These various moisturizing lotions also contain a variety of synthetic chemicals that can become free radicals.

Furthermore, many sunscreens available today effectively absorb UV-B rays, but let UV-A rays through. Because UV-A rays are quite dangerous out of balance with UV-B to an unhealthy body, the risk of skin cancer using these sunscreens is even higher than without any sunscreen protection. In a 2007 study from the University of California at San Diego, researchers (Gorham *et al.* 2007) reviewed 17 studies of sunscreen use and melanoma. For those studies performed in latitudes over 40 degrees from the equator where skin types are fairer, there was a more significant correlation between sunscreen use and skin cancer.

Many other skin lotions should also be considered toxic. An example is DEET, or N,N-Diethyl-meta-toluamide. DEET is an effective mosquito repellent, yes. But it also poisons us as well. Research has shown that DEET exposure causes impairments to cognition, mood issues and insomnia. Whatever we put on our skin is absorbed into the epidermal and subdermal tissues, and eventually, into the bloodstream, and in the case of DEET, into our central nervous system.

Other toxic chemicals are used for lubricants, moisturizers, exfoliants and masks. Ingredients to steer clear of include methylisothiazalone, DMDM hydantoin, octenylsuccinate (a neurotoxin), methylchloroisothiazalone and triclosan—an antibacterial ingredient that is suspected to be an endocrine disruptor. Common among most soaps and cleansers are sodium laureth sulfate and ceteareth, which can bond to carcinogen chemicals used in manufacturing, such as ethylen oxide and 1,4-dioxane.

Toxic Household Materials

The same researchers (Anderson and Anderson 2000) found that pulmonary irritation and decreased lung capacity results from the use of synthetic mattress pads. They identified respiratory irritants such as styrene, isopropylbenzene and limonene among polyurethane mattresses. When subjecting organic cotton mattresses to the same test, the results were quite the opposite. Increased respiratory rates and tidal breathing volumes were observed with organic fiber mattresses.

Fabric softener emission is also a dangerous source of air toxicity. Several known irritants and toxins are typically found in fabric softeners, including styrene, isopropylbenzene, thymol, trimethylbenzene and phenols. In yet another study, Anderson and Anderson subjected mice to five commercial fabric softener emissions for 90 minutes using laundry dryers. The results clearly illustrated that fabric softeners significantly irritate airways. These negative health effects were also seen resulting from emissions of clothing driers containing fabric softener pads.

The researchers (Anderson and Anderson 1999) also found that pulmonary toxicity resulted from commercial diapers, adding that a number of chemicals found in diapers were known pulmonary and sensory irritants.

Another potential indoor trigger category is propellants. Propellants are used in sprays and pump bottles to disperse fluids. While chlorofluorocarbons (CFCs) have been practically eliminated from aerosols, today's aerosols and pump sprays often involves the use of volatile organic compounds (VOCs). Noxious propellants such as isobutane, butane and propane will typically linger in the air for several minutes after spraying. They can be quite toxic.

Asbestos

Asbestos exposure has become less likely since the *Environmental Protection Agency* passed the *Asbestos Ban and Phase Out Rule* as part of the *Toxic Substances Control Act* in 1989—which was for the most part overturned in 1991 by the U.S. *Fifth Circuit Court of Appeals*. What remain are various specific bans such as those from the *Clean Air Act* and remnants of *Toxic Substances Control Act*, including some continued restrictions supported by Congressional rulings.

The CAA has stimulated various bans since 1973. The bottom line is that although paper- and cardboard-based asbestos has been banned along with certain spray-on versions, many products still contain asbestos. These include cement sheets, clothing, pipe wrap, roofing felt, floor tiles, shingles, millboard, cement pipe, and various automotive parts.

Beyond the banned items, there is no ban preventing manufacturers from using asbestos. The important thing to remember is that the EPA does not monitor manufacturers for their ingredients. In general, asbestos inclusion into today's building materials should be considered a given.

Formaldehyde

Formaldehyde has been shown to be a significant and prevalent toxin. Today so many building materials and furniture are built using formaldehyde. These include pressed wood, draperies, glues, resins, shelving, flooring, and so many other materials. The greatest source of formaldehyde appears to be those materials made using *urea-formaldehyde* resins. These include particleboard, plywood paneling, and medium density fiberboard.

Among these, medium density fiberboard—used to make drawers, cabinets and furniture tops—appears to contain the highest resin-to-wood ratio. Another sort of resin called *phenol-formaldehyde* or PF resin. PF resin apparently emits substantially less formaldehyde than the UF resins. The PF resin is easily differentiated from UF resin by its darker, red or black color. The incidental *off-gassing* of formaldehyde into the indoor environment from these resins results from sun, heat, sanding and demolition. As the formaldehyde slowly off gasses, it becomes a chemical toxin once in the body.

Other Building Materials

There are many other toxins in our building materials—including many yet to be discovered. Certainly, we can safely say that any kind of building or decomposition of a modern building will likely impart various hazardous chemicals, including but not exclusively asbestos and formaldehyde.

Polybrominated diphenyl ethers or PBDEs provide one example. PBDEs is an organobromine used as a fire retardant. It is used to make automobiles, polyurethane foams, furniture, electronic goods, textiles, airplanes and of course, building materials.

This means that the air during any kind of sanding, crushing, fire or demolition should be treated with extreme caution. Using a particle or gas mask is more than a good idea under these circumstances, though it should be noted that most particle masks do not form a tight enough bond with the face to filter much at all. Best is to use a gas filter or a mask with a rubber barrier that fits tightly onto the face.

With regard to off-gassing, prior to bringing in any type of new furniture or wood into the house, it is best to off-gas the product by setting it in the sunshine for a couple of days or at least for a full day. As the sun's resonating waves connect with the material, many of its toxins are disassociated and released. Not such a good thing for the environment, but at least it will disburse outside of our immediate breathing environment. Off-gassing can help us avoid more than a potent toxin.

Fresh paint can also be toxic. This is because paint typically contains VOCs.

'New Car Smell'

Many other indoor pollutants exist, depending upon the structure and condition of the environment. For example, automobiles, trains, planes, or buses can provide a whole range of triggers, from carbon monoxide to lead, formaldehyde and plasticizers—which can off-gas (also called *outgassing*), especially when the weather gets warmer.

This is especially the case for new cars. That 'new car smell' is the toxic off-gassing of a mixture of plasticizers, formaldehyde and other synthetics. In the case of older cars, air vents may be clogged with a number of molds, dust and bacteria, which may spray out whenever the "air" is turned on.

It might help to periodically clean out the filters of any car—especially older ones. In the case of a newer car, we might also consider leaving the windows cracked while parking in sunny locations between drives for a few weeks, to let the various materials outgas.

Radon

Radon is another indoor pollutant worth consideration as a toxin. It is estimated that almost 12% of American cancer deaths from lung cancer (about 19,000 deaths a year) result from radon exposure (Field *et al.* 2006).

Radon is caused by various soils and rocks from the earth. Increased radon exposure occurs when a house is not properly ventilated, especially in cold weather. Cold outside weather combined with an unventilated warm indoor environment creates an energy vacuum, drawing radon into the house and keeping it there. Houses without adequate coverage over ground soils may have greater radon exposure.

Sick Buildings

Over the last thirty years, researchers have become increasingly aware that certain buildings, especially older ones with older ventilation systems, can make people sick. This effect is often termed *sick building syndrome,* or SBS. The major symptoms reported in SBS include chronic fatigue, brain fog, headaches, allergies, nausea, chronic sore throat, bronchial congestion, and others.

Toxin overload becomes apparent in the case of toxins provided by older buildings, or buildings without sufficient ventilation or cleaning policies.

For example, research from the National Center for Healthy Housing (Jacobs *et al.* 2009) found that lower-income families tend to live in older homes, where there can be poor ventilation, more water leaks, more lead paint and greater moisture and mold levels. They found that these trends also relate to increased rates of respiratory illness, obesity and lead poisoning. They saw a clear association between respiratory disorders and home ventilation, home age, and the windows of homes. In other words, higher toxin exposure.

Researchers from the Vermont Department of Health's Division of Health Surveillance (Laney *et al.* 2009) studied a 2006 respiratory disorder cluster among workers who worked in a building that had water-damage. Physicians diagnosed increased incidence of sarcoidosis and asthma among the workers, and conducted pulmonary function tests.

As the researchers investigated the data, they found that adult respiratory disorders incidence in the office workers was 3.3/1,000 person-years prior to their working in the office, and 11.5/1,000 person-years after they began working in the building. Their respiratory disorders incidence tripled, in other words.

The workers were removed from the building while it was cleaned up.

In a study of school buildings (Sahakian *et al.* 2008), 309 school employees in two older elementary schools were tested. Excess dampness produced increased incidence of respiratory irritation, wheezing and rhinitis symptoms among the employees. The older, damper school of the two also produced more illness.

SBS is indicated when multiple workers or inhabitants of a building complain of one or more of these symptoms soon after beginning to work or live in the building. Sometimes, however, SBS can develop over time, or directly after or during an extreme change in the weather. A humid summer or heavy rainfall period, for example, may stimulate a growth in mold in the ventilation system. After a smoggy summer in a city or during a fire season, the ventilation system may become clogged with soot. Workers or occupants of the building need to speak up and request from management that filters and vents be periodically cleaned and flushed. The upholstery, walls and other parts of workplaces should also be cleaned periodically.

Occupational Airborne Toxins

Scientists from the University of Texas School of Public Health (McHugh *et al.* 2010) analyzed the data from the National Health and Nutrition Examination Survey (2001-2004) to determine the relative risks of toxicity in different occupations. They found that miners, health-care workers, and teachers have significantly higher rates of respiratory disorders than other occupations, including construction workers. Miners, for example had over four times the respiratory disorders incidence than construction workers. This of course relates to their exposure to indoor air pollutants at work.

Researchers from the National Institute for Occupational Safety and Health and the Centers for Disease Control (Greskevitch *et al.* 2007) investigated respiratory disease among agricultural workers using the 1988-1998 National Centers for Health Statistics' Multiple Cause of Death Data and the 1988-1994 Third National Health and Nutrition Examination Survey data (NHANES III). They studied mortality ratios for eleven respiratory illnesses in crop farm workers, livestock workers, farm managers, landscapers, horticultural workers, forestry workers, and fishery workers. Among the different occupations, the crop farm workers and livestock farm workers suffered significantly more deaths from respiratory conditions. Pneumonia with hypersensitivity was 10 to 50 times the normal levels. Landscapers and horticultural workers suffered more deaths from lung abscesses and COPD.

Wheeze and shortness of breath were also significantly elevated among the farm workers, especially among female farm workers. Respiratory disorders were heightened among agricultural workers, especially those who also smoked.

It is notable that these occupations each present particular toxins. In the case of miners, they are exposed to coal dust and soot, together with exhaust, with minimal ventilation. In the case of agricultural workers, landscapers and horticulture workers, they are exposed to chemical pesticides and herbicides. In the cases of teachers and healthcare workers, they are exposed to the contaminants that occupy their respective buildings and ventilation systems.

Exposure to specific toxins requires extensive ventilation and filtration systems. Whether these come in the form of protective breathing gear or building HVAC systems, the toxin exposures within a workplace must be minimized. Reducing exposure is, in fact, one of the driving purposes of the U.S. Occupational Safety and Health Administration (OSHA). Toxin exposure at the workplace has reached such significant levels that OSHA has put in place many regulations, such as Material Safety Data Sheets (MSDS), in efforts to protect workers from the effects of workplace toxins.

Why such an effort to protect workers from toxins? Today there are in the neighborhood of 100,000 different synthetic chemicals available in the marketplace. The chemical industry has produced many workplace chemicals for industrial uses over the past century, and many of these chemicals have been subsequently found to be carcinogenic or otherwise toxic. Keeping track of the effects and safeguards of each of these chemical toxins is a dizzying affair. Yet it is theoretically the responsibility of any business to make efforts to protect its workers from these toxins.

Here is a small list of occupations and their toxins:

Occupation	Exposures
Agricultural workers	Pesticides, herbicides
Plastics manufacturers	Plasticizers, VOCs, polymers
Painters	Paints/thinners (VOCs)
Drivers	Carbon, soot, formaldehyde, micro
Metal workers	Metallic dusts, heavy metals
Saw millers	Wood dust, preservatives
Janitorial and housekeepers	VOCs, cleaning chemicals
Bakers and food workers	Airborne food particles
Home builders	VOCs, formaldehyde, asbestos
Health workers	SBS, microorganisms, chemicals

Strategies to Reduce Toxin Exposure

By reducing our toxin exposure, we can dramatically lighten the burden on our immune systems, allowing our body's own detoxification systems to work more effectively. While this is not the total solution, reducing toxin exposure should not be overlooked. Below are some strategies to reduce our incoming toxins.

Know Your Toxins

One of the first things we can do is find out precisely what toxins are in our immediate environment. This means inspecting tags, reading labels and in general getting to know that materials that surround us in our home and work environments.

We should understand what is in our local drinking water. If on a municipal water supply, our local water district will likely list the results of their periodic tests. The EPA mandates that municipalities make this information available to the public, so there should be a website for our local water district.

We should also investigate the makeup and levels of our local air pollution levels are important. We might also find out what times of day the smog levels are higher and lower. Coordinating our exercise times and outdoor activities with lower smog periods is not a bad idea. A good place to start for those in the U.S. is the Environmental Protection Agency's local pollutant website:

http://www.epa.gov/epahome/commsearch.htm

By typing in our zip code into this database, we will be able to investigate the following information about our area:

Air pollution contents, levels and comparison to averages.

Locations of toxic spills, hazardous waste sites, or other areas, and any sites that have been categorized as an NPL—on the National Priorities List.

- ➢ Notifications of water quality issues.
- ➢ Sites of oil, natural gas or other mining operations nearby.
- ➢ Any toxic releases in area.
- ➢ Any sites subject to Superfund, Brownfields or other cleanup projects.
- ➢ Sites that have been subject to environmental enforcement nearby.

Outdoor Air Pollution Strategies

The best recommendation we find in some texts is simply to shut all the windows as much as possible. Is this really a solution? As we mentioned earlier, research has confirmed that indoor pollution is generally worse than outdoor pollution. What are we to do, then?

As we've discussed, ozone, particulate matter (soot) and carbon monoxide can contribute to and worsen toxicity.

Fresh Air

There is little doubt that city living increases toxicity. For example, a study done by the Arizona Health Care Cost Containment System (Smith *et al.* 2010) found that among 3,013 people, urban residents had a 55% greater likelihood of respiratory disorders than did rural residents.

Living around or at least visiting a natural setting such as a forest or beach has many advantages. For example, researchers from Japan's Chiba University (Park *et al.* 2010) conducted 24 field experiments using 280 subjects among 24 forests throughout Japan. In each of the tests, six subjects walked through a forest, while another six walked through a city. The next day the six that walked the city would walk the forest and vice versa. The research concluded that forest environments reduce stress-related cortisol levels, lower heart rate, reduce blood pressure, lower anxiety and increase reaction time. The researchers concluded that: *"These results will contribute to the development of a research field dedicated to forest medicine, which may be used as a strategy for preventive medicine."*

Other studies have confirmed these results. One study found that people living in natural environments had lower levels of stress than those living in urban environments (Ulrich *et al.* 1991). Another, from Emory University, found that natural environments improve health conditions (Frumkin 2001).

City Strategies

As much as we may want to, not everyone can pick up and move away from the city. In this case, focus can turn towards reducing immediate air pollutant exposure. We can make logical choices to reduce our exposure. This doesn't mean staying inside and closing all the windows either. It is important that we get enough sunshine and "fresh" air, and this requires us to go outside. We can simply use some common sense. For example, we can *avoid* the following:

- ➢ Running, walking or biking next to a freeway where soot and carbon monoxide levels are greatest.
- ➢ Hanging out downwind of a smokestack of an industrial plant known to throw toxins into the air.
- ➢ Sitting or standing downwind, or next to, an outdoor fire or gas stove for an extended period.
- ➢ Standing, sitting or walking next to someone spraying pesticides, herbicides or other chemicals.
- ➢ Frequenting tobacco-filled bars or other smoky places.
- ➢ Avoiding dusty areas such as construction sites, runways, race-tracks, rodeos and other events that stir up lots of airborne particulates.

In addition, there are a number of proactive things we can do to reduce our airborne toxins. As discussed earlier, breathing in through the nose helps to filter out some particulates and other foreigners. This also warms the air. As we discussed, cold air can dry the mucous membranes, and thinned mucous membranes expose our airways to more airborne toxins.

If we live in an urban area with poor air quality we might consider exercising or getting outside during the morning, when the air quality is typically better. As temperatures rise, immediate ozone levels increase. We might also consider exercising near a lake, river, or ocean. Polluted air around water tends to disperse more quickly in the presence of wind, humidity, pressure gradients, and temperature differences around the water.

Out and out wearing of a facemask is typically not practical—although during an extreme situation, it is not a bad idea. More subtle strategies include wearing a scarf during winter months, and covering our mouth and nose with it when outside. In colder climates, a fleece ski mask could also help filter out some particulates.

These are but a few ways to prevent burdening our immune system with airborne toxins—but again, these cannot be our only strategy. We must also undertake reducing the *other, more controllable* immune system burdens to the greatest degree possible. This may also mean increasing the amount of antioxidants we consume in our diet. And let's not forget that the more antioxidants we eat, the better our ability to remove toxins will be. We can add to this the other strategies discussed—herbs, diet, detoxification and so on.

Home Pollution Strategies

Americans spend over 90% of their lives indoors, and indoor air pollution averages double to five times worse than outdoor pollution levels. In some cases, indoor pollution can be tens, even hundreds of times higher than outdoor pollutant levels.

The issue here is ventilation. While older homes might exchange all the air in the house every couple of hours—even up to twice an hour—modern energy-efficient homes exchange air well over five times slower. The average, in fact, is about .25 times per hour, meaning that it would take four hours to exchange all the air in the home. This problem has been termed the *tight building syndrome*.

Previously, we discussed *sick building syndrome*. Tight building syndrome can result in sick building syndrome, assuming that a tight building is not properly ventilated, or ventilated with a clean ventilation system. Or, quite simply, keeping windows open throughout the house. While this might be frowned upon by city dwellers, most indoor air is still quite worse than even big city air. Plus, as we'll explain further, circulating air removes particulates and other toxins as it moves.

For example, University of Glasgow researchers (Wright *et al.* 2009) found that ventilation increases lung function, but does little to reduce dust mite populations. They tested the homes of 120 asthmatic adults—who were allergic to *Dermatophagoides pteronyssinus* dust mites—using mechanical heat recovery ventilation systems (MHRV). This was in addition to conventional allergen avoidance measures in an attempt to reduce dust mite populations. After one year, the peak expiratory flow among the ventilator group was significantly better than the non-ventilator group. However, the ventilation systems *did not* reduce the mite levels within the houses.

So it is not the number of dust mites: It is the composition of the air itself, determined by circulation. A good ventilation system will circulate air while sending it through a filter. A good filter can remove endotoxins that mites produce, as well as the molds, bacteria, soot and other debris that commonly reside in our indoor air.

As we discussed in depth earlier, indoor air pollution is caused by fungi-laden basements, formaldehydes from furniture, asbestos and other building chemicals, household chemicals, volatile organic compounds, smoking, moldy ventilation systems, moldy dust-mite ridden carpets, and so on.

Air Filtration

These toxins can help overload our immune systems, especially if overloaded by other toxins and/or pathogens. In other words, it would be better to remove as many of these as possible before we breathed them in.

Air purifiers: These can significantly remove toxins from the air, as they draw air through a filter and then push the air out. Studies have shown that air purifiers can significantly increase the quality of life among asthmatics (Brodtkorb *et al.* 2010).

Electric ion generating machines generate negative ions. Ionizers have been reputed to remove dust and bacteria, yet this remains controversial. While dust and soot may be attracted to negative ions, they are likely to remain airborne, or possibly end up on floors or furniture to be picked up again.

The amount of ions generated by these machines may also be of concern. While outdoor air may range from 500 to 5,000 negative ions per cubic centimeter, and indoor air may only have a couple hundred per cubic centimeter, negative ion generators can easily pump out from ten thousand to ten million negative ions per cubic centimeter. At these higher levels—especially over a million—negative ions can become irritating to mucous membranes. They can irritate the throat, the eyes, and the lungs. Quite simply, our bodies were not designed for this level of negative ions.

Furthermore, a Cochrane review (Blackhall *et al.* 2003) of six good quality studies concluded that ionizers exerted no significant effects upon respiratory health.

Ozone generators may be effective at removing bacteria, because bacteria require oxygen to live, and ozone depletes their oxygen levels. For this reason, a good ozone generator will often create a fresher smelling indoor environment. While ozone is not the same as smog, which has carbon or sulphur molecules connected to the molecules, ozone is an atmospheric response to smog, as ozone helps stabilize oxygen levels and clear out other molecules.

At the same time, higher ozone levels may also result in lung irritation and allergic response. As mentioned earlier, the FDA limits ozone generating machines in medical devices (used in hospitals and clinics) to emit no more than 50 parts per billion. The bottom line with both ionizers and ozone generators is that the atmosphere contains a fragile balance of components: It is not a random mixture. The level of ozone present in outdoor pollution reflects the atmosphere's cleansing process. In other words, the decision to use these machines should be made carefully, and the composition of fresh air is likely healthier than any machine-driven composition.

High-Efficiency Particular Arresting (HEPA) filters: It might be noted that neither the ozone nor ion generator systems have been shown to effectively remove dust, dander or allergens (unless the allergens are bacteria, which can be removed with ozone). A HEPA filter is a better strategy for removing dust, dander and other particulates. HEPA filters are designed to pick up over 99.9% of particulate sized .3 micron in size. Putting a HEPA filter on a simple air ducting system with a fan or heater will thus do wonders for removing dust, dander, and allergens.

Electrostatic air filters for forced air systems can be a good choice. These HEPA filters typically filter between ninety and a hundred percent of dander, mold, mites, dust, soot, and bacteria. Many of these filters come with the ability to clean and reuse, allowing us to clean them as often as needed—which should be at least monthly if use is constant.

Environmental filters are good alternatives, especially for cold urban environments. These draw in, filter and heat outdoor air. This maximizes circulation, ventilation and temperature control: The best of all worlds.

Pillowcase filters: This air filtration device is designed to filter the nighttime air through the pillowcase. One study (Stillerman *et al.* 2010) tested this with 35 adults who had allergic rhinoconjunctivitis and sensitivities to either dander or dust mites. The device was found to reduce 99.99% of allergen particulates greater than .3 microns within the patients' breathing zones. The patient group using the filtration device was found to have significantly fewer symptoms and better quality of lie than the placebo group.

Natural Air Sanitation

We can also restrict the level of indoor pollutants by choosing to use household products with natural ingredients free as possible from chemical preservatives. This means using natural flooring and furniture, natural fragrance-free soaps and cosmetics, and cotton clothing. This also means buying fewer plastic household goods and more natural fiber goods. Should we change our purchasing behavior, we may also alter the behavior of those companies manufacturing these items.

When it comes to freshening up stale indoor air, pressurized aerosol air fresheners are not the way to go. They may contain various synthetic fragrances, benzyl ethanols, naphthalene, and formaldehydes among other undesirables. Various micro-particles are also created by these aerosols.

As mentioned in the trigger chapter, many aerosols and pump sprays also contain noxious propellants—many of which are also volatile organic compounds (VOCs). These include butane and propane. Despite their demand in the marketplace, aerosols are not required for survival: Humankind did just fine without them for thousands of years. An effective disbursing method is a simple spray bottle. An active ingredient—say lemon juice—can be diluted with water and lightly sprayed through a room to freshen it up nicely. There are, of course, many other uses for such a common spray bottle—effectively replacing propellant aerosols.

Beware of perfumes and colognes that may reside in the bathroom or on family members. And be careful of fashion magazines and men's magazines that insert fragrances into their pages and advertisements. These perfumes might smell nice, but they can also contain toxins that can burden the immune system.

Candles may smell nice, but they are often made with synthetic fragrances, hydrocarbon-based paraffin waxes, and lead or other heavy metal wicks. The combination often releases unhealthy black soot into our air.

Beeswax candles with essential oils can provide good alternatives for the candle-loving household, combined, of course, with fresh air.

Healthy alternatives to toxic household cleaners include lemon, vinegar, borax and/or baking soda. Borax is a great scrubbing detergent for heavy household and yard cleaning jobs. Olive oil, lemon oil or beeswax make for good natural furniture polishes.

Cleaning surfaces with these will also significantly freshen indoor air as well. Rotting food and unclean surfaces create mildew and bacteria quite quickly. Fresh air is quite easy to achieve with clean surfaces. Dusting and wiping down flooring and walls with vinegar can be a good strategy. A small cup of vinegar or a box of baking soda placed in a corner can also absorb odors and airborne toxins. Non-septic friendly chlorine bleach or rubbing alcohol can be used sparingly to remove mold or other microorganisms.

As far as pesticides, there are also natural alternatives. These include clove oil, mints, orange oil, borax and others. Many pest control companies will now apply these alternatives upon request.

House Plants

A house full of indoor plants will do wonders for improving our indoor air quality. Placing between two and five plants in a hundred square foot room—depending upon the outside air—can significantly remove carbon and raise oxygen levels. Research from the *Mississippi Stennis Space Center* concluded that indoor plants absorbed and broke down formaldehydes, trichloroethylenes, benzenes and zylenes.

Better performing plants included the lady palm, the rubber plant, English ivy, and the areca palm plants. Toxin removal rates can range from 1,000 to 1,800 micrograms per hour. One study done in Norway (Fjeld *et al.* 1998) found 23% fewer complaints of fatigue and sinus congestion among workers working around plants.

Studies performed in Texas and at Washington State University found that cognition response and problem-solving were also significantly higher among people working around plants (Wolverton 1997).

It should be noted that potting soils of indoor plants can also harbor some molds, so care can be taken to dry out the soil between waterings, and keep some sunlight on the soil surface.

We can also create forests around our homes. This means planting and maintaining indigenous trees that provide oxygen, shade and soil health: Soils without good plant life and rooting systems become loose and dusty. Nearby outdoor plants can significantly decrease the carbon and toxins in our immediate circulating environment. This also means instead of tearing out trees and paving our courtyards, we can leave the trees or replant them. Living in a space surrounded by trees can also render more privacy, allowing us to keep our windows open more often.

Pros and Cons on Air Conditioning

Air conditioning offers benefits and downsides. On the benefit side, a good one can filter out particulates and some pollutants. This of course depends on the type of filter inside the air conditioner, and how often it is cleaned. And filters not cleaned frequently can build up with fungi and bacteria that can significantly infect our airspace.

Most air conditioners reduce humidity as well. The problem with this massive reduction in humidity is that it can dry out the mucosal membranes in our airways. This, along with the cold air provided by many air conditioners, can lead to or worsen respiratory disorders.

Swamp coolers provide filtering and cooling, but add humidity. This can help keep the airways and skin hydrated. However, swamp coolers can easily get infected with molds and bacteria: So they have to be cleaned periodically, at least seasonally.

Practically every air conditioner creates condensation, which results in small droplets of water dripping around the unit or inside the unit. This can encourage fungi and bacteria growth around the walls and ventilation ducts of the system.

Air conditioning artificially cools down body temperature and airways. While this might be considered a good thing when it is hot outside, artificially cooling the body also stresses the body and the airways. The body must work harder to heat and humidify the air before it hits the lungs. This can stress the turbinates, the airway mucosal membranes, and the immune system. Remember the research we laid out earlier that confirms colder, dryer air can increase airway hypersensitivity.

Also note that car air-conditioning systems typically intake air from around the car—full of traffic exhaust. The air can also contain exhaust from the car itself, or combustion byproducts from the engine. While screened through a filter, this air still contains toxins. We can periodically refresh the car's indoor air by stopping and rolling down the car windows.

Air filters in car air conditions can also become filled with fungi and bacteria, so they can be periodically cleaned. Generally, people do not clean their car air filters. So it is safe to say that any older car has a significant build up of mold and other toxins within its air conditioner system and filters.

Noting these issues, it is probably more sustainable to simply minimize air conditioning and utilize fans when possible. Opening the car windows while driving also provides a fan of sorts. Fanned air on the skin helps cool the skin down without chilling the air. Remember that circulated air is typically cleaner than the same type of air when stagnant.

A fan strategy also allows our bodies to better acclimate to the outdoor temperatures. This is healthier for the body. Our bodies have cooling mechanisms that include sweating and relaxing. Both of these are healthy strategies. Sweating removes waste and toxins from the body, and relaxing takes pressure off the adrenal glands. We can conclude that sweating a little and relaxing a bit can reduce toxicity.

Natural Materials

Using nature's materials for floors, walls and furniture is also a good strategy. This means using stone, ceramic, wood, wool, cotton and so on. Practically every synthetic piece of furniture, wall covering or floor covering contains a host of chemicals, including formaldehyde, VOCs, insecticides, asbestos and fire retardants. While retarding fires is certainly commendable, these can also make us sick in the worst case, and add to our toxin load in the best case. Besides, stone can be a pretty good fire retardant.

Stone, ceramic tile or wooden floors can also be easily cleaned with vinegar and baking soda to safely eliminate dust and allergens. Wood can also be polished and cleaned with olive oil. Nowadays, most walls are sheet rock, which often contains chalks and asbestos that can slowly build up in the airways. Replacing them with wood siding is a possible strategy.

Outgassing

Outgassing (or off-gassing) any new materials we buy is a good idea, regardless. To outgas a material, we can simply set it in the sun for a day before using it. This is a good idea for any new piece of furniture, wall covering, and anything else that may have been coated in VOCs or formaldehydes during manufacturing. Plastics may also be outgassed, but outgassing plastic in direct sunlight can also release additional monomer plasticizers.

Outgassing a new car might also be considered. That "new car smell" is more than just a nice smell. Leave the car in the sun for a few days or weeks with the windows open. For best results, always keep car windows cracked.

Ventilation

Air travels in currents. These currents are electromagnetic. Airflows will thus grab hold of air pollutants and channel them away. Air works much as water does, as it uses electrostatic forces to remove toxins. This means that our freshest air will be the air that flows through our environment. Stagnated air is polluted air. Moving air is typically cleaner and provides the best means to minimize toxicity. Circulating air also has the greatest tendency of maintaining normal atmospheric composition, humidity and pressure values.

Therefore, if possible, we might consider keeping our windows open at all times, even in the wintertime. When it is cold outside, we can crack the window barely—just enough to allow for some airflow. Fans can do the rest.

Work and School Pollution Strategies

Work and school environments are toxin traps. Why? Because they bring people and limited ventilation systems together under the same roof. They also host a number of toxins in building materials, carpets, desks, chairs, production materials, manufacturing exhaust, and whatever anyone brings in to work or school. This of course includes animal dander, dust mites, microorganisms and mold attached to people's clothing, hair and skin as they venture into the building.

This was illustrated in the New Zealand research discussed earlier, where cat allergens were found throughout schools, workplaces, theaters and airplanes.

While there is no way to eliminate these potential toxins, we can certainly take measures to lower our exposure, since as a whole, toxins from the workplace and school do contribute to our overall toxic load and burden upon our immune system. Furthermore, exposure to workplace toxicity in the form of manufacturing wastes, cleaners, gases and other chemical toxins can single-handedly make a person downright sick.

A number of policies and strategies that can reduce our toxin exposure among workplaces and schools:

Hazardous Materials: Workplaces and schools typically utilize various chemicals and cleaning materials. Some workplaces use hazardous materials on a daily basis. These should be handled with care, to make sure that exposures are minimized.

According to United States Occupational Safety Code, *Manufacturer's Safety Data Sheets* (MSDS) are required for every chemical used by consumers, workers or cleaning professionals. These should be carefully read over to make sure that the material is being used in accordance with the MSDS. This means that enough ventilation is supplied. For most hazardous materials, this is the greatest risk: Hazardous materials are frequently used without the proper ventilation. These toxins can also cause illness and death, depending upon the chemical and exposure level.

HVAC: Our school and workplace should have a heating, ventilating and air conditioning system (also called HVAC) that is adequate for the population, space and environmental conditions. The more people, space and toxins present, the better the HVAC system needs to be. In the United States, these are typically determined by local, state or county building codes. When a building is designed, its HVAC must comply with the building code in place.

The standard codes are determined by The *American Society of Heating, Refrigerating and Air Conditions Engineers* (ASHRAE), who have developed the standards that most municipalities abide by. For example, the 1989 standards (6.2-1989) called for 15-20 cubic feet of fresh air to be brought in per minute (CFM) and per person occupying an indoor space. This means, for example, that an office with 10 people must have a system that pumps in 150-200 cubic feet of fresh air per minute.

This same calculation can be done for any school or other space.

In addition, building codes have changed over the years with respect to insulation. This means that if the building has been built in the past few decades, the building codes are tighter, and there will be likely less ventilation in general. This puts an extra strain on the HVAC system.

Windows are certainly a form of ventilation, but they should not be included in this calculation, because during cold or hot weather, the windows are often closed (though they should not be).

Any building needs to be checked with current code to make sure that the HVAC system matches the use and occupancy of the building. The building specifications designed by the architect before the building was built can easily be different from the building's current use. There may be many more workers or children in the building than originally specified for example. Or if the HVAC was designed for office space, but the building is now used as manufacturing space, for example, the HVAC requirements will be different—depending upon what is being produced, and the municipality. So the company owners or school administrators must be reminded to assure their workers or parents that the workplace's/school's HVAC systems are compliant with current codes. This should also be reviewed for any apartment or condominium.

HVAC systems also should also be periodically cleaned. This includes the drip pans and ducting. These can build up with molds and other microorganisms, and infect their occupants. As we discussed earlier, cases have shown that extreme weather changes (from cold to warm or wet) can dramatically affect the HVAC system ducting in terms of mold and microorganisms—significantly infecting the building's occupants.

Flooring: Carpeting in workplaces and schools is particularly problematic. This is because they attract bacteria, molds, dander, allergens and other toxins quickly. Cleaning carpets is typically expensive and difficult. Wood, stone or concrete floors clean easier and can be disinfected more easily, as we've discussed.

Furniture: Chairs and sofas in the work place are susceptible to mold, toxin and allergen build-up as they age, and formaldehydes when newer. Therefore, they need to be periodically cleaned or replaced. Wooden furniture or furniture with cleanable surfaces and moisture barriers are preferred.

Windows: From an individual perspective, sitting or working close to an openable window is suggested in any workplace or school classroom. Any time there is an offensive odor or concern about indoor air quality, the window should be opened and left open until the risk has subsided. Hotel rooms can also be checked for openable windows before they are reserved. A closed-in room with a dirty HVAC system can practically produce illness in itself.

Keeping the house on the dry side. Water feeds molds and fungi. Look for leaks into the windowsills, basements and house corners.

Chemicals: Our houses and work places are best clear of pesticides, fragrances, incense, and other chemicals. If bugs are a problem, try borax or traps.

Household and workplace cleaners should be natural. These include baking soda, vinegar, lemon and borax. These are all, to relative degrees, also antimicrobial.

Tubs and bathrooms should be cleaned of molds and fungi frequently, before mold forms. Mold grows in moist, dark places, so those areas of the bathroom should be cleaned more frequently than areas exposed to sunshine.

Fans: Fans are a valuable and inexpensive addition to any room. These can help blow offensive air out the door or window, for example. Fans, in fact, are better strategies than air conditioning, because they do not artificially cool the body down—as we've discussed. In the opinion of this author, every workplace and school should be equipped with fans.

Carbon monoxide and NO$_2$ strategies include venting any gas appliance to the outdoors, making sure there are no leaks, using the right fuels for each appliance; using an exhaust fan over a gas appliance; using certified wood stoves; having stoves inspected and cleaned; opening fireplace flues (vents to the outside); and opening the garage door before starting the car.

Air purifiers: Small air purifiers can significant help a person working in a workplace with questionable air. These can be placed right on the desk. These can significantly help remove particulates, mold and allergens from our immediate breathing airspace.

Regular Cleaning: This is a requisite for any workplace, school or apartment building. Common areas should be cleaned at least weekly. Floors and walls should be sanitized. Good natural cleaners include vinegar, lemon, borax and baking soda. Chlorine or rubbing alcohol can be used sparingly to disinfect. Furniture requires regular dusting and sanitization, and HVAC systems and ducts require regular cleaning.

Wearing a mask when we are using any chemical that might contain VOCs or other breathable toxins. Best strategy is to not use these types of chemicals at all, but sometimes we might have to. The mask should have an outside rubber seal. Paper masks do very little to prevent breathing in toxins.

Strengthened Immunity: No matter how clean we get our workplaces and schools, there will always be lots of toxins. While these strategies can help remove toxin exposure, we still need to strengthen our immunity and tolerance. Hygiene, after all, has its place. But it cannot replace a strong immune system. This means following through with other strategies outlined in this text.

Major Toxins and Sources

Source	Toxins
Air pollutants	Lead, mercury, carbon monoxide, sulfur, arsenic, nitrogen dioxide, ozone…
Animals	Dried skin, bacteria, waste excreted from animal (dander)
Carpets, rugs	Molds, dander, lice, PC-4, latex
Cigarette/Cigar/Pipe Smoke	Carbon monoxide, nicotine, aldehydes, ketones, soot, formaldehyde, others
Cosmetics	Aluminum, phosphates and chemicals
Spray cans	Propellants, other chemicals
Foods/Additives	Food colors, preservatives, trans fats, pesticides, arachidonic acids, acrylamide, phytanic acid, artificial flavors, refined sugars and much, much more
House	Radon, formaldehyde, pollen, dust, mold, dander, pesticides, cleaning products, asbestos, lead, paint, endotoxins
Household chemicals	Cleaners, pesticides, herbicides, paints
Insects	Endotoxins from dust mites, cockroaches and other insects
Laundry soaps	Fragrances, detergents, surfactants
Microorganisms	Mold, bacteria, viruses, parasites
Mattresses/pillows	Endotoxins, molds, formaldehyde
Paints	Lead, arsenic, VOCs, adhesives
Pets	Dander, up to 240 infectious diseases & parasites (65 from dogs/39 from cats)
Pharmaceuticals	Many-see short list on pages 112-113
Water	Chorine byproducts, pesticides, pharmaceuticals, many others
Pollinating plants	See pollen list on page 104
Pools and spas	Chlorine byproducts such as trihalomethanes (THMs), various carbonates
Soaps and Shampoos	Fragrances, detergents, surfactants
Stoves, Fireplaces	Carbon monoxide, NO_2, arsenic, soot
Work and school environments	SBS, practically all of the above

Chapter Three

The Physiology of Detoxification

One of the problems with many cleansing programs is that they attempt to force the body into a cleanse. These protocols might use a combination of herbal supplements, fasting, and laxatives to stimulate an immediate cleanse. This is not always so healthy, however. Sometimes the body can overreact to these, producing toxemia. Yes, we may be able to stimulate some detoxification, but at what cost? And is it a long-term solution?

The cleansing protocol we are recommending in this text is altogether different. This protocol utilizes *the body's own detoxification systems* to efficiently and effectively remove pathogens and toxins that are invading our bodies.

The core strategy is to first reduce the burden upon our immune systems by reducing toxin exposure, combined with using diet and lifestyle tools that will stimulate the body's immune system. These two steps can almost immediately remove a condition of systemic inflammation that may be plaguing the body and slowing down the process of toxin removal.

Once systemic inflammation is reduced and the immune system is stimulated, our protocol then maintains this strengthened immune system. By incorporating painless strategies into our lives on an ongoing basis, we can maintain the 'edge' with the immune system. This will result in continued efficiency in toxin removal.

To understand how this program works, we should review the basics of the immune system, according to the latest research.

When a toxin enters our body, our immune system immediately begins to reject it. This is because the living immune system recognizes the foreigner immediately. How does this happen? In this chapter, we'll show how the body's natural detoxification system works. This will help us understand how we can better utilize and even stimulate the immune system later.

The immune system is located throughout the body. We find immune cells on the skin, in the blood, in the lungs, in the bones and in every organ system. We also find the immune system within trillions of probiotic bacteria scattered around the body.

The immune system has a number of intelligent abilities. The first is recognition. The immune system has the facility to recognize molecules that endanger the body's welfare. The immune system also maintains memory. The immune system can remember the identity of a toxin or pathogen by virtue of recognizing its antigens (byproducts or molecular structure). This is the rationale for vaccination. Vaccination exposes the body to a small amount of a particular pathogen so the immune system will develop the tools and the memory to recognize its antigens, so that the body can respond appropriately the next time it is exposed to the same pathogen.

The immune system is incredible in its ability to maintain specificity and diversity. These characteristics allow the immune system to respond to literally millions, if not billions of different antigens. Moreover, each particular antigen requires a completely different response.

The immune system is an intelligent scanning and review system intended to gauge whether a particular molecule, cell or organism belongs in the body. This is determined through a complex biochemical identification system. We might compare this system to an iris scan, often used as a password entry system. Utilizing a database of information, the immune system checks molecular structures against this database. If the molecular structure isn't recognized, or matches a structure considered foreign, the immune system launches an attack. This attack is referred to as an immune response or an inflammatory response.

Despite significant research in the areas of vaccination, antibiotics, and inflammation, modern medical science is still perplexed with the autoimmune syndrome. A massive list of degenerative diseases are now considered autoimmune, including irritable bowel syndrome, Crohn's, asthma, allergies, fibromyalgia, lupus, urinary tract disorders and many, many others. Physicians also classify most types of arthritis as autoimmune disorders. Why can't the immune system repair these disorders, as it does with most other types of injuries? What has gone wrong with the immune system in these cases? How about in a body that is overwhelmed with toxins?

Chemical toxins also invade the body via the digestive tract, the nose and sinuses, the genitals, the lungs, the skin, the ears and even the eyes. Microbial infections can also be caused by normal residents of the body, should they grow beyond their typical populations. These include *H. pylori*, *E. coli* and *Candida albicans*. These are also considered by the body as toxins, because these foreigners must be cleared from the body or otherwise controlled.

There are four processes the body uses to guard against and remove toxins:

Non-specific Immunity: The Barriers

The first is called the *non-specific* immune response. This utilizes a network of biochemical barriers that work synergistically to prevent infectious agents from getting into the body. The barrier structures include the ability of the body to shut down its orifices. We can close our eyes, mouths, noses and ears to prevent invaders or toxins from entering the body. Within these lie further defensive structures: Nose hairs, eyelashes, lips, tonsils, ear hair, pubic hair and hair in general are all designed to help screen out and filter invaders. Most of the body's passageways are also equipped with tiny cilia, which assist the body evacuate invaders by brushing them out. These cilia move rhythmically, sweeping back and forth, working caught pathogens outward with their undulations. The surfaces of most of the body's orifices are also covered with a mucous membrane. This thin liquid membrane film contains a combination of biochemicals and cells that prevent invaders from penetrating any further.

These mucous membranes lining the passageways accomplish this with a combination of immune cells, immunoglobulins and colonies of probiotics.

The digestive tract is equipped with another type of sophisticated defense technology. Should any foreigners get through the lips, teeth, tongue, hairs, mucous membranes, cilia and sneak down the esophagus, they then must contend with the digestive fire of the stomach. The gastrin, peptic acid and hydrochloric acid within a healthy stomach keep a pH of around two. This is typically enough acidity to kill or significantly damage many bacteria. However, a person can mistakenly weaken this protective acid by taking antacids or acid-blockers. In this case, the stomach's ability to neutralize pathogens will be handicapped. In addition, a number of microorganisms are accustomed to acidic environments, and still others can tuck away into clumps of food—especially food that has not been chewed well enough.

Humoral Immunity: Toxin Attackers

The second form of immune response involves a highly technical strategic attack that first identifies the invader's weaknesses, followed by a precise and immediate offensive attack to exploit those weaknesses. This is often called humoral immunity. More than a billion different types of antibodies, macrophages and other immune cells mobilize and execute specific attack plans. As an immune cell scans a particular invader, it may recognize a particular biomolecular or behavioral weakness within the toxin or pathogen. Upon recognizing this weakness, the immune system will devise a unique plan to exploit this weakness. It may launch a variety of possible attacks, using a combination of specialized B-cells (or *B-lymphocytes*) in conjunction with specialized antibodies.

Cruising through the blood and lymph systems, the antibodies and/or B-cells can quickly sense and size up invading microbes. Often this will mean the antibody will lock onto or bind to the invader to extract critical molecular information. This process will often draw upon databases held within certain helper B-cells that memorize vulnerabilities. The specific vulnerability is often revealed by molecular structures of pathogenic cell membranes. Each pathogen will be identified by these unique structures or antigens. The B-cell then reproduces a specific antibody designed to record and communicate that information to other B-cells through biochemical transception. This allows for a constant tracking of the location and development of pathogens, allowing B-cells to manage and constantly assess the response.

Cell-Mediated Immunity: Detoxing the Cells

The third process used by the immune system is the cell-mediated immune response. This also incorporates a collection of smart white blood cells, called T-cells. T-cells and their surrogates wander the body scanning the body's own cells. They are seeking cells that have become infected or otherwise damaged by microbes or toxic free radicals. Infected cells are typically identified by special marker molecules (antigens) that sit atop their cell membranes. These antigens have particular molecular arrangements that signal roving T-cells of the damage that has occurred within the cell. Once a damaged cell has been recognized, the cell-mediated immune system will launch an inflammatory response against the cell. This response will typically utilize a variety of cytotoxic (cell-killing) cells and helper T-cells. These types of immune cells will often directly kill the damaged cell by inserting toxic chemicals into it. Alternatively, the T-cell might send signals into the damaged cell, switching on a self-destruct mechanism within the cell.

Probiotic Immunity: The Protectors

The fourth and most powerful part of the immune system takes place among the body's probiotics. This is the backbone of the living immune system, because our probiotics drive many of our immune processes.

The human body can house more than 32 billion beneficial and harmful bacteria and fungi at any particular time. When beneficial bacteria are in the majority, they constitute up to 70-80% of the body's immune response. This takes place both in an isolated manner and in conjunction with the rest of the immune system.

Probiotic colonies work with the body's internal immune system to organize strategies that prevent toxins and pathogenic microorganisms from harming the body. Probiotics will communicate and cooperate with the immune system to organize cooperative strategies. They will stimulate the body's immune cells, activating the cell-mediated response, the humoral response, and indirectly, the body's exterior barrier mechanisms through immunoglobulin stimulation. As we will see in the research, they stimulate T-cells, B-cells, macrophages and NK-cells with smart messages that promote specific immune responses. They also activate cytokines and phagocytic cells directly to coordinate their intelligent immune response.

Probiotics can also quickly identify harmful bacteria or fungal overgrowths and work directly to eradicate them. This process may not directly involve the rest of the immune system. Even still, the immune system will be notified of any probiotic offensives. The immune system will support the process by breaking up and escorting dead pathogens out of the body.

Probiotics produce chemical substances that destroy invading microorganisms. Probiotics make up our body's own antibiotic system. Because probiotics are extremely intelligent and want to survive, they have developed various strategies to defend their homeland (our body). It is a territorial issue. Invading bacteria threaten their homes and families. Probiotics also learn how to fight newer bacteria species and new bacteria strategies. While static pharmaceutical antibiotics are counteracted by smart super-bugs, probiotics can alter their antibiotic strategies as needed. Our continued survival illustrates their intelligence.

Probiotics produce antimicrobial biochemicals that manage, damage or kill pathogenic microorganisms. In some cases, they will simply overcrowd the invaders with biochemistry and populations to limit their growth. In other cases, they will secrete chemicals into the fluid environment to eradicate large populations. In still other cases, they will insert specific chemicals into the invaders, which will directly kill them. Probiotic mechanisms are quite complex and variegated to say the least.

Dr. Mechnikov hypothesized that the beneficial effects of lactobacilli arise from the lactic acid they excrete. Indeed, the lactic acid produced by *Lactobacillus* and *Bifidobacteria* species sets up the ultimate pH control in the gut to repel antagonistic organisms. Lactic acids are not alike, however. There are different lactic acid molecular structures, and combinations with other chemicals. For example, some probiotics produce an L(+) form of lactic acid and other probiotics may produce the D(-) from. Many probiotic strains also produce a molecular combination with hydrogen peroxide called lactoperoxidase.

Probiotics also produce acetic acids, formic acids, special lipopolysaccharides, peptidoglycans, superantigens, heat shock proteins and bacterial DNA—all in precise portions to nourish each other, inhibit challengers and/or benefit the host.

Precision and proportion is the key. For example, some bifidobacteria secrete a 3:2 proportion of acetic acid to lactic acid in order to barricade certain pathogenic microbes.

Probiotics also secrete a number of key nutrients crucial to its host's (our body) immune system and metabolism, including B vitamins pantothenic acid, pyridoxine, niacin, folic acid, cobalamin and biotin, and crucial antioxidants such as vitamin K.

Probiotics also produce antimicrobial molecules called bacteriocins. *Lactobacillus plantarum* produces lactolin. *Lactobacillus bulgaricus* secretes bulgarican. *Lactobacillus acidophilus* can produce aciophilin, acidolin, bacterlocin and lactocidin. These and other antimicrobial substances equip probiotic species with territorial mechanisms to combat and reduce pathologies related to *Shigella*, *Coliform*, *Pseudomonas*, *Klebsiella*, *Staphylococcus*, *Clostridium*, *Escherichia* and other infective genera. Furthermore, antifungal biochemicals from the likes of *L. acidophilus*, *B. bifidum*, *E. faecium* and others also significantly reduce fungal outbreaks caused by *Candida albicans* (Shahani *et al.* 2005).

These types of antimicrobial tools give probiotics the ability to counter the mighty *H. pylori* bacterium—known to be at the root of a majority of ulcers. *H. pylori* inhibition has been observed in studies on *L. acidophilus* DDS-1, *L. rhamnosus GG*, *L. rhamnosus Lc705*, *Propionibacterium freudenreichii* and *Bifidobacterium breve Bb99*, as we will see later.

Furthermore, probiotics will specifically stimulate the body's own immune system to attack pathogens. For example, scientists from Finland's University of Turku (Pessi *et al.* 2000) gave nine atopic dermatitis children

Lactobacillus rhamnosus GG for four weeks. They found that serum cytokine IL-10 levels specific to the infection increased following probiotic consumption.

Whatever the strategy, smart probiotic microorganisms work collectively and synergistically with the other three components of our immune system. Our probiotic system works within the non-specific immune system to help protect the body from invasions. Probiotics live within the oral cavity, the nasal cavity, the esophagus, around the gums, and in pockets of our pleural cavity (surrounding our lungs). They dwell within our stomach, within our intestines, within the vagina and around the rectum, and amongst other pockets of tissues. This means that for microbes to invade the bloodstream, they must first get through legions of probiotic bacteria that populate those entry channels—assuming a healthy body of course.

Probiotics participate deeply in immune activity. In one study, the probiotic organism *Bifidobacterium lactis* HN019 or a placebo was given to 30 healthy elderly volunteers (average age 69 years old) for nine weeks. The probiotic group had significant increases among total T-cells, helper T-cells (CD4+), activated (CD25+) T-cells, and natural killer T-cells. Cytotoxic capacity among mononuclear and polymorphonuclear phagocytes and tumor-cell killing activity among natural killer cells also increased among the probiotic group (Gill *et al.* 2001).

Probiotics modulate the inflammatory Th1/Th2 system. Illustrating this, yogurt with *Bifidobacterium longum* BB536 or plain yogurt was given to 40 patients with Japanese cedar pollinosis for 14 weeks. Peripheral blood mononuclear cells from the patients indicated that *B. fragilis* microorganisms induced significantly more helper TH cell type2 cytokines such as interleukin [IL]-6, and fewer Th1 cytokines such as IL-12 and interferon (Odamaki *et al.* 2007).

Probiotics utilize cytokine communications to transmit intelligent information to the body's network of white blood cells. Illustrating this, Scientists from the Slovak Institute of Cardiovascular Diseases (Hlivak *et al.* 2005) gave a placebo or probiotic *Enterococcus faecium* M-74 to human volunteers for 60 weeks. Peripheral blood analysis indicated significant decreases in cytokines sICAM-1, CD54 on monocytes, and CD11b on lymphocytes after one-year. These are related to anti-adhesion strategies following inflammatory responses to artery damage.

In order to better understand the relationship between probiotics and our immune system, let's discuss the other players among the body's immune system and their interaction with our probiotic populations.

The Cleansing Cells

The immune system produces at least five different types of white blood cells. Each is designed to identify and target specific types of pathogens. After identification, they will either initiate an attack with other components, or directly begin their attack. The main types are lymphocytes, neutrophils, basophils, monocytes and macrophages. Each plays an important role in the pathogen-identification and inflammatory process. Lymphocytes are the body's self-specific immune response team.

The primary lymphocytes are the T-cells (thymus cells) or B-cells (bone marrow cells). These cells and their specialized proteins work together to strategically attack and remove invaders. Then they memorize the strategy in preparation for a future invasion.

All white blood cells are initially assembled by stem cells in the bone marrow. Following their release, T-cells undergo further differentiation and programming in the thymus gland. B-cells undergo a similar process of maturity before release from the spleen. Both T-cells and B-cells circulate via lymph nodes, the bloodstream and among tissue fluids. Both also have a number of special types, including memory cells and helper cells to identify and memorize invaders.

B-cells look for foreign or potentially harmful pathogens moving freely. These might include toxins or microbes. Once identified, B-cells will stimulate the production of a particular type of antibody protein, which is designed to destroy or break apart the foreigner. There are several different types of B-cells. Most are monoclonal, which means they will adjust to the specific type of invader. Some B-cells are investigative and surveillance oriented. They are focused on roaming pathogens. Once activated, they can then damage these invading pathogens using a variety of biochemical secretions or physical activities. B-cells that circulate and surveil the bloodstream are often called plasma B-cells. Others—like memory B-cells—record previous invasions for future attacks.

T-cells, on the other hand, are oriented toward the body's own cells. They are focused upon internal cellular problems, toxin absorption, or those pathogens that have invaded cells.

There are different types of T-cells. Each is programmed in the thymus to look for a different type of problem, and each has the capability of destroying different types of cells and infections. Many T-cells simply respond to a pathogen that has invaded the cell by destroying the cell itself—this is the *killer* T-cell. It does this by inserting special chemicals into the cell or submitting instructions for the cell to kill itself. Cell death is called apoptosis, and T-cells capable of killing our cells are called cytotoxic T-cells and natural killer T-cells.

T-cells work through a communication system of cytokines to relay instructions and information amongst the various T-cells. Prominent cytokine communications thus take place between helper T-cells, natural killer cells and cytotoxic T-cells.

The initial scanning of an infected cell by a helper T-cell utilizes electromagnetic scanning just as the B-cells do. The T-cell's support network also includes delta-gamma T-cells. Delta-gamma T-cells are stimulated by specific molecular receptors on cell membranes. In general, helper T-cells communicate previous immune responses, memorize current ones, and pass on strategic information on the progress of pending attack plans.

The helper T-cell scan surveys the cell's membrane for indications of either microbial infection or some sort of genetic mutation due to a virus or toxin. This antigen scan might reveal invasions of chemical toxins, protozoa, worms, fungi, bacteria and viruses that have intruded or deranged the cell. The scanning helper T-cell immediately communicates the information by releasing their tiny coded protein cytokines. These disseminate the information needed to coordinate macrophages, NK-cells and cytotoxic T-cells for attack.

Most cells contain tumor necrosis factor or TNF—a sort of self-destruct switch. When signaled from the outside by a T-cell, TNF will initiate a self-destruct and the cell will die.

Under some circumstances, entire groups of cells or tissue systems may be damaged. Macrophages may be signalled to cut off the blood supply to kill these deranged or infected cells.

The two primary helper T-cell types are the Th1 and the Th2. The Th1 T-cell focuses on the elimination of bacteria, fungi, parasites, viruses, and similar types of invaders. The Th2 cells, on the other hand, are focused upon allergic and antibody responses. The Th2 is thus explicitly involved in the responses of inflammation and allergic reaction. This is important to note, because research has revealed that stress, chemical toxins, poor dietary habits and lack of sleep tend to suppress Th1 levels and increase Th2 levels. With an abundance of Th2 cells in the system, the body is prone to respond more strongly to allergens and toxins, causing problems like hay fever and allergies. This is why we sometimes see people who are under physical or emotional stress overreacting with hives, psoriasis and other allergic-type responses.

Neutrophils are white blood cells that circulate within the blood stream, looking for abnormal behavior among various cells and tissues. Once they identify a problem, they will signal a mass assembly and begin the process of cleaning the area. This typically involves inflammation, as they work to break down and remove debris.

Neutrophils are also coordinated by probiotics. Researchers from the Liver Failure Group and The Institute of Hepatology at the University College London's Medical School (Stadlbauer et al. 2008) found in a study of 20 liver failure patients that neutrophil function and cytokines were significantly modulated by the probiotic Lactobacillus casei Shirota. Starting neutrophil phagocytic capacity was significantly lower than healthy controls (73% versus 98%) before probiotic treatment. Neutrophil phagocytic capacity after probiotic treatments were equal between the cirrhosis patients and the healthy volunteers at the end of the study—while the placebo group's neutrophil capacity did not change. In addition, endotoxin-stimulated TNF-receptors 1 and 2 and interleukin-10 (IL-10) levels were significantly lower among the probiotic group. The scientists concluded: "Our data provide a proof-of-concept that probiotics restore neutrophil phagocytic capacity in cirrhosis, possibly by changing IL10 secretion and TLR4 expression."

Monocytes are like the neolithic ancestors of the attack soldiers. After being produced in the marrow, monocytes differentiate into either macrophages or dendrite cells. The macrophages are particularly good at engulfing and breaking apart pathogens. Dendritic cells are interactive cells that stimulate certain responses. They may, for example, isolate and present a pathogen to the T-cells. Dendritic cells also stimulate the production of those special inter-white blood cell communication proteins called cytokines.

Coordinating the Cleanse

As mentioned, cytokines are communication devices that allow different immune cells to communicate. These typically come with complex names like interleukin (IL), transforming growth factor (TGF), leukemia inhibitory factor (LIF), and tumor necrosis factor (TNF). There are five basic types of cell communication: intracrine, autocrine, endocrine, juxtacrine and paracrine.

Autocrine communication takes place between two different types of cells. This message can be a biochemical exchange or an electromagnetic signal. The other cell in turn may respond automatically by producing a particular biochemical or electromagnetic message. We might compare this to leaving a voicemail on someone's message machine. Once we leave the message, the machine signals that the message has been received and will be delivered. Later the machine will replay the message. The immune system uses this type of autocrine message recording process to activate T-cells. Once the message is relayed, the T-cell will respond specifically with the instructed activity.

A paracrine communication takes place between neighboring cells of the same type, to pass on a message that comes from outside of the tissue system. Tiny protein antennas will sit on cell membranes, allowing one cell to communicate with another. This allows cells within the same tissue system to respond in a coordinated manner.

Juxtacrine communications take place via smart biomolecular structures. We might call these structures relay stations. They absorb messages and pass them on. An example of this is the passing of inflammatory messages via immune cell cytokines.

An intracrine communication takes place within the cell. First, an external message may be communicated into the cell through an antenna sitting on the cell's membrane. Once inside the cell, the message will be communicated around cell's organelles to initiate internal metabolic responses.

The endocrine message takes place between endocrine glands and individual cells. The endocrine glands include the pineal gland, the pituitary gland, the pancreas, adrenals, thyroid, ovary and testes. These glands produce endocrine biochemicals, which relay messages directly to cells. Their messages stimulate a variety of metabolic functions within the body. These include growth, temperature, sexual behavior, sleep, glucose utilization, stress response and so many others. One of the functions of the endocrine glands relevant to disease is the production of inflammatory co-factors such as cortisol, adrenaline and norepinephrine. These coordinate and initiate instructions that stimulate inflammatory processes.

Probiotics utilize these systems to communicate with the body's various cells. They utilize paracrine and juxtacrine communications to pass on messages about the location, type and weaknesses of invading organisms. These messages are then compared with the programmed history within helper T-cells and helper B-cells. This creates a coordinated response. For example, the immune system might launch phagocytic cells to help attack the pathogens a probiotic colony may be battling.

Scientists from the Nagoya University Graduate School of Medicine's Department of Surgery (Sugawara et al. 2006) found in a study of 101 patients that supplementation with probiotics increased NK activity and lymphocyte counts. Pro-inflammatory IL-6 cytokines decreased significantly among the probiotic group. Serum IL-6, white blood cell counts, and C-reactive protein also significantly decreased among the probiotic group.

Furthermore, probiotics have the ability to *uniquely modify* cytokines depending upon the condition and disease of the person. Illustrating this, a probiotic drink with either placebo or a probiotic combination of *Lactobacillus paracasei* Lpc-37, *Lactobacillus acidophilus* 74-2 and *Bifidobacterium animalis* subsp. *lactis* DGCC 420 (*B. lactis* 420) was given to 15 healthy adults and 15 adults with atopic dermatitis. After 8 weeks, CD57(+) cytokines levels increased significantly among the healthy group taking probiotics, while CD4(+)CD54(+) cytokines decreased significantly among the AD patients who were taking the probiotics, compared with the placebo group and compared to the levels at the beginning of the trial (Roessler *et al.* 2008).

Attaching Toxins

Immunoglobulins are proteins that are programmed for a particular type of response in the presence of particular pathogens in different areas and maturity. IgA immunoglobulins line the mouth and digestive tract, scanning for pathogens that might infect the body. IgDs sense infections and activate B-cells. IgEs attach to foreign substances and launch histamine responses—typically associated with allergic responses. IgGs cross through membranes, responding to growing pathogens that have already invaded the body. IgMs are focused on new intrusions that have yet to grow enough to garner the attention of the IgGs.

Each of these general immunoglobulin categories contain numerous subtypes geared to different types of pathogens and responses. Other immunoglobulin proteins also exist. Some of these aid macrophages and lymphocytes in identifying specific pathogens.

An element of immunoglobulins is the CD glycogen-protein complex. CD stands for cluster of differentiation. CDs are molecules that sit on top of immune cells to navigate and steer their behavior. They will sit atop T-cells, B-cells, NK-cells, granulocytes and monocytes, identifying pathogens and infected cells. They often negotiate and bind to pathogens. This allows the lymphocyte to proceed to attack the pathogen, often by inserting a toxic chemical that destroys the pathogen or the cell hosting it.

CDs are identified by their molecular structure: This is also referred to as a ligand. The specific molecular arrangement (or CD number) will also match a specific type of receptor at the membrane of the cell or pathogen. Each CD number will produce a bonding relationship with a certain receptor structure on the cell to allow the accompanying immunoglobulin or lymphocyte to have interactivity with the pathogen. This gives the immunoglobulin or lymphocyte an access point from which to attack the pathogen.

Immunoglobulins and CDs are also tools probiotics utilize to define or influence appropriate responses for the immune system. Probiotics stimulate IgAs through CDs, for example, when they discover a pathogen has invaded parts of the body's entry passageways.

CDs are also utilized by our body's probiotics to define the cells and tissue systems that have been damaged by toxins, bacteria, or viruses. Probiotics will respond appropriately, signalling back and forth with the immune system. This signalling often stimulates particular inflammatory and injury-healing responses.

Illustrating this, Finnish scientists (Ouwehand *et al.* 2009) gave healthy elderly volunteers lactitol (a milk sugar) with *Lactobacillus acidophilus* or a placebo. The group given the probiotics showed a significant modification of pro-inflammatory IgA and PGE2 levels. The researchers also noticed that levels of bifidobacteria in the stool of the elderly subjects were similar to those of a young person—as usually bifidobacteria colonies are reduced among the elderly. They also observed improved spermidine levels—an enzyme involved in DNA synthesis. These improvements suggested increased mucosal and intestinal immunity and probiotic content among the probiotic group.

In a study of 105 pregnant women, University of Western Australia scientists (Prescott *et al.* 2008) found that *Lactobacillus rhamnosus* and *Bifidobacterium lactis* stimulated higher levels of cytokine IFN-gamma, higher levels of TGF-beta1, and higher levels of breast milk IgA. Plasma of their babies had lower CD14 levels, and greater CB IFN-gamma levels. These indicated improvements in immune response stimulated by the probiotics.

In another example, researchers from the Turku University Central Hospital in Finland (Rinne *et al.* 2005) gave 96 mothers either a placebo or *Lactobacillus rhamnosus* GG before delivery and continued the supplementation in their infants after delivery. At three months of age, immunoglobulin IgG-secreting cells among breastfed infants supplemented with probiotics were significantly higher than the breastfed infants who received the placebo. In addition, IgM-, IgA-, and IgG-secreting cell counts at 12 months were significantly higher among the breastfed infants who supplemented with probiotics, compared to breastfed infants receiving the placebo.

In yet another example, researchers from the Teikyo University School of Medicine in Japan (Araki *et al.* 1999) gave *Bifidobacterium breve* YIT4064 or placebo to 19 infants for 28 days. Rotavirus shedding in the feces of the probiotic group was significantly reduced compared to the placebo group. IgA levels also significantly changed among the probiotic group.

Inflammatory Toxin Removal

Most people think of inflammation as bad. Especially when they see that so many disease conditions involve inflammation. Rather, inflammation simply coordinates the various immune players into a frenzy of healing responses. Part of the response is to purge the area of toxins.

Our body's immune system launches inflammatory cells and factors that heal injury sites and prevent bleed-outs. This process is often stimulated by leukotrienes and prostaglandins.

Leukotrienes are molecules that identify problems and stimulate the immune system. They pinpoint and isolate areas of the body that require repair. Once they pinpoint the site of repair, one type of leukotriene will initiate inflammation, and others will assist in maintaining the process. Once the repair process proceeds to a point of maturity, another type of leukotriene will begin slowing down the process of inflammation.

This smart signalling process takes place through the biochemical bonding formations of these molecules. Leukotrienes are paracrines and autocrines. They are paracrine in that they initiate messages that travel from one cell to another. They are autocrine in that they initiate messages that encourage an automatic and immediate response—notably among T-cells, engaging them to remove bad cells. They also help transmit messages that initiate the process of repair through the clotting of blood and the patching of damaged tissues.

Leukotrienes are produced from the conversion of essential fatty acids (EFAs) by an enzyme produced by the body called arachidonate-5-lipoxygenase (sometimes called LOX). The central fatty acids of this process are arachidonic acid (AA), gamma-linolenic acid (GLA), and eicosapentaenoic acid (EPA). Lipoxygenase enzymes produce different types of leukotrienes, depending upon the initial fatty acid. The important point of this is that the leukotrienes produced by arachidonic acid stimulate inflammation, while the leukotrienes produced by EPA halt inflammation. The leukotrienes produced by GLA, on the other hand, block the conversion process of polyunsaturated fatty acids to arachidonic acid.

Prostaglandins are also produced through an enzyme conversion from fatty acids. Like leukotrienes, prostaglandins are messengers that transmit particular messages to immune cells. Their messaging is either paracrine or autocrine. Prostaglandins are critical parts of the process of injury repair. They also initiate a number of protective sequences in the body, including the transmission of pain and the clotting of blood.

Prostaglandins are produced by the oxidation of fatty acids by an enzyme produced in the body called cyclooxygenase—also called prostaglandin-endoperoxide synthase (PTGS) or COX. There are three types of COX, and each convert fatty acids to different types of prostaglandins. The central fatty acid that causes inflammation again is arachidonic acid. COX-1 converts AA to the PGE2 type of prostaglandin. COX-2, on the other hand, converts AA into the PGI2 type of prostaglandin.

The central messages that prostaglandins transmit depend upon the type of prostaglandin. Prostaglandin I2 (also PGI2) stimulates the widening of blood vessels and bronchial passages, and pain sensation within the nervous system. In other words, along with stimulating blood clotting, PGI2 signals a range of responses to assist the body's wound healing at the site of injury.

Prostaglandin E2, or PGE2, is altogether different from PGI2. PGE2 stimulates the secretion of mucus within the stomach, intestines, mouth and esophagus. It also decreases the production of gastric acid in the stomach. This combination of increasing mucus and lowering acid production keeps healthy stomach cells from being damaged by our gastric acids and the acidic content of our foods. This is one of the central reasons NSAID pharmaceuticals cause gastrointestinal problems: They interrupt the secretion of this protective mucus in the stomach.

This means that the COX-1 enzyme instigates the process of protecting the stomach, while the COX-2 enzyme instigates the process of inflammation and repair within the body. In the case of autoimmune disease, the COX-2 process often lies at the root of pain and swelling.

Cyclooxygenase also converts ALA/DHA and GLA to prostaglandins. Just as lipoxygenase converts ALA/DHA and GLA to anti-inflammation leukotrienes, the conversion of ALA/DHA and GLA by cyclooxygenase produces prostaglandins that either block the inflammatory process or reverse it. This means that a healthy diet with plenty of GLA and ALA/DHA fats will balance inflammation response. ALA is found in walnuts, soybeans, flax, canola, pumpkin seeds and chia seeds. The purest form of DHA is found in certain algae, and the body produces EPA from DHA. Fish and krill also get their DHA up the food chain from algae. GLA is found in borage, primrose oil and spirulina.

Probiotics are often involved in the production of intermediary fatty acids used for these LOX and COX conversions, producing anti-inflammatory effects. To illustrate this, scientists from the University of Helsinki (Kekkonen *et al.* 2008) measured lipids and inflammation markers before and after giving probiotic *Lactobacillus rhamnosus* GG to 26 healthy adults. After three weeks of probiotic supplementation, the subjects had decreased levels of intermediary inflammatory fatty acids such as lysophosphatidylcholines, sphingomyelins, and several glycerophosphatidylcholines. Probiotics also reduced inflammatory markers TNF-alpha and CRP in this study.

The arachidonic acid conversion process that produces prostaglandins also produces thromboxanes. Thromboxanes stimulate platelets in the blood to aggregate. They work in concert with platelet-activating factor or PAF. Together, these biomolecules drive the process of clotting the blood and restricting blood flow. This is good during injury healing, but the inflammatory process must also be slowed down as the injury heals.

Probiotics help modulate that process. In the research from Poland's Pomeranian Academy of Medicine (Naruszewicz *et al.* 2002) mentioned earlier, scientists found that giving *Lactobacillus plantarum* 299v to 36 volunteers resulted in a 37% decrease in inflammatory F2-isoprostanes. Isoprostanes are similar to prostaglandins, formed outside of the COX process.

The probiotic and immunoglobulin immune system work together to deter and kill particular invaders—hopefully before they gain access to the body's tissues. Should these defenses fail, they can stimulate the humoral immune system in a strategic attack that includes identifying antigens and recognizing their weaknesses. B-cells and probiotics coordinate through the stimulation of immunoglobulins and clusters of differentiation (CDs).

This progression also stimulates an activation of neutrophils, phagocytes, immunoglobulins, leukotrienes and prostaglandins. Should cells become infected, they will signal the immune system using paracrines located on their cell membranes. Once the intrusion and strategy is determined, B-cells will surround the pathogens while T-cells attack any infected cells. Natural killer T-cells may secrete chemicals into infected cells, initiating the death of the cell.

Leukotrienes immediately gather in the region of toxicity or infection, and signal to T-cells to coordinate efforts in the process of repair. Prostaglandins initiate the widening of blood vessels to bring more T-cells and other repair factors (such as plasminogen and fibrin) to the site. Histamine opens the blood vessel walls to allow all these healing agents access to the injury site to clean it up.

Prostaglandins also stimulate substance P within the nerve cells, initiating the sensation of pain. At the same time, thromboxanes, along with fibrin, drive the process of clotting and coagulation in the blood, while constricting certain blood vessels to decrease the risk of bleeding.

Depending upon the toxin or invader, the inflammation response will also accompany an H1-histamine response. As mentioned earlier, histamine is primarily produced by the mast cells, basophils and neutrophils after being stimulated by IgE antibodies. This opens blood vessels to tissues, which stimulates the processes of sneezing, watering of the eyes and coughing.

These measures, though sometimes considered irritating, are all stimulated in an effort to remove the toxin and prevent its re-entry into the body.

As histamine binds with receptors, one of the resulting physiological responses is alertness (also why antihistamines cause drowsiness). These are natural responses to help the body and mind remain vigilant in order to avoid further toxin intake.

At the height of the repair process, swelling, redness and pain are at their peak. The T-cells, macrophages, neutrophils, fibrin and plasmin all work together to purge the allergen from the body and repair the damage.

As macrophages continue the clean up, the other immune cells begin to retreat. Antioxidants like glutathione will attach to and transport the byproducts—broken down toxins and cell parts—out of the body. As this proceeds, prostaglandins, histamines and leukotrienes are signaled to reverse the inflammation and pain process.

One of the central features of the normalization process is the production of bradykinin. Bradykinin slows clotting and opens blood vessels, allowing the cleanup process to accelerate. A key signalling factor is the production of nitric oxide (NO). NO slows inflammation by promoting the detachment of lymphocytes to the site of infection or toxification, and reduces tissue swelling. NO also accelerates the clearing out of debris with its interaction with the superoxide anion. NO was originally described by researchers as endothelium-derived relaxing factor (or EDRF)—because of its role in relaxing blood vessel walls.

The body produces more nitric oxide in the presence of good nutrition and lower stress. Probiotics also play a big role in nitric oxide production in a healthy body. Lactobacilli such as *L. plantarum* have in fact been shown to remove the harmful nitrate molecule and use it to produce nitric oxide (Bengmark *et al.* 1998). This is beneficial to not only reducing inflammation: NO production also creates a balanced environment for increased tolerance.

Low nitric oxide levels also happen to be associated with a plethora of conditions, including diabetes, heart failure, high cholesterol, ulcerative colitis, premature aging, cancers and many others. Low or abnormal NO production is also seen among lifestyle factors such as smoking, obesity, and environmental air pollution.

In cases of toxicity from air pollutants, the cough reflex may be enlisted to help clear toxins. Irritated sites in the airways and lungs stimulate coughing, but this is also attenuated by a neural cough center located within the brainstem and within the cerebral cortex, where coughing is often initiated, suppressed or modified by consciousness. The cough reflex is, as put by Dr. John Christopher, *"a result of nature's effort to expectorate mucous from the lungs, after which breathing becomes easier."*

In other words, the stimulus for chronic coughing is the build-up of mucous in the airways. While incidental coughing might follow the inhalation of some smoke or other toxin, a chronic cough is stimulated by a build-up of thickened mucous in the airways.

And why is there this build up of mucous? Because the immune system is undergoing the inflammatory process by flushing out broken-down cells, broken down toxins, and even live infections. This thickened mucous is like the composition of flushed toilet water after a bowel movement: *it is full of crap.*

The Toxic Allergic Response

An overload of toxins and subsequent systemic inflammation can stimulate a state of hypersensitivity within the body. In this state, the body is on high alert. This makes the body respond out of proportion to the actual threat. In other words, the body overwhelmed with toxins will over-react, just as an overworked person might blow up at an innocent remark by a co-worker.

Let's review the various hypersensitivity responses and see how they are connected to toxicity.

Atopic Hypersensitivity

This response occurs when IgE antibodies bind to an allergen. Antigens include air pollutants, pollen, dust mite allergens, and dander. An allergen can also be any food the immune system has become sensitized to. When this binding between an antigen and IgE takes place, the bound IgE will set off the release of inflammatory mediators from white blood cells called mast cells, basophils and/or neutrophils. The mediators released by these immune cells include histamine, prostaglandins and leukotrienes. Depending upon the location and type of mast/basophil/neutrophil cells, these mediators can spark an inflammatory response within the airways, and/or other tissues, including the sinuses, skin, joints, intestines and elsewhere.

This response can be further broken down into two stages: sensitization and elicitation.

Sensitization: The allergen sensitization process takes place when a potential antigen happens to come into contact with a type of immune cell called a progenitor B-cell. As part of their immune system responsibilities, these B-cells will break apart the allergen proteins into smaller parts—often called *epitopes*. These will become attached to hystocompatibility complex class II complex molecules.

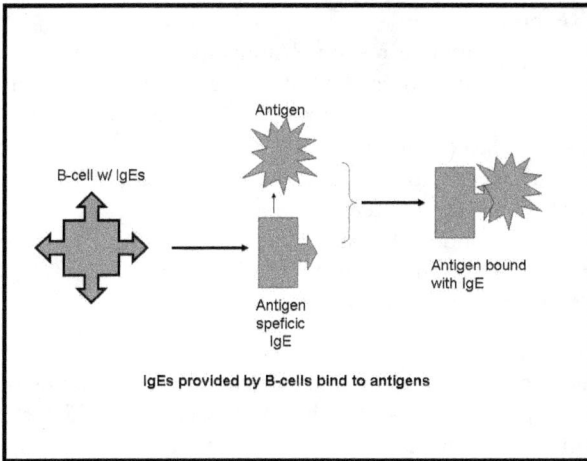

IgEs provided by B-cells bind to antigens

The T-cell hystocompatibility complex is transferred onto the surface of the B-cell, which binds to a particular allergen. Once upon the B-cell surface, T-helper cells take notice of this foreign particle stuck to the B-cell. The T-helper cell cytokine CD4 receptors trigger a response, and this stimulates the production of the IgE immunoglobulins. These particular IgE immunoglobulins are now sensitized to the particular epitope of the antigen in the future.

Elicitation: Once sensitized, the IgE associates with the specific IgE receptors that lie on the surface of the neutrophil, basophil or mast cells. Within these cells are packages called granules.

The granules are stock full of a variety of inflammatory mediators. The most notorious of these are the leukotrienes and histamines that are released into the bloodstream and lymph. These drive much of the symptoms of inflammation, including but not limited to hives, coughing, watery eyes, uritica, sinusitis and others.

The below diagram illustrates elicitation:

Cytotoxic Responses

In this type of immune response, antigens have penetrated the tissues, and the immune system is on a state of alert as it responds to kill these cells. This typically takes place through an antigen binding to IgG or IgM immunoglobulins in a delayed immune and inflammatory response. This response can happen concurrently to allergic responses; though it is most often a delayed response. This type of inflammatory response can last several days.

Should the red blood cells be involved in the antigen absorption, hemolysis (the destruction of red blood cells) and anemia (a lack of red blood cells) may result. These can in turn cause more inflammatory responses.

Systemic Inflammation Responses

Systemic and chronic inflammation creates hypersensitivity of the airway passages due to the immune system being stressed and on high alert status. In this situation, the immune system is overloaded by infection(s), chemical toxicity, or a diet that constantly exposes the body to toxins. One or a combination of these effects generally produces a whole-body diseased state. In such a state, the body will overreact to an exposure to stress in the airways. These triggers can be as simple as exercise, cold air, smoke or fragrance.

This type of systemic inflammatory status is evidenced by high C-reactive protein in the body. CRP levels are easily determined through blood analysis. We'll discuss some of the research that illustrates this later.

Immune Complex Responses

Here the allergen-bound antibody complex actually penetrates cell tissues and injures them. This can occur within the airway epithelial cells, intestinal cells, liver, or virtually anywhere around the body. Here the damage to the cells immediately stimulates the inflammatory response, regardless of whether there is an allergen trigger involved or not. Whatever is damaging the cells is considered a direct threat.

In some instances, these immune complexes can severely change alveoli permeability, vascular permeability and/or intestinal permeability, producing imbalances in respiration, circulation and digestion—sometimes even simultaneously.

This type of response is also often a delayed response, occurring hours or even a day or two after exposure to the toxin or allergen.

This alerted immune complex condition will also stimulate mast cells, basophils and/or neutrophils, resulting in continued degranulation of histamine, prostaglandins and leukotrienes, which in turn produce hypersensitivity to the foreigner.

Delayed T-Cell Responses

While the immune complex response may generate an immediate T-cell response once cells and tissues are damaged, a delayed T-cell response will occur over a period of time—as T-cells continue to destroy damaged airway cells. Here airway epithelial cells become damaged, and the T-cells are removing those damaged cells with an inflammatory response.

This type of response is the driving factor behind airway remodeling. In airway remodeling, the epithelial cell network that lines the airways become inflamed, damaged and chronically irritated. They are swollen and hyperreactive on an ongoing basis, in other words.

This same general condition can exist within the epithelial layers of many parts of the body. On the skin, this is seen as eczema. In the intestines, it is seen as colitis or Crohn's disease. In the sinuses, it is called sinusitis. In the urinary tract, it is called interstitial cystitis. In the stomach and lower esophagus, it is called GERD.

This response is also often attributed to autoimmunity, which is explained as the immune system attacking healthy cells. This notion is incorrect, however, because the immune system is not attacking healthy cells. The immune system is removing cells that have been damaged. Once these epithelial cells are damaged, T-cells stimulate the immune response to clear out the damaged cells. In other words, it is an inflammatory immune response to cellular and tissue toxicity.

The Thymus Gland: Programming the Warriors

One of the most important players in the body's purging of toxins is the thymus gland. The thymus gland is located in the center of the chest, behind the sternum. The thymus is one of the more critical organs of the lymphatic system. Some have compared the thymus gland of the lymphatic system to the heart of the circulatory system.

The thymus gland is not a pump, however. The thymus activates T-cells and various hormones that modulate and stimulate the immune and autoimmune processes. The thymus converts a type of lymphocyte called the thymocyte into T-cells or natural killer cells. These activated T-cells are released into the lymph and bloodstream ready to protect and serve. Within the thymus, the T-cells are infused with CD surface markers—which identify particular types of problematic cells or invading organisms. The CD markers define their mission.

In other words, the thymus codes the T-cells with receptors that will bind to particular toxins and the cells that have been invaded or damaged by toxins. The types of cells or toxins they bind to or identify are determined by the major histocompatibility complex, or MHC determinant. During the process of converting thymocytes to T-cells, their receptors are programmed with MHC combinations. This allows them to tolerate particular frailties within the body while attacking what the body considers to be true invaders (Kazansky 2008).

Therefore, it is the MHC that gives the T-cell the ability to identify the difference between *self* and *non-self* parts of the body. A non-self identification will produce an immunogen—a factor that stimulates an immune response. Once the immunogen is processed, it stimulates the inflammatory cascade.

The thymus gland develops and enlarges from birth. It is most productive and at its largest during puberty. From that point on, depending upon our diet, stress and lifestyle, our thymus gland will shrink over the years. By forty, an immunosuppressed person will often have a tiny thymus gland. In elderly persons, the thymus gland is often barely recognizable. For some, the thymus is practically non-functional.

Throughout its productive life, the thymus gland processes T-cells with the appropriate MHC programming. If the thymus gland is functioning, it will continue to produce T-cells with MHC programming that reflects the body's current status. The revised programming will accommodate the various genetic changes that can happen to different cells around the body as we age and adapt to our changing environment. With a shrunken and non-functioning thymus, however, its ability to re-program T-cells with a new MHC—enabling them to identify the body's cells that have adapted—is damaged. The T-cells will have to keep working off the old MHC programming. This means the T-cells will not be able to properly identify self versus non-self.

Herein we find at least part of the solution to the mystery of autoimmune disease.

Probiotics, on the other hand, stimulate a healthy thymus gland. Illustrating this, medical researchers from the University of Bari (Indrio *et al.* 2007) gave a placebo or a probiotic combination of *Bifidobacterium breve* C50 and *Streptococcus thermophilus* 065 to 60 newborns in a randomized, placebo-controlled study on thymus size. Thymus size was significantly larger in the probiotic group compared to the standard formula (placebo) group after the probiotic treatment period.

Liver: Filtering and Breaking Down Toxins

The liver is the body's most important detoxifying organ. The liver is a blood filtering mechanism, where it screens out many toxins. The liver also produces numerous enzymes and proteins that break down and otherwise metabolize toxins.

The liver sits just below the lungs on the right side under the diaphragm. Partially protected by the ribs, it attaches to the abdominal wall with the falciform ligament. The ligamentum teres within the falciform is the remnant of the umbilical cord that once brought us blood from mama's placenta. As the body develops, the liver continues to filter, purify and enrich our blood. Should the liver shut down, the body would die within hours.

Into the liver drains nutrition-rich venous blood through the hepatic portal vein together with some oxygenated blood through the hepatic artery. A healthy liver will process almost a half-gallon of blood per minute. The blood is commingled within well cavities called sinusoids, where blood is staged through stacked sheets of the liver's primary cells—called hepatocytes. Here blood is also met by interspersed immune cells called kupffers. These kupffer cells attack and break apart bacteria and toxins. Nutrients coming in from the digestive tract are filtered and converted to molecules the body's cells can utilize. The liver also converts old red blood cells to bilirubin to be shipped out of the body. Filtered and purified blood is jettisoned through hepatic veins out the inferior vena cava and back into circulation.

The liver's filtration/purification mechanisms protect our body from various infectious diseases and chemical toxins. After hepatocytes and kupffer cells break down toxins, the waste is disposed through the gall bladder and kidneys. The gall bladder channels bile from the liver to the intestines. Recycled bile acids combine with bilirubin, phospholipids, calcium and cholesterol to make bile. Bile is concentrated and pumped through the bile duct to the intestines. Here bile acids help digest fats, and broken down toxins are (hopefully) excreted through our feces. Assuming we have healthy probiotic colonies within the intestines.

The liver produces over a thousand biochemicals the body requires for healthy functioning. The liver maintains blood sugar balance by monitoring glucose levels and producing glucose metabolites. It manufactures albumin to maintain plasma pressure. It produces cholesterol, urea, inflammatory biochemicals, blood-clotting molecules, and many others.

Interspersed within the liver are functional fat factories called stellates. These cells store and process lipids, fat-soluble vitamins such as vitamin A, and secrete structural biomolecules like collagen, laminin and glycans. These are used to build some of the body's toughest tissue systems.

We know that our livers become burdened from the avalanche of toxins pelting our bodies. Today our diets, water and air are full of plasticizers, formaldehyde, heavy metals, hydrocarbons, DDT, dioxin, VOCs, asbestos, preservatives, artificial flavors, food dyes, propellants, synthetic fragrances and more. Every single chemical requires the liver to work harder.

Frankly, most livers are now overloaded and beyond their natural capacity. What happens then? Generally, two things. First, the hepatocytes collapse from overtoxification, causing genetic mutation, cell death, and liver exhaustion. Secondly, their weakened condition opens hepatocytes to diseases from infectious agents such as viral hepatitis.

Liver disease—where one or more lobes begin to malfunction—can result in a life-threatening emergency. Cirrhosis is a common diagnosis for liver disease, often caused by years of drinking alcohol or taking prescription medications. During its downfall into cirrhosis, the sub-functioning liver can also cause jaundice, high cholesterol, gallstones, encephalopathy, kidney disease, clotting problems, heart conditions, hormone imbalances and many others. As cirrhosis proceeds, it results in the liver cells' massive die-off and subsequent scarring, causing the liver to begin to shutdown.

While most of us have heard about the damage alcohol can have on the liver, many do not realize that pharmaceuticals and even some supplements can also be extremely toxic to the liver. The liver must find a way to break down these foreign chemicals. Many pharmaceuticals require a Herculean effort simply because the liver's various purification processes were not designed for these foreign molecules. As liver cells weaken and die their enzymes leak into the bloodstream. Blood tests for AST and ALT enzymes can reveal this weakening of the liver.

We must therefore closely monitor the quantity and types of chemicals we put into our body. Eliminating preservatives, food dyes and pesticides in our foods can be done easily by eating whole organic foods. We can eliminate exposures to many environmental toxins mentioned above by simply replacing them with natural alternatives.

A number of herbs help detoxify and strengthen the liver. These include goldenseal, dandelion, milk thistle and others.

Probiotics also play a large role in liver disease. When pathogenic bacteria get out of control in the intestines, they can overload the liver with endotoxins—their waste products. The bombardment of endotoxins onto the liver produces a result similar to alcohol or pharmaceuticals: When complex proteins (such as found in animal products) are putrefied by pathogenic bacteria, one of the metabolites is excessive ammonia. Ammonia is toxic to the liver.

In addition, urea is metabolized by pathogenic bacteria such as *Clostridium* spp., resulting in ammonia and carbon dioxide. Liver cells are damaged by this onslaught of endotoxins and metabolites produced by pathogenic bacteria.

In a study from scientists at the G.B. Pant Hospital in New Delhi (Sharma *et al.* 2008), 190 cirrhosis patients were given a combination of probiotics for one month. The probiotic group experienced a 51.6% improvement in symptoms, as measured by psychometric testing and blood ammonia levels.

Respiration: Purging Foreigners

Our lungs provide one of the body's most effective means of detoxification, as well as an active filtering mechanism that screens out toxins.

With every breath, we purge the body of toxins. The epithelial cells of our airways house sub-mucosal ducts that push toxins out to the mucous membranes. As we breathe out and as our mucous is channeled out, we send these toxins out.

In addition, the lungs filter and prevent the body from inheriting more toxins. As air moves through the nostrils through to the *pharynx*, the *larynx* and the *trachea*, it passes over a mucous membrane lined with tiny hairs called *cilia*. These cilia capture foreign particles with a web of sticky mucous. After being stuck, the particles are gathered up within the mucous. The tiny cilia hairs will undulate the mucous and foreign particles towards exit points like the throat, nostrils and mouth. At these points, the particles can be sneezed or coughed out as phlegm, blown out through the nose, or swallowed down into the acidic abyss of the stomach.

More offensive particles like bacteria and viruses are attacked by the macrophages and probiotics that line the mucous membranes. They break down the foreigners and escort their parts out of the body. These may travel out with the mucous, or be absorbed into the lymph or blood and pushed out through urine, sweat or the colon.

About 97% of our incoming oxygen is delivered to the cells by hemoglobin molecules. After being escorted through the micro-capillaries to the cells, the oxygen disassociates from the hemoglobin. Only about 20% of oxygen disassociates from hemoglobin while we rest. More disassociates as needed. The rest stays in the bloodstream, on standby. This standby oxygen effectively alkalizes the blood, inhibiting oxidative radicals with the presence of O_2.

Cellular respiration proceeds in a process called *oxidative phosphorylation*. Here the two-phosphate ADP combines with oxygen and another phosphate atom to form a triple phosphate (ATP) structure. The resulting electromagnetic energy produced is held within the phosphate-oxygen bond. Once in ATP form, glucose interacts with one of the phosphates to release ADP, glucose 6-p along with heat and energy for metabolism. The process releases energy as the phosphoryl is transferred, producing a cyclic process of exchange between ADP (adenosine diphosphate) and ATP (adenosine triphosphate), which utilizes oxygen to feed the process.

The Krebs ATP/ADP cycle process releases kinetic energy and heat, along with carbon dioxide and other important byproducts such as cyclic AMP (which helps regulate the cell membrane). As carbon dioxide is released, the CO_2 combines with water to form carbonic acid. Carbonic acid releases hydrogen acid (H+) and blood bicarbonate (HCO_3) into the bloodstream. This creates an acidic environment, which means there are more H+ ions.

The freed H+ ions will then combine with dissociated hemoglobin. As this H+ rich hemoglobin and bicarbonate blood reach the alveoli capillaries, hemoglobin releases the H+, which reforms carbon dioxide (CO_2) as it reacts with the bicarbonate. Hemoglobin is then ready for another oxygen molecule and the CO_2 is ready to diffuse back through to the alveoli and out through the lungs to the atmosphere.

Should there not be enough oxygen available for the cell's energy needs; the cells will produce energy without the use of oxygen. This process has about 5% of the efficiency of aerobic respiration, however. This is called *anaerobic glycolysis*, and NAD+ and NADH become the vehicles for energy exchange instead of ATP and ADP.

During heavy exercise or breathing deficiencies, the blood will become laced with heavier doses of carbonic acid and carbonates, acidified with H+ hemoglobin. This acidic situation can become toxic to the tissue systems if it remains too long without clearance.

This lack of oxygen also increases anaerobic glycolysis. The problem with anaerobic glycolysis is that instead of easily-exchanged byproducts like carbon dioxide, glycolysis produces acidic lactates and other radicals that can buildup in the bloodstream. They are also difficult to clear. Muscle fatigue is often attributed to lactic acid buildup in the bloodstream and muscle tissues. But it is the significant acids (H+) produced by anaerobic glycolysis—creating acidosis—that produces muscle soreness. Thus, the faster we can alkalize the blood and tissues, the faster our muscle recovery will be.

Should exhalation not be able to deplete this acidic environment in the blood, one of the first locations of damage will be to the walls of the blood vessels and alveoli. The acidic radicals look for stability as they borrow atomic elements from the molecules making up these tissues. This leaves these tissues damaged and in need of repair.

This later process of energy production in the absence of oxygen (oxygen debt) produces many more acids than does the Krebs cycle. The result is a bloodstream subject to acidosis, which corresponds to overexertion.

The bottom line is that better and more complete breathing helps detoxify the bloodstream and keep the blood in more of a radical-free alkaline state.

The Respiratory Cilia

The bronchial epithelial cells of the airway passages are also equipped with microscopic hairs called cilia (see previous and next drawing). The cilia act like tiny brooms: They undulate towards the exits—the sinuses, mouth and pharynx. The little hairs "sweep" out the mucous, together with toxins and dead cell parts caught in the mucous membrane.

The ciliary hairs lining the airways beat rhythmically with the expansion and release of the lungs. This expansion and contraction increases the mucous surfactant as well.

Should toxin particles remain airborne, they will also likely be moved out through breathing and rhythmic ciliary hair undulations in healthy airways.

The membrane and ciliary hair move in slow waves—very similar to what we see among kelp beds as they move with undulating ocean waves. This wave-like action of the ciliary hairs acts as an effective transport system.

This transport mechanism—the clearing of toxins and cell parts out of the area by the cilia—is called the *mucociliary clearance apparatus*. This is a self-cleaning system of the airways: Should these 'automatic sweepers' become caught in the thick mucous of a toxin-rich and/or ionically imbalanced mucous membrane—they become ineffective.

The mucociliary clearance apparatus explains how we will gather an accumulation of phlegm within the throat and sinuses. Most of us clear our throats or blow our noses without a second thought. Little do we realize that much of that phlegm is the result of the cilias' self-cleaning undulations that sweep out toxins and mucous. This sweeping mechanism also helps prevent polluted air and particles from being absorbed into our blood. Those particles not tossed out with the breath or mucous get phagotized (broken down) and swept out. Or they may be transported to the blood or lymph and escorted out of the body through the colon, urinary tract or sweat glands.

However, should the mucosal fluid not be healthy and ionically balanced, thickened mucous will build up within the mucosal membrane. This will overwhelm and in effect *drown* the ciliary hairs—making them far less effective for removing toxins and toxin-rich mucous.

The cilia are stabilized by being seated in a thin pool of thicker mucous, with another layer of thinner mucous on top. The thinner mucous towards the surface of the mucous membrane allows the hairs to undulate faster near and at the surface of the mucous membrane.

It is essential that these cilia are healthy, vibrant, and free of toxin-debris. This is why, as we'll explain, that tar and soot from smoking and pollution can wreck such havoc on the lungs. The tops of the cilia—and mucous— become jammed up in this gummy residue.

Cilia must also have a warm temperature in a moist atmosphere. Should cold, dry air get into the passages where these sensitive airway cilia dwell, they may shut down or become uncoordinated. The ultimate temperature for productive cilia is about 98.6 degrees F with 100% relative humidity. This doesn't mean that outdoor temperatures must be that. A temperature of nearly 100 degrees F with 100% humidity would be practically unbearable.

Rather, the cilia are kept warm and moist by the combination of body heat, the warming of the air as it travels through the sinus turbinates, and the secretion of warm mucous in the airways.

Inflammation also involves reactive oxygen species. Indications of this during systemic inflammation include higher levels of superoxide anions and thiobarbituric acid-reactive products (TBARs), as well as hydrogen peroxide. This is because one of the main inflammatory byproducts of superoxide reactions is hydrogen peroxide (H_2O_2).

Research has illustrated that those with inflammatory conditions generate more hydrogen peroxide when they breathe out than normal people. In one study, asthmatics breathed out 26 times the levels of hydrogen peroxide as healthy subjects did. They also found that TBAR levels among asthmatics were 18 times the levels of healthy subjects (Antczak *et al.* 1997).

Inflammatory eosinophils—evidenced by higher eosinophil cationic protein (ECP) levels—are also significantly higher in inflammatory conditions. ECP can damage microorganisms such as viruses and bacteria, along with our body's cells. ECP damages cells by forming pores in the cell membranes, which produce a type of cell membrane damage called *permeability alteration.*

Research has indicated that ECP builds up in the airways and epithelial tissues in an inflammatory condition. While ECP is a defense measure in the case of infection, an overload of ECP damages the epithelial cells.

The build-up of ECP is simply part of an inflammatory process that occurs as part of an immune response: A deranged immune response that medical researchers call hyperreactivity.

Mucosal Membranes: Preventing Toxin Incursion

Mucous membranes cover just about every region of epithelial cells, including our skin, nose, throat, mouth, airways, digestive tract, urinary tract, vagina and other surfaces. Some surfaces, such as the skin, have very thin mucosal membranes. Other surfaces, such as the digestive tract and airways, have thick mucosal membranes.

The mucosal membrane is a thin layer of glycoproteins (mucin), mucopolysaccharides, special enzymes, probiotics, immune cells and ionic fluid. The ionic fluid provides a transporter medium, which escorts a host of elements back and forth between the epithelial cells and the surface of the mucosal membrane. These elements include chloride ions, sodium ions, oxygen, nitrogen, carbon dioxide, hydrogen carbonate and others.

Some of these—such as the sodium, bicarbonate and chloride ions—provide the transport mechanisms into the cells and tissues of the skin surfaces. These travel through openings or pores among the cells, attached to nutrients, oxygen and other elements—transporting them in, in other words.

Certainly, the body is choosy about what kinds of elements it will allow into the epithelial cells and tissues. There are countless toxins, microorganisms, debris allergens and other foreigners that the body wants kept out.

We might compare this to how oil lubricates and protects an engine from overheating and dirt. In a well-maintained car, good motor oil will be circulated through the rods and cylinders. The oil doesn't just allow the steel parts to move with minimal friction: The motor oil also helps keep the engine clean, and prevents dirt and other contaminants from clogging up the system. Imagine what would happen if a car were to run without oil for a few miles? The engine would surely seize up, and likely would break down completely. While this is a crude example, there are several elements that are consistent.

So just how does the body keep these invaders from penetrating the body's internal and external surfaces? The short answer is the mucosal membranes. This is why these membranes contain a host of immune cells. These include immunoglobulins such as IgA, B-cells, T-cells and others that are looking to trap foreigners before get any further. Once they find a foreigner, they will take it apart using a one of many immune system strategies.

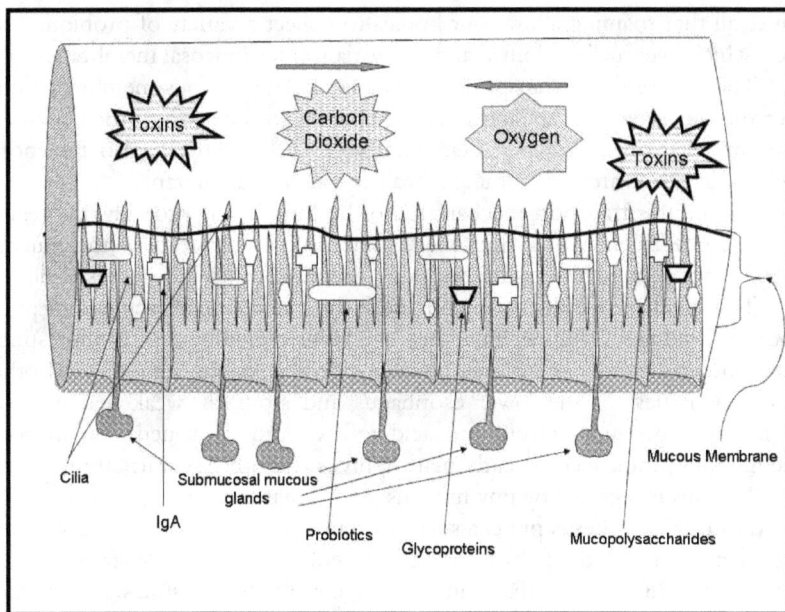

Airway Mucosal Membranes and Cilia

The mucous membranes are living structures. Probiotics populate our mucosal membranes, and are an important part of the "wall" of protection provided by these membranes. Tiny protective probiotic bacteria will inhabit all healthy mucosal membranes, including the skin. Like the immune system, these bacteria are trained to protect their territory. If an invading microorganism enters the mucosal membrane, the probiotics will lead an attack on them, with the immune cells in close pursuit.

The chemistry of the mucosal membrane also buffers and calms immune response. The mucosal membrane will help transport components such as corticosteroids from the adrenals to squelch inflammatory immune responses among our epithelial tissues. In other words, a healthy mucosal membrane is *calming* to our digestive tract, airways, skin and so on.

Other than our skin, which has been covered by placenta fluid, our mucosal membranes are raw and not well developed at birth. Gradually, as probiotics begin to colonize the sinuses, mouth and intestines—the mucosal membranes begin to mature. This maturity, as we'll discuss in detail, requires a host of nutrients as well as strong probiotic populations in order to populate the mucosal membranes. As this colonization occurs, the body's epithelial cells and mucous glands provide their balance of chemistry and protective attributes.

This is the basis for the hygiene theory, a product of many studies showing that infants and children that are allowed to roam the floors, parks, soils, and those among larger families have stronger immune systems. This is because all that roaming allows our bodies to collect a variety of probiotic species, which eventually colonize and territorialize our mucosal membranes.

Then there is the transporter mechanism. The mucous membranes utilizes this surfactant quality and ionic capabilities to transport nutrients among the epithelial cells, allowing them to function efficiently. It also transports toxins out of the area—assuming a healthy mucosal membrane.

Should this transport mechanism not be functioning properly, the region can become laden with a thickened, toxic mucous. Instead of the mucous membranes keeping these surfaces clean, the mucous itself becomes toxic.

This thickened mucous membrane is typical in hyperreactive airway responses among COPD, asthma, and hay fever conditions. In the intestines, the condition produces irritable bowel syndrome, colitis, Crohn's and other intestinal issues. In the lower esophagus and stomach, weakened mucosal membranes produces ulcers and acid reflux. And weakened skin mucosal membranes produce eczema, dermatitis, hives and other skin irritations.

Mucous is secreted by tiny mucous glands that lie within goblet cells scattered throughout these epithelia surfaces. They are called goblets because they are shaped like little goblet glasses, except their upper surface extends through the (internal) surfaces in tiny fingers. In the intestines and airways, they are called microvilli. On skin and other surfaces, they are become pores. They function almost identically with respect to their production of mucous.

The goblet cells and their end points both produce mucin through a process of contraction and glycosylation within the Golgi apparatus of the cells. This glycosylation of proteins produces the glycoproteins that are the mainstay in mucin.

The mucosal goblet cells of the respiratory tract are also similar to the gastric cells of the stomach and duodenum. The difference here is that these produce mucous fed by the pyloric glands in addition to the highly acidic gastrin. As we'll be discussing more at length throughout the remainder of the text, this similarity between the goblet cells, the villi and the gastric/pyloric cells facilitates an understanding of the mystery of GERD-related respiratory disorders.

The mucous membrane fluids can also become dehydrated if the ions that open the pores are blocked. Here the pores may be blocked due to an imbalance of ion chemistry in the sub-mucosal membrane. Tests have shown that chlorine and bicarbonate anions stimulate the opening of the pores that bring liquids into the mucous membrane. The mucin proteins produced by the submucosal membrane glands have to be diluted with these ion fluids to give the mucous membrane the right balance of stickiness and fluidity.

Among dehydrated mucosal membranes, the mucous is thickened and not fluid enough to provide its surfactant and transport functions.

In addition, exposure to toxins, pathogenic microorganisms, cold air and any number of other triggers can stimulate the production of mucous by the goblet cells. In a healthy body, this stimulates the quick removal of the toxin or invader, as the excess mucous is swept out by the cilia or other drainage facilities of the surface.

However, should the body be immunosuppressed or otherwise over-whelmed by the invasion, the goblet cells will over-produce mucous, which can swamp the epithelial surfaces with dead cell parts and toxins. When these surfaces are drowning in mucous, the removal process is deficient. The lack of mucous transport, combined with the need to remove toxins, produces inflammation as the immune system must engage to remove the toxins.

The Adrenals: The Moderators

The body's two adrenal glands are part of our endocrine system. The outer cortex is stimulated by master hormones from the hypothalamus and pituitary gland, while the inner medulla is stimulated directly with nerves. The adrenals produce an array of hormones, many of which are related to in-flammation and/or stress.

For example, the medulla produces epinephrine and norepinephrine, and other catecholamines. Epinephrine (as well as norepinephrine) relaxes the smooth muscles of the airways and constricts the blood vessels, increases the heart rate, increases metabolism, dilates the pupils and halts digestive activity, all in an effort to reduce inflammation and respond to inflammation and stress.

This multi-organ adrenal response might seem beneficial, but it also comes with a double-edged sword: Epinephrine and norepinephrine also significantly slow the rate of mucous secretion by submucosal glands that feed the mucous membranes.

This effect can be quite dangerous to the highly-stressed individual, be-cause the decreased mucous membranes also leave our lungs and digestive tracts open to irritation from toxins and environmental changes.

The adrenal glands also produce important steroids. Two of the most critical are cortisol and aldosterone.

Aldosterone is a mineralocorticoid. It and other mineralocorticoids are produced by the outer shell, or cortex, of the adrenal gland. Aldosterone and other mineralocorticoids adjust and balance the body's levels of sodium, potassium and other minerals; as well as alter sodium ion channels among various cells. These are critical to the acid/alkaline status of the blood and body fluids, and the body's ability to remove toxins through the kidneys, sweat glands and colon. Aldosterone is a critical player in maintaining blood pressure as well, and this affects the performance of respiration.

Aldosterone also balances the use and availability of cortisol and corti-sone, because many aldosterone receptors also bind with cortisol. This means that a balanced production of these two steroids (cortisol is a glucocorticoid) by the adrenals is critical to the detoxification efforts of the body—along with the body's ability to balance inflammation with efforts to heal the body.

This means that adrenal glands stimulated by stress and inflammation repeatedly for long periods begin to wear down. As mentioned earlier, this is called adrenal exhaustion. When this happens, the adrenal glands produce inconsistently deficient levels of theses critical steroids and catecholamines.

This creates drastic imbalances within the body, affecting the body's ability to respond to toxins, inflammation and stress. Signs of adrenal exhaustion include being easily fatigued, overstressed and over-reactive to toxins and environmental changes. Adrenal exhaustion is typical in an immune system over-responding with hyper-inflammation.

The Intestines: Sorting Toxins and Nutrients

What do the intestines have to do with cleansing and toxicity? Plenty.

This relates to the fact that the digestive tract protects against the penetration of toxins into our bloodstreams and tissues. When intestinal villi and their junctions are damaged, endotoxins (the poop and byproducts of pathogenic bacteria) and other toxins can get into the bloodstream—overloading the immune system and producing systemic inflammation.

The intestines utilize non-specific, humoral, cell-mediated and probiotic immunity to protect intestinal tissues from larger peptides, toxins and invading microorganisms.

This is all packaged nicely into what is referred to as the *intestinal brush barrier*. The intestinal brush barrier is a complex mucosal layer of mucin, enzymes, probiotics and ionic fluid—sealed by villi separated by tight junctions.

The intestinal mucosal membrane forms a protective surface medium over the intestinal epithelium. It also provides an active nutrient transport mechanism for nutrients and toxins. This mucosal layer is stabilized by the grooves of the intestinal microvilli. It contains glycoproteins, mucopolysaccharides and other ionic transporters, which attach to amino acids, minerals, vitamins, glucose and fatty acids—carrying them across intestinal membranes.

This mucosal layer is policed by billions of probiotic colonies, which help process and identify incoming food molecules; excrete various nutrients; and control toxins and pathogens.

The Healthy Intestinal Wall

The breakdown of the mucosal membrane causes it to thin. This depletes the protection rendered by the mucopolysaccharides and glycoproteins, probiotics, immune IgA cells, enzymes and bile. This thinning allows toxins and macromolecules that would have been screened out by the mucosal membrane to be presented to the intestinal cells.

In its entirety, the brush barrier is a triple-filter that screens for molecule size, ionic nature and nutrition quality. Much of this is performed via four screening mechanisms existing between the intestinal microvilli: tight junctions, adherens junctions, desmosomes, and colonies of probiotics. The tight functions form a bilayer interface between cells, controlling permeability. Desmosomes are points of interface between the tight junctions, and adherens junctions keep the cell membranes adhesive enough to stabilize the junctions. These junction mechanisms together regulate permeability at the intestinal wall.

This mucosal brush barrier creates the boundary between intestinal contents and our bloodstream. Should the mucosal layer chemistry become altered, its protective and ionic transport mechanisms become weakened, allowing toxic or larger molecules to be presented to the microvilli junctions. This contact can irritate the microvilli, causing a subsequent inflammatory response. Research illustrates that this is a contributing cause of irritable bowel syndrome (IBS).

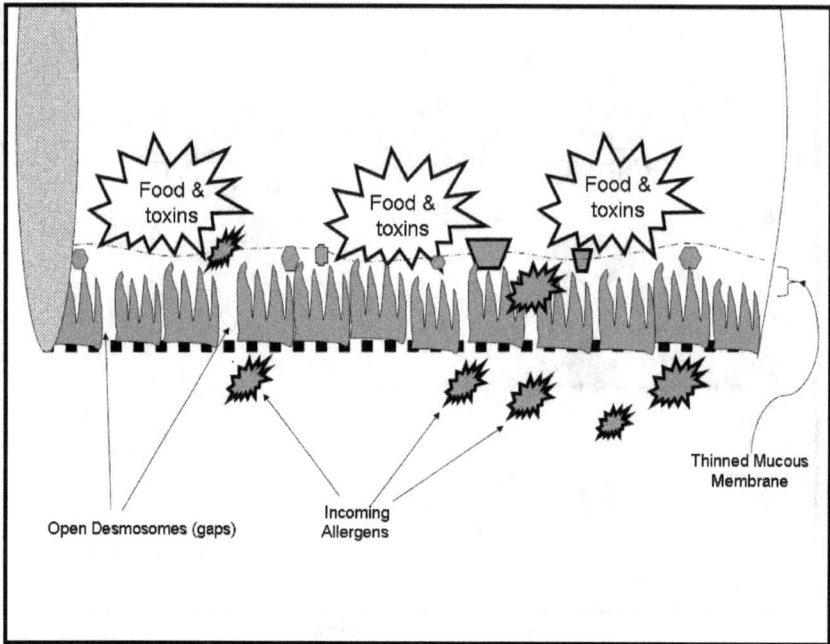

The Unhealthy Intestinal Wall

Should the mucous membrane thin, these mechanisms become irritated, producing an inflammatory immune response that causes the desmosomes and tight junctions to open. These gaps allow toxins and food macromolecules to enter the blood, where they can become allergens and contribute to systemic inflammation. Scientists call this condition *increased intestinal permeability*.

The Intestinal Permeability Index

How do scientists and physicians test for increased intestinal permeability? Intestinal permeability is typically measured by giving the patient indigestible substances with different molecular sizes. Urine samples then show relative levels of these, illustrating degrees of intestinal permeability. For example, alcohol-sugar combinations such as lactulose and mannitol are often used. These indicate intestinal permeability because of their different molecular sizes. A few (typically 5-6) hours after ingestion, the patient's urine is tested to measure the quantities of these two molecules in the urine.

Because lactulose is a larger molecule than mannitol, greater permeability will be indicated by high lactulose levels in the urine relative to mannitol levels. Intestines with normal permeability will have little lactulose absorption.

These relative levels create a ratio between lactulose and mannitol, which scientists call the L/M ratio. This L/M ratio is used to quantify intestinal permeability. When the lactulose-to-mannitol ratio is higher, more permeability exists. When it is lower, less (more normal) intestinal permeability exists. Higher levels are compared using what many researchers call the *Intestinal Permeability Index.*

Other large molecule substances are also sometimes used to detect intestinal permeability using the same protocol of measuring recovery in the urine over a period of time. These other substances include polyethylene glycols of various molecular weights, horseradish peroxidase, EDTA (ethylenediamine-tetraacetic acid), CrEDTA, rhamnose, lactulose, and cellobiose. Because these substances are not readily metabolized in the intestine or blood, and have large molecular sizes, they can also give accurate readings on the relative intestinal permeability.

The Probiotics: Guarding their Territory

Yes, we did discuss probiotics earlier. But this section is to emphasize the critical role that probiotics play in the process of protection against toxins and toxin removal. They temper and balance the immune system, reducing hypersensitivity responses.

Probiotics increase IgA levels and reduce IgE allergic response. As we discussed earlier, IgA blocks toxins before they can enter the tissues and bloodstream.

Illustrating this, Finnish scientists (Ouwehand *et al.* 2009) gave healthy elderly volunteers *Lactobacillus acidophilus* or a placebo. The probiotics modulated IgA and PGE2 levels. The probiotics also improved spermidine levels— an enzyme involved in DNA synthesis. The researchers concluded that these improvements suggested increased mucosal and intestinal immunity among the probiotic group.

In a study of 105 pregnant women, University of Western Australia scientists (Prescott *et al.* 2008) found that *Lactobacillus rhamnosus* and *Bifidobacterium lactis* stimulated higher levels of cytokine IFN-gamma, higher levels of TGF-beta1, and higher levels of breast milk IgA. Plasma of their babies had lower CD14 levels, and greater CB IFN-gamma levels. These indicated that the probiotics strengthened immunity and moderated hypersensitivity.

Researchers from the Teikyo University School of Medicine in Japan (Araki *et al.* 1999) gave *Bifidobacterium breve* YIT4064 or placebo to 19 infants for 28 days. IgA levels significantly increased among the probiotic group.

Researchers from the Turku University Central Hospital in Finland (Rinne *et al.* 2005) gave 96 mothers either a placebo or *Lactobacillus rhamnosus* GG before delivery and continued the supplementation in their infants after delivery. At three months of age, immunoglobulin IgG-secreting cells among breastfed infants supplemented with probiotics were significantly higher than the breastfed infants who received the placebo. In addition, the non-hypersensitivity IgM-, IgA-, and IgG-secreting cell counts at 12 months were significantly higher among the breastfed infants who supplemented with probiotics, compared to the breastfed infants receiving the placebo.

Probiotics help modulate the inflammatory processes. In research from Poland's Pomeranian Academy of Medicine (Naruszewicz *et al.* 2002), scientists found that giving *Lactobacillus plantarum* 299v to 36 volunteers resulted in a 37% decrease in inflammatory F2-isoprostanes. Isoprostanes are similar to prostaglandins, formed outside of the COX process.

Probiotics also stimulate a healthy thymus gland. Illustrating this, medical researchers from the University of Bari (Indrio *et al.* 2007) gave a placebo or a probiotic combination of *Bifidobacterium breve* C50 and *Streptococcus thermophilus* 065 to 60 newborns. The thymus glands of the probiotic group were significantly larger compared to babies who consumed the standard (placebo) formula.

Scientists from the Nagoya University Graduate School of Medicine (Sugawara *et al.* 2006) found in a study of 101 patients that supplementation with probiotics increased NK activity and lymphocyte counts. Pro-inflammatory IL-6 cytokines also decreased significantly among the probiotic group. Serum IL-6, white blood cell counts, and C-reactive protein also significantly decreased among the probiotic group.

Furthermore, probiotics have the ability to *uniquely* modify cytokines— relative to the condition of the person. Illustrating this, a probiotic drink with either placebo or a probiotic combination of *Lactobacillus paracasei* Lpc-37, *Lactobacillus acidophilus* 74-2 and *Bifidobacterium animalis* subsp. *lactis* DGCC 420 (*B. lactis* 420) was given to 15 healthy adults and 15 adults with atopic dermatitis. After eight weeks, CD57(+) cytokines levels increased significantly among the healthy group taking probiotics, while CD4(+)CD54(+) cytokines decreased significantly among the atopic patients taking the probiotics (Roessler *et al.* 2008).

Researchers from Poland's Pomeranian Academy of Medicine (Naruszewicz *et al.* 2002) gave *Lactobacillus plantarum* 299v or placebo to 36 healthy volunteers for six weeks. Monocytes isolated from probiotic subjects had significantly reduced adhesion to endothelial cells, and the probiotic group had a 42% reduction in pro-inflammatory cytokine interleukin-6. No changes were observed among the placebo group.

Probiotics are often involved in the production of critical intermediary fatty acids used in LOX and COX enzyme conversions, producing anti-inflammatory effects. To illustrate this, scientists from the University of Helsinki (Kekkonen *et al.* 2008) measured lipids and inflammation markers before and after giving probiotic *Lactobacillus rhamnosus* GG to 26 healthy adults. After three weeks of probiotic supplementation, the subjects had decreased levels of intermediary inflammatory fatty acids such as lysophosphatidylcholines, sphingomyelins, and several glycerophosphatidylcholines. Probiotics also reduced hyper-inflammatory markers TNF-alpha and CRP in this study.

Within the intestines, probiotics attach to and dwell in between the villi and microvilli. This allows them to not only keep pathogenic bacteria from infecting those cells: It also allows them to monitor food molecule size of nutrients being presented to the intestinal wall for absorption. This helps prevent the body from absorbing molecules that are too large or not sufficiently broken down. As we will discuss further, large, atypical molecules that have entered the bloodstream will stimulate an inflammatory and allergic response. This is because these larger molecules are not recognized by the immune system.

Oral probiotics will vigorously defend the areas around the gums and teeth. The problem arises when our diets become overly sugary. As we will discuss later in more detail, probiotics require complex oligosaccharides like inulin, FOS (fructooligosaccharides) and GOS (galactooligosaccharides) for food sources. They do not thrive from simple sugars like glucose and sucrose. Pathogenic bacteria, on the other hand, typically thrive from these simple sugars. In fact, they can grow quite quickly, and may immediately begin to outnumber the probiotic populations, causing caries and gum infections.

These pathogenic bacteria, if unchallenged by oral probiotics, can also leak their endotoxins into the bloodstream, causing carotid artery damage.

Probiotic Defense Mechanisms

The following table is a list of activities of probiotics proven in the research. The author's book, *Probiotics: Protection Against Infection* provides the specific research and references on these mechanisms:

Allergies	reduce Th1/ Th2 ratio; decrease Th2 levels; lower TGF-beta2; increase IgE
Anorexia nervosa	increase appetite; increase assimilation; increase lymphocytes
Antibiotics	produce antibiotic and antifungal substances (such as acidophillin and bifidin) that repel or kill pathogenic bacteria, adjusting to pathogen and resistance
B-cells	modulate and redirect B-cell activity
Bile	break down bile acids
Biochemicals	secrete lactic acids, lactoperoxidases, formic acids, lipopolysaccharides, peptidoglycans, superantigens and others to manage pH and repel pathogens.
Bladder cancer	reduce recurrent bladder cancer incidence and inhibit new tumors
Blood pressure	reduce hypertension; inhibit ACE
Calcium	increase serum calcium; decrease parathyroid hormone
Cancer (general)	reduce mutagenicity; increase natural killer tumoricidal activity; increase survival rates
Candida overgrowth	control populations; reduce overgrowths
CD cell orientation	modulate and direct particular CD cells depending upon condition, including CD56, CD8, CD4, CD25, CD69, CD2, others

Cell degeneration	slow cellular degeneration and associated diseases among elderly persons
Colds and Influenza	reduce infection frequency; reduce infection duration; reduce symptoms; prevent complications; decrease worker sick days
Colic	reduce crying time; decrease infection; increase stool frequency; decrease bloating and indigestion
Colon cancer	reduce recurrence; increase survival rates; reduce beta-glucosidase; inhibit cell abnormality and mutation; increase IL-2
Constipation	increase bowel movement frequency; ease colon and impacted feces
Control pathogens	compete with pathogenic organisms for nutrients, thus checking their growth
C-reactive protein	reduce levels in blood
Cytokines	stimulate the body's production of various cytokines, including IL-6, IL-3, IL-5, TNF alpha, and interferon
Dental caries	reduce and control cavity-causing bacteria
Digestion	reduce gas, nausea and stress-related gastrointestinal digestive difficulty
Digestive difficulty	secrete digestive enzymes; help break down nutrients from fats; proteins and other foods
Diverticulosis	reduce polyps and strengthen intestinal wall mucosa
Ear infections	hasten otitis media healing response; prevent infections
EFAs	manufacture essential fatty acids, including important short-chained FAs, and help body assimilate EFAs
Fiber digestion	aid in soluble fiber fermentation, yielding fatty acids and energy
Food poisoning	increase resistance to food poisoning; battle and remove pathogenic organisms; reduce diarrhea and other symptoms
Glucose metabolism	improve glucose control
Gum disease	reduce gum infections; deplete gingivitis
H. pylori	reduce H. pylori infections; reduce ulcers
HIV/AIDS	stimulate immune system; reduce symptoms; reduce co-infections; increase survival rates
Hormones	balance and stimulate hormone production
Hydrogen peroxide	manufacture H2O2 - oxygenating/antiseptic
IBS	decrease bloating, pain, cramping
Immunoglobulins	modulate IgA, IgG, IgE, IgM to weakness
Inflammation	modify prostaglandins (E1, E2), IFN-gamma, re-

	duce CRP; modulate TNF-alpha; increase IgA; slow inflammatory response as needed
Intestinal Permeability	protect against IIPS; block penetration of toxins; work cooperatively with villi and microvilli; attach to mucosa; improve barrier function
Intestine walls	protect walls of intestines against toxin exposure and colonization of pathogens
Iron absorption	increase iron assimilation; increase hemoglobin count
Keratoconjunctivitis	decrease burning, itching and dry eyes
Kidney stones	reduce urine oxalates; reduce blood oxalates
Lipids/Cholesterol	reduce LDL, triglycerides and total cholesterol; increase HDL
Liver	stimulate liver cells (hepatocytes); stimulate liver function; reduce cirrhosis symptoms; reduce liver enzymes
Liver cancer	stimulate immune response; decrease infection and complications after surgery
Lung cancer	increase survival rates; reduce chest pain and other symptoms
Mental state	improve mood; stimulate positive mood hormones like serotonin and tryptophan
Milk digestion	aid dairy digestion for lactose-intolerant people; produce lactase
Monocytes	increase oxidative burst capacity
Mucosa	coat intestines, stomach, oral, nasal and vagina mucosa, providing protective barrier
NF-kappaB	modulate activity to condition
NK-cells	stimulate natural killer cell activity
Nutrition	manufacture biotin, thiamin (B1), riboflavin (B2), niacin (B3), pantothenic acid (B5), pyridoxine (B6), cobalamine (B12), folic acid, vitamin A and/or vitamin K; aid in assimilation of proteins, fats and minerals
Pancreatitis	reduce pancreas infection (sepsis); reduce necrosis; speed healing
pH control	produce a number of other acids and biochemicals, modulating pH (see biochemicals)
Phagocytes	increase phagocytic activity as needed
Phytonutrients	convert to bioavailable nutrient forms
Premature births and Low birth weights	speed growth; reduce infection; improve immune response; increase nutrition
Protein assimilation	break down amino acid content; inhibit assimilation of allergic polypeptides
Respiratory infections	inhibit pneumonia; reduce duration of infection; inhibit bronchitis; inhibit tonsillitis

Rotavirus infections	speed healing times; prevent infection; ease abdominal pain; eradicate infective agents
Spleen	stimulate spleen activity
Stomach cancer	inhibit tumors; reduce *H. pylori* overgrowths
T-cells	modulate T-cell activity to condition
Th1 - Th2	decrease Th2 activity; increase Th1 (increases healing and decreases allergic response)
Thymus	increase thymus size and activity
Toxins	break down toxins; inhibit assimilation of heavy metals, chemicals, and endotoxins
Ulcers	control *H. pylori*; speed healing; improve mucosa; moderate acids; reduce pain
Vaccination	increase vaccine effectiveness
Vaginosis/Vaginitis	reduce infection; re-establish healthy pH; reduce odor

This summary of primarily randomized, double-blinded, and placebo-controlled human clinical research is by no means a complete list of all the probiotic effects that have been found by researchers. Furthermore, medical scientists have only chosen a small portion of probiotics' possible health benefits for controlled human research. The effects shown in these studies illustrate a variety of other possible benefits for specific infections and diseases. As we can see from probiotics' ability to specifically stimulate the immune system, there are many other possible applications for probiotics in medicine. The research has only begun.

The bottom line is that our body's probiotics head up the living immune system. At least 70% of the immune system *is* probiotic. Consider this carefully: If the intestine's probiotics were decimated by either a lethal bacteria infection or a course of antibiotics, *we would lose nearly three quarters of our gut's immune system.*

Chapter Four

Nutritional Cleansing

In this chapter we'll discuss strategies to arm and boost the body's own cleansing and detoxification systems. This protocol is not a 'shock and awe' system where we force the body into a full-body purge. As we've discussed, this can be unhealthy, and downright dangerous.

The strategy we offer is to lighten the burden off the immune system by removing as many toxins as practical, while boosting the body's immunity with a combination of nutrition, herbs and lifestyle changes.

Here we will lay out the foods that we should incorporate into our diets. Certainly it may be difficult for some to completely give up eating certain foods. And certainly, some of those foods may be toxic to our body (such as deep-fried foods) because they release lipid peroxidation into our bodies). Still, this protocol does not necessarily require us to fully give up our current diets—though it might be healthier to do so.

Rather, this protocol is about *adding* certain foods and nutrients to our diet. We can incorporate these foods as best we can, while making selections among the foods that we outline here. In other words, we can add the foods and nutrients that are more available to us, and can more easily be blended into our diets.

For this reason, this book will not outline extensive recipes. Recipes can be awfully restrictive. And restrictive diets do not last long. Rather, this chapter will lay out a number of foods in each category, and the reader can choose the foods to add to their current recipes. This may require a bit of substitution for some, but there are many natural food recipe books on the market today that will outline how to have most of the standard dishes we might eat today, but with the foods we outline here.

It should be added that doing this will have an interesting effect: Because most of the foods outlined here are tasty and delicious when added to our recipes, and because they have a positive benefit upon our moods, our immunity and our energy levels, it is likely that we will naturally add more and more of these foods to our diet. As we do that, we will experience even more of the benefits that these living foods provide—without having to undergo either a restrictive diet or a maddeningly disciplined protocol.

What are Cleansing Nutrients?

There are a variety of fad diets and gimmicks out there, some using incredibly restrictive protocols and clever approaches. One of these is the raw food diet. In fact, many raw food advocates have called their foods "living foods" to indicate that they are 'alive' with enzymes and various nutrients.

We in no way criticize the raw food diet. Certainly this diet is incredibly healthy, and someone who can maintain such a diet should be commended for their discipline and determination to be healthy.

However, we are not recommending the raw food diet here simply because it is too restrictive, and very few people can maintain such a diet for long. In addition, there are many foods that are better when they are minimally cooked. This of course includes grains, beans and a variety of vegetables that have fibers that need to be softened in order to adequately digest them and extract their nutrients.

Our definition of 'living' is somewhat different than raw foods. 'Living foods' in this text refers to:

- ✓ Foods that are cultured or fermented with probiotic microorganisms, whether yeasts or probiotic bacteria.
- ✓ Foods that are mixed with cultured or fermented foods.
- ✓ Grains or beans that have been sprouted.
- ✓ Plant-based foods that have been harvested whole and prepared as whole foods, with minimal cooking and processing.
- ✓ Supplements that contain probiotics and/or plant-based whole foods that have been minimally cooked or processed.

While the strict definition of 'living' should eliminate those foods that are no longer alive—such as are cultured foods with live probiotics—it is essential that we be practical. Certainly many animals—deer for example—can cruise through a forest and directly eat from living plants, few of us have the luxury of being able to eat as we walk through the woods. Modern humans are stuck with having others collect and harvest our foods before storing them and shipping them to our local food stores.

A diet high in living foods will:

- ➤ increase antioxidant levels
- ➤ increase detoxification
- ➤ lower the burden on the body's immune system
- ➤ provide a host of bioavailable nutrients
- ➤ provide fiber, reducing LDL lipid peroxidation
- ➤ increase liver activity and strengthen of the liver
- ➤ alkalize and help purify the blood
- ➤ provide the body with trace and macro minerals
- ➤ lower inflammation
- ➤ increase our body's resident probiotics

All of these effects work together to cleanse the body of toxins and reduce the body's toxic burden. When the body's toxic burden is reduced, our immune system's ability to remove toxins is increased. This is the secret to a life-long purification: A long-term reduction of toxins.

Mushrooms for Detoxification

Edible mushrooms offer a significant tool to cleanse out toxins and boost our immunity. We can include delicious mushrooms like Shiitake, Buttons or Chanterelles into our dishes, and we can also take mushroom supplements with Reishi (*Ganderma lucidum*), Hoelen (*Wolfiporia extensa*), Maitake (*Grifola frondosa*), Shiitake (*Lentinula elodes*), Turkey Tails (*Coriolus versicolor or Trametes versicolor*), Agaricus (*Agaricus blazeil*), Cordyceps (*Cordyceps sinensis*) and Lion's Mane (*Hericium erinaceus*). All of these significantly stimulate the immune system, and their constituents bind to toxins within our bodies.

The Agaricus species is the most popular eating mushroom, and this species contains the button mushroom. But there are many, many others. Scientists have cataloged some 50,000 mushrooms, and identified less than 20,000 different mushroom species. Some estimate there may be over 150,000 mushroom species within the Fungi kingdom, which likely encompasses more than 1.5 million total species. Biologists have described less than 5% of Fungi species.

Over 600 mushroom species have been documented to stimulate the immune system. However, the ones mentioned above have received the most attention. Research on these mushrooms have revealed their effects as being antimicrobial, cholesterol-lowering, anti-inflammatory, anti-oxidant, anti-mutagenic, anti-tumor, adaptogenic and immunostimulating.

Cancer has been a significant area of research. A number of these mushrooms have been shown to inhibit cancer cell line growth, for example. American researchers were awakened by Dr. Tetsuro Ikekawa's groundbreaking epidemiological study showing significantly lower cancer rates among Japanese mushroom growers between 1972 and 1986. The research since then has shown significant anticarcinogenic properties among most of the mushrooms mentioned above. While most clinical research to date has been adjunctive to conventional therapies for ethical reasons, human studies have consistently confirmed animal and laboratory models. By August of 2008, there were 4,087 mushroom studies and scientific papers filed with the U.S. National Library of Medicine.

These mushrooms are incredible radical scavengers. For example, lion's mane mushroom has been shown to reduce the risk of Alzheimer's and senility. The mushroom appears to stimulate nerve growth factor, a substance that has can reduce dementia and benefit Alzheimer's patients.

A immune-boosting compound called AHCC—Active Hexose Correlated Compound—has been is derived from shiitake mushroom and their sub-species. This has been shown to stimulate the activity of white blood cells. Further research showed they stimulated interferon (IFN-y) and tumor necrosis factor (TNF-a) as well.

Much of the dramatic immunity effects of mushrooms are due to their polysaccharides and polysaccharide-protein complexes. Laboratory research has isolated multiple polysaccharide types within each species. Twenty-nine unique polysaccharides have been isolated in Maitake, for example.

Mushroom polysaccharides are primarily glucans with different glycosidic linkages, including 1->3 and 1->6 beta glucans, and 1->3 alpha glucans. The complex branching and even helical nature of mushroom glucans appears to be significant. Schizophyllan polysaccharides with (1,3)-b-glucans with 1,3-b-d-linked glucose with 1,6-b-d-glucosyl side groups have been described as "stiff triple-stranded" helices in laboratory research, for example. Schizophyllan (SPG) is an active macrophage stimulator, increasing T cell and NK cell activity and inhibiting various infective agents.

Various immunostimulatory effects have been also attributed to polysaccharide-protein complexes such as PSK (krestin), PSP, lentinan and others. While many varieties contain different levels of the various beta glucans, many researchers believe it is their unique protein sequencing that differentiates effects among species.

Medicinal mushrooms also contain a variety of nutrients. Many mushrooms contain significant amounts of protein. Shiitake can be as much as 17% protein while oyster mushrooms can be 30% protein by weight. Several also contain vitamin B complexes. Most edible mushrooms also contain a variety of macro-minerals and trace elements. Shiitake also can contain as much as 126 mg of calcium, and 247 mg of magnesium per serving, for example. Reishi also contains magnesium, calcium, zinc, iron, copper and trace minerals. Many are good sources of selenium.

Maitake and a number of other mushrooms also contain ergosterols (provitamin D2), along with phosphatidylcholine and phosphatidylserine. Shiitake, Reishi and Maitake have been known to increase from less than 500 IU of D2 in indoor growing conditions to 46,000 IU, 2760 IU, and 31,900 IU respectively, following six to eight hours of sunlight exposure (Stamets 2005).

Various anti-oxidants have been isolated among popular mushroom varieties. Constituents such as ganoderic acid (*G. lucidum*), cordycepic acid (*C. sinensis*), linzhi (*G. frondosa*), agaric acid (several), sizofilan and sizofiran (*S. commune*), galactomannan (*C. sinesis*), and various triterpenoids (several) can actively reduce oxidative radicals and stimulate the immune system.

The density of these in mushrooms is quite incredible. Reishi has over 100 ethanol-soluble triterpenoids. Most of these are antioxidant, and many are anti-inflammatory agents.

Some of the mechanisms of mushrooms to safely stimulate the immune system and produce long-term cleansing benefits are quite complicated. For example, differently branched beta glucans have been observed stimulating immune cells in different ways. For example, certain beta glucans from Maitake will stimulate T-cell production, while differently bonded-chain beta glucans from *Agaricus blazei* stimulate natural killer (NK) cells. Others stimulate B-cells, T-helper cells, lymphokine activated killer cells [LAK], macrophages; and the cytokines interferon gamma, interleukin-2, -12 and tumor necrosis factor [TNF].

Mushrooms significantly detoxify heavy metals inside our bodies, and in their natural environments. Their proteins will bind to certain heavy metals within the soil. These same metabolites become active within the body when eaten, and thus help chelate minerals in our bodies.

For this reason, Cordyceps, reishi, *Agaricus blazei* and maitake have been used in China to reduce effects of heavy metal and radiation poisoning.

Mushrooms can be eaten fresh, frozen, drank as teas, cooked with sauces or eaten as supplements. Parts used include the fruiting body (cap and stem) and the mycelia (colonizing rooting network).

While each form will stimulate our immune system, fresh or freeze-dried are preferable. Some supplements are hot-water extracted, and some are alcohol extracted. Hot water extracts likely retain more constituents, although alcohol can extract specific medicinal constituents as well.

Living Antioxidant Foods

When we harvest a fresh plant-based food and eat it with minimal storage, processing and cooking, we are deriving significant benefits from the living organism that produced the food. Because living organisms defend themselves against toxins throughout their lives, by eating fresh whole foods or whole foods minimally cooked, our bodies can utilize the same elements the plant utilized to protect itself against toxins.

This in turn stimulates our immune systems, and also provides direct free radical protection. This is because antioxidants are designed to neutralize toxins.

As we've discussed, a plethora of research has confirmed that damage from free radicals is implicated in many health conditions. Free radicals from toxins damage cells, cell membranes, organs, blood vessel walls and airways—producing systemic inflammation—as the immune system responds to an overload of tissue damage.

Free radicals are produced by synthetic chemicals, pathogens, trans fats, fried foods, red meats, radiation, pollution and various intruders that destabilize within the body. Free radicals are molecules or ions that require stabilization. They reach stabilization by 'stealing' atoms from the cells or tissues of our body. This in turn destabilizes those cells and tissues—producing damage.

Antioxidants serve to stabilize free radicals before our cells and tissues are robbed—by donating their own atoms. A diet with plenty of fruits and vegetables supplies numerous antioxidants. Although antioxidants cannot be considered treatments for any disease, many studies have proved that increased antioxidant intake supports immune function and detoxification. These effects allow the immune system to respond with greater tolerance.

Antioxidant constituents in plant-based foods are known to significantly repeal free radicals, strengthen the immune system and help detoxify the system. These include *lecithin* and *octacosanol* from whole grains; *polyphenols* and *sterols* from vegetables; *lycopene* from tomatoes and watermelons; *quercetin* and *sulfur/allicin* from garlic, onions and peppers; *pectin* and *rutin* from apples and other fruits; *phytocyanidin flavonoids* such as *apigenin* and *luteolin* from various greenfoods; and *anthocyanins* from various fruits and oats.

Some sea-based botanicals like kelp also contain antioxidants as well. Consider a special polysaccharide compound from kelp called *fucoidan*. Fucoidan has been shown in animal studies to significantly reduce inflammation (Cardoso *et al.* 2009; Kuznetsova *et al.* 2004).

Procyanidins are found in apples, currants, cinnamon, bilberry and many other foods. The extract of *Vitis vinifera* seed (grapeseed) is one of the highest sources of bound antioxidant *proanthocyanidins* and *leucocyanidines* called *procyanidolic oligomers* or PCOs. Pycnogenol® also contains significant levels of these PCOs. Blueberries, parsley, green tea, black currant, some legumes and onions also contain PCOs and similar proanthocyanidins.

Research has demonstrated that PCOs have protective and strengthening effects on tissues by increasing enzyme conjugation (Seo *et al.* 2001). PCOs have also been shown to increase vascular wall strength (Robert *et al.* 2000).

Oxygenated carotenoids such as *lutein* and *astaxanthin* also have been shown to exhibit strong antioxidant activity. Astaxanthin is derived from the microalga *Haematococcus pluvialis*, and lutein is available from a number of foods, including spirulina.

Most of these phytonutrients specifically modulate the immune system. For example, the flavonoids *kaempferol* and *flavone* have been shown to block mast cell proliferation by over 80% (Alexandrakis *et al.* 2003). Sources of kaempferol include Brussels sprouts, broccoli, grapefruit and apples.

Furthermore, *resveratrol* from grapes and berries modulate nuclear factor-kappaB and transcription/Janus kinase pathways—which strengthens immunity. Good sources of resveratrol include peanuts, red grapes, cranberries and cocoa (wine is not advisable for cleansing as we'll discuss later).

Nearly every plant-food has some measure of phytonutrients discussed above and more. These phytonutrients alkalize the blood and increase the detoxification capabilities of the liver. They help clear the blood of toxins.

Foods that are particularly detoxifying and immunity-building include fresh pineapples, beets, cucumbers, apricots, apples, almonds, zucchini, artichokes, avocados, bananas, beans, collard greens, berries, casaba, celery, coconuts, cranberries, watercress, dandelion greens, grapes, raw honey, corn, kale, citrus fruits, watermelon, lettuce, mangoes, mushrooms, oats, broccoli, okra, onions, papayas, parsley, peas, whole grains, radishes, raisins, spinach, tomatoes, walnuts, and many others.

These plant-based foods are also our primary source of soluble and insoluble fiber. Diets with significant fiber help clear the blood and tissues of toxins, and lipid peroxidation-friendly LDL cholesterol. Fiber is also critical to a healthy digestive tract and intestinal barrier. Fiber in the diet should range from about 35 to 45 grams per day according to the recommendations of many diet experts. Six to ten servings of raw fruits and vegetables per day should accomplish this—which is even part of the USDA's recommendations. This means raw, fibrous foods should be present at every meal.

Good fibrous plant sources also contain healthy *lignans* and *phytoestrogens* that help balance hormone levels, and help the body make its own natural corticoids. Foods that contain these include peas, garbanzo beans, soybeans, kidney beans and lentils.

Plant-based foods provide these immune-stimulating factors because these vary same factors make up the plants' own immune systems. For example, the red, blue and green flavonoid pigments in plants and fruits help protect the plant from oxidative damage from radiation. The proanthocyanidins in grains like oats, for example, help protect the oat plant from crown rust caused by the *Puccinia coronata* fungus. So the same biochemicals that stimulate immunity in humans are part of plants' immune systems.

These same whole food phytonutrients also neutralize oxidative radicals in our bodies—the reason they are called antioxidants. How do we know this? Scientists can measure the ability of a particular food to neutralize free radicals with specific laboratory testing. One such test is called the *Oxygen Radical Absorbance Capacity Test* (ORAC). This technical laboratory study is performed by a number of scientific organizations that include the USDA, as well as specialized labs such as Brunswick Laboratories in Massachusetts.

Research from the USDA's Jean Mayer Human Nutrition Research Center on Aging at Tufts University has suggested that a diet high in ORAC value may protect blood vessels and tissues from free radical damage that can result in inflammation (Sofic *et al.* 2001; Cao *et al.* 1998). These tissues, of course, include the airways. Research has confirmed that consuming 3,000 to 5,000 ORAC units per day can have protective benefits.

ORAC Values (100 grams) of Selected (raw) Fruits (USDA, 2007-2008)

Cranberry	9,382		Pomegranate	2,860
Plum	7,581		Orange	1,819
Blueberry	6,552		Tangerine	1,620
Blackberry	5,347		Grape (red)	1,260
Raspberry	4,882		Mango	1,002
Apple (Granny)	3,898		Kiwi	882
Strawberry	3,577		Banana	879
Cherry (sweet)	3,365		Tomato (plum)	389
Gooseberry	3,277		Pineapple	385
Pear	2,941		Watermelon	142

There is tremendous attention these days on two unique fruits from the Amazon rain forest and China called *açaí* and *goji berry* (or wolfberry) respectively. A recent ORAC test documented by Schauss *et al.* (2006) gives açaí a score of 102,700 and tests documented by Dr. Paul Gross gives goji berries a total ORAC of 30,300. However, subsequent tests done by Brunswick Laboratories, Inc. gave these two berries 53,600 (açaí) and 22,000 (goji) total-ORAC values.

In addition, we must remember that these are the dried berries being tested in the latter case, and a concentrate of acai being tested in the former case. The numbers in the chart above are for fresh fruits. Dried fruits will naturally have higher ORAC values, because the water is evaporated—giving more density and more antioxidants per 100 grams.

For example, in the USDA database, dried apples have a 6,681 total-ORAC value, while fresh apples range from 2,210 to 3,898 in total-ORAC value. This equates to a two-to-three times increase from fresh to dried. In another example, fresh red grapes have a 1,260 total-ORAC value, while raisins have a 3,037 total-ORAC value. This comes close to an increase of three times the ORAC value following dehydration.

Part of the equation, naturally, is cost. Dried fruit and concentrates are often more expensive than fresh fruit. High-ORAC dried fruits or concentrates from açaí or gogi will also be substantially more expensive than most fruits grown domestically (especially for Americans and Europeans). Our conclusion is that local or in-country grown fresh fruits with high total-ORAC values produce the best value. Local fresh fruit offers great free radical scavenging ability, support for local farmers, and pollen proteins we are most likely more tolerant to.

By comparison, spinach—an incredibly wholesome vegetable with a tremendous amount of nutrition—has a fraction of the ORAC content of some of these fruits, at 1,515 total ORAC. Spinach, of course, contains many other nutrients, including proteins lacking in many high-ORAC fruits.

Dehydrated spices can have incredibly high ORAC values. For example, USDA's database lists ground Turmeric's total ORAC value at 159,277 and oregano's at 200,129. However, while we might only consume a few hundred milligrams of a spice per day, we can eat many grams—if not pounds—of sweet colorful fruit every day.

Quercetin Foods

A number of foods and herbs that reduce inflammation and toxicity contain quercetin. This is no coincidence. Multiple studies have shown that quercetin inhibits the release inflammatory mediators histamine and leukotrienes. Foods rich in quercetin include onions, garlic, apples, capers, grapes, leafy greens, tomatoes and broccoli. In addition, many of the herbs listed earlier contain quercetin as an active constituent. Many of the herbs listed in the herbal section also contain quercetin. Onions, garlic and apples contain some of the highest levels.

Quercetin stimulates and balances the immune system. In an *in vivo* study, four weeks of quercetin reduced histamine levels and allergen-specific IgE levels. More importantly, quercetin inhibited anaphylaxis responses (Shishehbor *et al.* 2010).

Cairo researchers (Haggag *et al.* 2003) found that among mast cells exposed to allergens and chemicals in the laboratory, quercetin inhibited histamine release by 95% and 97%.

Over the past few years, an increasing amount of evidence is pointing to the conclusion that foods with quercetin slow inflammatory response and autoimmune derangement. Researchers from Italy's Catholic University (Crescente *et al.* 2009) found that quercetin inhibited arachidonic acid-induced platelet aggregation. Arachidonic acid-induced platelet aggregation is seen in allergic inflammatory mechanisms.

Researchers from the University of Crete (Alexandrakis *et al.* 2003) found that quercetin can inhibit mast cell proliferation by up to 80%. Onions have also been shown *in vivo* tests to reduce bronchoconstriction.

Organic foods contain higher levels of quercetin. A study from the University of California-Davis' Department of Food Science and Technology (Mitchell *et al.* 2007) tested flavonoid levels between organic and conventional tomatoes over a ten-year period. Their research concluded that quercetin levels were 79% higher for tomatoes grown organically under the same conditions as conventionally-grown tomatoes.

Root Foods

It is no coincidence that many antioxidants are roots, such as ginger, turmeric, onions garlic, beets, carrots, turnips, parsnips and others. These root foods are known for their ability to alkalize the bloodstream and stimulate detoxification. They are also known to help rejuvenate the liver and adrenal glands.

Beets, for example, contain, among other nutrients, betaine, betalains, betacyanin and betanin. They also contain generous portions of folate, iron and fiber. One of the primary fibers in beets is pectin, which is also found in apples. Pectin has a unique soluble and insoluble fiber content that maximizes the attachment of radical-producing LDL cholesterol in the intestines. Pectin also attaches to many other toxins, drawing them out of the body as well.

Meanwhile, betaine is known as stimulating liver health. Betaine has been shown to reduce liver injury (Okada et al. 2011). Betaine is also considered healthy for the bile ducts, because it helps draw out toxins. Beets are delicious foods that can be grated into salads, juiced, steamed, baked and simply eaten raw. Red beets are typically considered the healthiest, but pink and white beets also contain betaine.

We should note that while beets contain significant amounts of betaine, other betaine-rich foods include broccoli, spinach and some whole grains.

Each of the root foods listed above contain unique constituents that support liver health and detoxification.

Fermented Soy Foods

Soy foods have been shown in numerous studies to reduce breast cancer risk, reduce cholesterol, reduce the risk of heart disease, increase artery health, reduce allergies and reduce the risk of bone fractures (Messina 2010).

In addition, several large epidemiological studies done in the 1990s found that those populations that ate higher levels of tofu in their diets had lower levels of heart disease and many cancers.

Washington state researchers (Lerman et al. 2010) found that people with higher LDL cholesterol levels and cardiovascular disease experienced a reduction of LDL cholesterol and smaller particle size, greater HDL cholesterol, lower apolipoprotein levels and lower homocysteine levels. Remember that LDL cholesterol is related to lipoperoxidation, which is what causes artery disease leading to heart attacks and strokes. And lower apolipoprotein levels and lower homocysteine levels mean lower levels of systemic inflammation.

These benefits come from one of soy's isoflavones, genistein. Researchers from Northwestern University's Feinberg School of Medicine, in association with the American Lung Association Asthma Clinical Research Centers (Smith *et al.* 2004) studied asthma severity in 1,033 adolescents and adults. They found that 250 micrograms per 1,000 Kcal per day of the soy isoflavone genistein significantly increased forced expiratory volumes and peak expiratory volumes.

Because some soy nutrients (such as raffinose) can be difficult for some to digest, soy's best antioxidant benefits come when soy is cultured or fermented. Cultured soy foods such as tofu and tempeh thus provide easily assimilable sources of soy.

Greenfoods

A greenfood is a category of foods that are considered nutritionally superior than the typical fruits and vegetables. Greenfoods include the wheat grasses, sprouts, algaes, and sea vegetables.

Greenfoods provide practically every nutrient imaginable, including enzymes, minerals, trace elements, essential and non-essential amino acids, vitamins, antioxidants and various phytonutrients. Many will provide over 1,000 nutrients.

A big benefit of greenfoods is their alkalinity. This gives them the ability to neutralize radicals and lipid peroxides.

Much of this alkalinity comes from greenfoods' bioavailable mineral content. Many of these minerals are also are colloidal. They tend to be hydrophobic, and maintain a positive electrical charge—rendering them alkaline.

Cereal Grasses

Wheat grass is the young grass of the wheat species, *Triticum aestivum*. In addition to a plethora of vitamins, minerals, amino acids, phytonutrients, metabolic enzymes—including superoxide dismutase and cytochrome oxidase—wheat grass maintains up to 70% chlorophyll.

Early research by Dr. Charles Schnabel, Dr. George Kohler and Dr. A.I. Virtanen in the 1925-1950 era found that cereal grasses like wheatgrass achieved their highest nutrient content at around 18 days—right before the first jointing.

Wheat grass can increase blood hemoglobin levels. Wheat grass tablets decreased blood transfusion needs by 25% among 20 children requiring frequent blood transfusions in a recent study.

Barley grass maintains similar properties. Research has found that barley grass is a potent free radical scavenger; significantly reduces total cholesterol and LDL-cholesterol; and inhibits LDL oxidation. Barley grass juice powder can have 14 vitamins, 18 amino acids, 15 enzymes, 10 antioxidants, 18 minerals and 75 trace elements.

Another cereal grass is Kamut grass. The khorasan wheat has higher protein levels than most wheat varieties, and contains higher zinc, selenium and magnesium content. Selenium is known for stimulating glutathione activity as we've discussed.

Sprouts

Sprouts and their powders are nutritional powerhouses. They have exponential nutritional value, well above the nutrient content of their seeds or the fully-grown plants. This was confirmed in 1970s experiments by former Hippocrates Health Institute Director of Research, Viktoras Kulvinskas, M.S. Kulvinskas, who found that ascorbic acid levels in soybean sprouts increased from zero to 103 milligrams per 100 grams by day six—about the ascorbic acid content found in lime juice. These levels fall off significantly within days.

Each plant has a different nutrient peak. Ascorbic acid content in broad bean sprouts—used to cure scurvy during World War I—peaks in three days, after which the levels fall off.

Many believe that sprouts produce this greater antioxidant content to defend themselves against threats from the soil.

Great nutritional sprouts include wheat grass sprouts, barley, oats, beans, broccoli and cabbage. The latter two provide a class of nutrients called glucosinolates. These glucosinolates yield sulfur compounds and indole-3 carbinols. Both have shown to have significant anticarcinogenic and anti-inflammatory effects in the body.

Seed selection is critical. A good quality seed will germinate at least 50%. Heirloom seeds often germinate at much higher rates.

Sea Grasses

Kelps might be called seaweeds, but these phytonutrient powerhouses are anything but weeds. About 1,500 species of sea kelps flourish, many in the North Pacific and North Atlantic oceans.

Most kelps are stationary, and sustainably harvested in the wild. This means they must be allowed to regrow to guarantee future harvests. *Ascophyllum nodosum* kelp contains an impressive array of vitamins—more than many vegetables. They include over 60 essential minerals, amino acids and vitamins. They also contain growth promoters, according to kelp researchers.

Most kelps also contain fucoidan, a sulfated polysaccharide. Laboratory studies have indicated fucoidan has anti-tumor, anticoagulant and anti-angiogenic effects. It down-regulates Th2 (inhibiting allergic response), inhibits beta-amyloid formation (implicated in Alzheimer's), inhibits proteinuria in Heymann nephritis and decreases artery platelet deposits.

Other kelps include dulse, sargassi seaweed, *Undaria pinnatifida,* sea palm and others.

Spirulina

Spirulina use dates back to the Aztecs. A good source of carotenoids, vitamins (including vegan B12 according to independent laboratory tests) and minerals, spirulina contains all essential and most non-essential amino acids, with up to 65% protein by weight. It also contains antioxidant phytonutrients such as zeaxanthin, myxoxanthophyll and lutein. It also will contain antioxidant carotenoids, vitamins and minerals.

Spirulina also contains phycobiliprotein, a unique blue pigment anti-inflammatory and antioxidant. Research has showed that phycobiliproteins can protect the liver and kidney from toxins. They are also anti-viral, and stimulate the immune system.

In one study from the University of California-Davis, 12 weeks of 3000 milligrams of Hawaiian spirulina per day significantly increased hemoglobin concentration and mean corpuscular hemoglobin among 30 adults over the age of 50. IDO (indoleamine 2,3-dioxygenase) enzyme activity—a sign of increased immune function—was also higher among the subjects.

Chlorella

More than 800 published studies have verified the safety and efficacy of *Chlorella pyrenoidosa*. Chlorella's reputation of drawing out heavy metals and other toxins make it a favorite among health practitioners.

Chlorella maintains considerable vitamins minerals, and phytonutrients—including chlorella growth factor (CGF), known to stimulate cell growth. It is also a complete protein, with about 60% protein by weight and every essential and non-essential amino acid. Clinical studies have shown that chlorella stimulates T-cell and B-cell activity and contributes to the improvement of fibromyalgia, ulcerative colitis and hypertension. Another study showed that chlorella increases IgA levels and lowers dioxin levels in breast milk.

Chlorella's tough cell wall must be broken down mechanically to allow these nutrients' bioavailability. Our digestive enzymes cannot digest these outer cell walls. For this reason, quality chlorella growers will pulverize this tough outer cell wall.

Haematococcus and Astaxanthin

Another greenfood algae is *Haematococcus pluvialis,* known for its high astaxanthin content. Astaxanthin is a strong carotenoid similar to beta-carotene. For this reason, astaxanthin is one of the most powerful natural antioxidants known. It also has anti-inflammatory effects, and has been used for eye health, joint healthy, muscle soreness, cardiovascular health, and skin health. It can also protect against damage from UV radiation.

Blue-Green Algae from Klamath Lake

Aphanizomenon flos-aquae or AFA, grows on the pristine waters of Klamath Lake in Oregon. Commercial AFA harvesting began in the early 1980s. This rich volcanic Klamath Lake gives AFA a good source of protein and all the essential and non-essential amino acids. It also has many vitamins, minerals and phytonutrients. AFA contains about 60% protein by weight, and at least 58 minerals at ppm levels, along with significant chlorophyll content.

One of the more exciting phytonutrient compounds discovered in AFA is phenylethylamine (PEA). PEA has been called the 'love molecule,' as it serves to increase positive moods. PEA is also found in chocolate. AFA has significantly more PEA, however.

Aloe Vera

While aloe has long been known for its skin irritation and wound healing abilities, science on its internal use is still emerging.

Aloe is now used for gastrointestinal health, immune support and cardio-vascular health, as well as the health of the skin and mucosal membranes.

Aloe may also help prevent kidney stones. A study published in the *Journal of the Thailand Medical Association* found that 200 grams of fresh aloe gel a day significantly decreased urinary oxalate excretion.

In addition, a study from London's Queen Mary School of Medicine on 44 active ulcerated colitis patients found that internal aloe use resulted in clinical improvement. And double-blind, randomized research using Aloecorp's Qmatrix processed aloe has shown that it reduces oxidative stress markers and stimulates the immune system.

Aloe can be taken as a juice or a gel.

About Juicing

Juicing has been advocated for many years by a number of health experts and nutritionists. Many have promoted juicing for detoxification and cleansing. This is not the case here.

However, juicing is a suboptimal way to glean the benefits of fruits and vegetables. This is because it is the combination of the antioxidant nutrients and the soluble and insoluble fibers in fruits and vegetables that give them their true cleansing benefits.

The moral here is that natural fiber with antioxidants renders more cleansing benefits than do antioxidants alone. While antioxidants do attach and bind to toxins and neutralize radicals such as lipid peroxides, fiber attaches to LDL cholesterol in the intestines, which prevents them from becoming lipid peroxides in the first place. Fibers also attach to numerous other radicals and toxins within the intestines, flushing them out through the colon. *This prevents their entry into the bloodstream.*

While juicing is somewhat practical for hard fiber vegetables like carrots, the best strategy for most other fruits and vegetables is to make smoothies. This is basically putting the whole fruit or vegetable into a blender (after peeling in the case of oranges and the like, although orange peels are also a great cleansing nutrient), mixing with some water, a greenfood powder, and perhaps some kefir or yogurt, and then blending them up into a fruit/vegetable smoothie. For thinner consistency, simply add more water, and for thicker consistency, less water.

While juice can also be added to our smoothies, juices are not recommended in the living cleanse diet. This is because juices have been separated from their fibers, and this makes the juice not wholesome. Furthermore, many commercial juices are pasteurized or flash-pasteurized, rendering many of the enzymes and antioxidants useless, and often denatured. Furthermore, the sugars in pasteurized juices can turn to more simplified versions, rendering them unstable and acidic upon consumption and subject to becoming radicals within the body.

This denaturing can easily be observed. Simply pour some pasteurized filtered orange juice into a glass. Now peel an orange and put into the blender. Pour that into a glass next to the juice glass. Now take a gulp of the juice, and then take a gulp of the orange smoothie. You will taste the difference. As you let the juice slide past your throat, take an extra swallow and see if you do not sense the acidification of the juice on the epithelia of the throat/esophagus. Now do the same with the smoothie. The smoothie will go down, uh, okay, *smooth.*

Fats for Cleansing

The types of fats we eat relate directly to detoxification because some fats result in more radicals and other fats result in fewer radicals. As a result, some fats are pro-inflammatory while others are anti-inflammatory.

Here we refer to the anti-inflammatory fats as being *cleansing* because these come from low-processed plant-sources that maintain high levels of what the plant utilized for its own metabolism, development and procreation (as most healthy plant fats come from the seeds of plants). A few of the healthy fats come from algae sources, as we'll discuss.

The fat balance of our diet is critical to cleansing because our cell membranes are made of different lipids and lipid-derivatives like phospholipids and glycolipids. An imbalanced fat diet therefore can lead to weak cell membranes, which leads to cells that have restricted or inconsistent pores. The cell membrane pores allow nutrients in to the cells and waste out of the cells. Unhealthy fats also lead to weaker cell membranes that are more prone to damage by oxidative radicals—producing more cell damage and more toxicity in the body.

An example of this is the International Study of Asthma and Allergies in Childhood (ISAAC) conducted among eight Pacific countries, which included Samoa, Fiji, Tokelau, French Polynesia and New Caledonia. The research found that margarine consumption was one of the leading predicating factors in current asthma and wheezing among children.

Furthermore, they found that the risk factors for increased rhinoconjunctivitis included the regular consumption of meat products, butter and margarine among others. Allergic eczema was also associated with regular meat consumption and butter consumption among others.

Here is a quick review of the major fatty acids and the foods they come from:

Major Omega-3 Fatty Acids (EFAs)

Acronym	Fatty Acid Name	Major Dietary Sources
ALA	Alpha-linolenic acid	Walnuts, soybeans, flax, canola, pumpkin seeds, chia seeds
SDA	Stearidonic acid	hemp, spirulina, blackcurrant
DHA	Docosahexaenoic acid	Body converts from ALA; also obtained from certain algae, krill and fish oils
EPA	Eicosapentaenoic acid	Converts in the body from DHA

Major Omega-6/7 Fatty Acids (EFAs)

Acronym	Fatty Acid Name	Major Dietary Sources
LA	Linoleic acid	Many plants, safflower, sunflower, sesame, soy, almond especially
ARA	Arachidonic acid	Meats, salmon
PA	Palmitoleic acid (7)	Macadamia, palm kernel, coconut
GLA	Gamma-linolenic acid	Borage, primrose oil, spirulina

Major Omega-9 Fatty Acids

Acronym	Fatty Acid Name	Major Dietary Sources
EA	Eucic acid	Canola, mustard seed, wallflower
OA	Oleic acid	Sunflower, olive, safflower

Major Saturated Fatty Acids

Acronym	Fatty Acid Name	Major Dietary Sources
Lauric	Lauric acid	Coconut, dairy, nuts
Myristic	Myristic acid	Coconut, butter
Palmitic	Palmitic acid	Macadamia, palm kernel, coconut, butter, beef, eggs
Stearic	Stearic acid	Macadamia, palm kernel, coconut, eggs

Essential fatty acids (EFAs) are fats the body does not form. Eaten in the right proportion, they can also lower inflammation and speed healing. EFAs include the long-chain polyunsaturated fatty acids—and the shorter chain linolenic and linoleic polyunsaturates. EFAs include omega-3s and omega-6s. The omega-3s include alpha linolenic acid (ALA), docosahexaenoic acid (DHA) and eicosapentaenoic acid (EPA). EPA and DHA are found in algae, mackerel, salmon, herring, sardines, sablefish (black cod). The omega-

6s include linoleic acid, (LA), palmitoleic acid (PA), gamma-linoleic acid (GLA) and arachidonic acid (ARA). The term *essential* was originally given with the assumption that these types of fats could not be assembled or produced by the body—they must be taken directly from our food supply.

This assumption, however, is not fully correct. While it is true that we need *some* of these from our diet, our bodies can readily convert LA to ARA, and ALA to DHA and EPA as needed. Therefore, these fats can be considered essential in the sense that they are not generated by the body, but we do not necessarily have to consume each one of them.

Monounsaturated fats are high in omega-9 fatty acids like oleic acid. A monounsaturated fatty acid has one double carbon-hydrogen bonding chain. Oils from seeds, nuts and other plant-based sources have the largest quantities of monounsaturates. Oils that have large proportions of monounsaturates such as olive oil are known to lower inflammation when replacing high saturated fat in diets. Monounsaturates also aid in skin cell health and reduce atopic skin responses.

Monounsaturated fatty acids like oleic acid have been shown in studies to lower heart attack risk, aid blood vessel health, and offer anti-carcinogenic potential. They are typical among Mediterranean diets, which have been shown to reduce heart disease risk and cancer risk—related to their lower levels of lipid peroxidative radicals. The best sources of omega-9s are olives, sesame seeds, avocados, almonds, peanuts, pecans, pistachio nuts, cashews, hazelnuts, macadamia nuts, several other nuts and their respective oils.

Polyunsaturated fats have at least two double carbon-hydrogen bonds. They come from a variety of plant and marine sources. Omega-3s ALA, DHA and EPA simply have longer chains with more double carbon-hydrogen bonds. ALA, DHA and EPA are known to lower inflammation and increase artery-wall health. These *long-chain* omega-3 polyunsaturates are also considered critical for intestinal health.

The omega-6 fatty acids are the most available form of fat in the plant kingdom. Linoleic acid is the primary omega-6 fatty acid and it is found in most grains and seeds.

Saturated fats have multiple fatty acids without double bonds (the hydrogens "saturate" the carbons). They are found among animal fats, and tropical oils such as coconut and palm. Milk products such as butter and whole milk contain saturated fats, along with a special type of healthy linoleic fatty acid called CLA or *conjugated linoleic acid.*

The saturated fats from coconuts and palm differ from animal saturates in that they have shorter chains. This actually gives them—unlike animal saturates—an antimicrobial quality.

Medium chain fatty acids like coconut and palm oils have been shown in human studies to lower lipoprotein-A concentrations in the blood while having fibrinolytic (plaque and clot reduction) effects (Muller et al. 2003).

Trans fats are oils that either have been overheated or have undergone hydrogenation. Hydrogenation is produced by heating while bubbling hydrogen ions through the oil. This adds hydrogen and repositions some of the bonds. The "trans" refers to the positioning of part of the molecule in reverse—as opposed to "cis" positioning. The cis positioning is the bonding orientation the body's cell membranes work best with. Trans fats have been known to be a cause for increased radical species in the system; damaging artery walls; contributing to inflammation, heart disease, high LDL levels, liver damage, diabetes, and other metabolic dysfunction (Mozaffarian *et al.* 2009). Trans fat overconsumption slows the conversion of LA to GLA.

Conjugated linoleic acid (CLA) is a healthy fat that comes from primarily from dairy products. CLA is also a trans fat, but this is a trans fat the body works well with—it is considered a healthy trans fat.

Researchers from St Paul's Hospital and the University of British Columbia (MacRedmond *et al.* 2010) gave 28 overweight adults 4.5 g/day of CLA or a placebo for 12 weeks in addition to their medications. After the twelve weeks, those in the CLA group experienced significantly better lung function compared to the placebo group. The CLA group also experienced a significant reduction of weight and BMI compared with the control group. The CLA group also had lower leptin/adiponectin ratios—associated with balanced metabolism.

Other research has also found that CLA can to reduce lipid peroxidation and provide better balance among lipids (Noone et al. 2002).

Arachidonic acid (ARA): ARA is considered an essential fatty acid, and research has shown that it is vital for infants while they are building their intestinal barriers. However, ARA is pro-inflammatory and stimulates pro-inflammatory mediators like leukotrienes. Too much of it as we age thus burdens our immune systems, pushing our bodies towards systemic inflammation and slower detoxification.

Red meats provide the highest levels of arachidonic acid. Because arachidonic acid stimulates the production of pro-inflammatory prostaglandins and leucotrienes in an enzyme conversion process, too much ARA leads to a greater level of toxicity, producing more inflammation.

Interestingly, carnivorous animals cannot or do not readily convert linoleic acid (found in many common plants) to arachidonic acid, but herbivore animals do convert linoleic acid to arachidonic acid, as do humans. This conversion—on top of a red meat-heavy diet—produces high arachidonic acid levels. In contrast, a diet that is balanced between plant-based monounsaturates, polyunsaturates and some saturates (such as the Mediterranean diet) will balance arachidonic acids with the other fatty acids.

Gamma linolenic acid (GLA): A wealth of studies have confirmed that GLA reduces or inhibits the inflammatory response. Leukotrienes produced by arachidonic acid stimulate inflammation, while leukotrienes produced by GLA block the conversion of polyunsaturated fatty acids to arachidonic acid.

This means that GLA lowers inflammation, and promotes a healthy immune system.

A healthy body will convert linoleic acid into GLA readily, utilizing the same delta-6 desaturase enzyme used for ALA to DHA conversion. From GLA, the body produces *dihomo-gamma linolenic acid,* which cycles through the body as an eicosinoid. This aids in skin health, healthy mucosal membranes, and down-regulates inflammatory hypersensitivity.

In addition to conversion from LA, GLA can also be obtained from the oils of borage seeds, evening primrose seed, hemp seed, and from spirulina. Excellent food sources of LA include chia seeds, seed, hempseed, grapeseed, pumpkin seeds, sunflower seeds, safflower seeds, soybeans, olives, pine nuts, pistachio nuts, peanuts, almonds, cashews, chestnuts, and their respective oils.

The conversion of LA to GLA (and ALA to DHA) is reduced by trans fat consumption, smoking, pollution, stress, infections, and various chemicals that affect the liver.

Docosahexaenoic acid (DHA) obtained from algae, fish and krill, has significant therapeutic and anti-inflammatory effects according to the research. DHA is also associated with stronger cell membranes, and lower levels of lipid peroxidation.

It appears that the anti-inflammatory effects of DHA in particular relate to a modulation of a gene factor called NF-kappaB. The NF-kappaB is involved in signaling among cytokine receptors. With more DHA consumption, the transcription of the NF-kappaB gene sequence is reduced. This appears to reduce inflammatory signaling (Singer *et al.* 2008).

DHA readily converts to EPA by the body. EPA degrades quickly if unused in the body. It is easily converted from DHA as needed. Our bodies store DHA and not EPA.

Because much of the early research on the link between fatty acids and inflammatory disease was performed using fish oil, it was assumed that both EPA and DHA fatty acids reduced inflammation. Recent research from the University of Texas' Department of Medicine/Division of Clinical Immunology and Rheumatology (Rahman *et al.* 2008) has clarified that DHA is primarily implicated in reducing inflammation. DHA was shown to inhibit RANKL-induced pro-inflammatory cytokines, and a number of inflammation steps, while EPA did not.

The process of converting ALA to DHA and other omega-3s requires an enzyme produced in the liver called delta-6 desaturase. Some people—especially those who have a poor diet, are immune-suppressed, or burdened with toxicity such as cigarette smoke—may not produce this enzyme very well. As a result, they may not convert as much ALA to DHA and EPA.

For those with low levels of DHA—or for those with problems converting ALA and DHA—low-environmental impact and low toxin content DHA from microalgae can be supplemented. Certain algae produce significant amounts of DHA. They are the foundation for the DHA molecule all the way up the food chain, including fish. This is how fish get their DHA, in other words. Three algae species—*Crypthecodinium cohnii, Nitzschia laevis* and *Schizochytrium spp.*—are in commercial production and available in oil and capsule form.

Microalgae-derived DHA is preferable to fish or fish oils because fish oils typically contain saturated fats and may also—depending upon their origin—contain toxins such as mercury and PCBs (though to their credit, many producers also carefully distill their fish oil). However, we should note that salmon contain a considerable amount of arachidonic acid as well (Chilton 2006).

Thus, the DHA derived from fish sources, because it requires increased levels of filtering and processing to remove PCBs and mercury, would not be considered a living source of DHA, as it is too far removed from the living source. Algae-derived DHA is a wholesome source, as it is derived directly from living algae. Algae-derived DHA also does not strain sensitive fishery populations.

Algal-DHA also decreases pro-inflammatory arachidonic acid levels. One study (Arterburn *et al.* 2007) measured pro-inflammatory arachidonic acid levels within the body before and after supplementation with algal DHA. It was found that arachidonic acid levels decreased by 20% following just one dose of 100 milligrams of algal DHA.

For those who consider fish the superior source of DHA: In a study by researchers from The Netherlands' Wageningen University Toxicology Research Center (van Beelen *et al.* 2007), all three species of commercially produced algal oil showed equivalency with fish oil in their inhibition of cancer cell growth. Another study (Lloyd-Still *et al.* 2007) of twenty cystic fibrosis patients concluded that 50 milligrams of algal DHA was readily absorbed, maintained DHA bioavailability immediately, and increased circulating DHA levels by four to five times.

In terms of DHA availability, algal-DHA is just as good as fish. In a randomized open-label study (Arterburn *et al.* 2008), researchers gave 32 healthy men and women either algal DHA oil or cooked salmon for two weeks. After the two weeks, plasma levels of circulating DHA were bioequivalent.

Alpha-linolenic acid (ALA) is the primary omega-3 fatty acid the body can most easily assimilate. Once assimilated, the healthy body will convert ALA to omega-3s, primarily DHA, at a range of about 7-40%, depending upon the health of the liver. One study of six women performed at England's University of Southampton (Burdge *et al.* 2002) showed a conversion rate of 36% from ALA to DHA and other omega-3s. A follow-up study of men showed ALA conversion to the omega-3s occurred at an average of 16%.

We should include that ALA, which comes from plants, has been shown to halt or slow inflammation processes, similar to DHA. In studies at Wake Forest University (Chilton *et al.* 2008), for example, flaxseed oil produced anti-inflammatory effects, along with borage oil and echium oil (the latter two also containing GLA).

Furthermore, flaxseed has been recommended specifically for toxicity and inflammation for centuries. This is not only because of its omega-3 levels: it is also because flaxseed contains mucilage, which helps strengthen our mucosal membranes.

The healthy fat balance: In a meta-study by researchers from the University of Crete's School of Medicine (Margioris 2009), numerous studies showed that long-chain polyunsaturated omega-3s tend to be anti-inflammatory while omega-6 oils tend to be pro-inflammatory.

This, however, simplifies the equation too much. Most of the research on fats has also shown that most omega-6s are healthy oils. Balance is the key.

Research has illustrated that reducing animal-derived saturated fats reduces inflammation, cardiovascular disease, high cholesterol and diabetes (Ros and Mataix 2008). All of these relate to toxicity, because as we've discussed, lipid peroxidation lies at the root of these conditions.

The relationships became clearer from a study performed at Sydney's Heart Research Institute (Nicholls *et al.* 2008). Here fourteen adults consumed meals either rich in saturated fats or omega-6 polyunsaturated fats. They were tested following each meal for various inflammation and cholesterol markers. The results showed that the high saturated fat meals increased inflammatory activities and decreased the liver's production of HDL cholesterol; whereas (good) HDL levels and the liver's anti-inflammatory capacity were increased after the omega-6 meals.

What this tells us is that the omega-3/omega-6 story is complicated by the saturated fat content of the diet and subsequent liver function. High saturated fat diets increase (bad) LDL (lipid peroxidation) content and reduce the anti-inflammatory and antioxidant capacities of the liver. Diets lower in saturated fat and higher in omega-6 and omega-3 fats encourage antioxidant and anti-inflammatory activity.

We also know that diets high in monounsaturated fats—such as the Mediterranean diet—are also associated with significant anti-inflammatory effects. Mediterranean diets contain higher levels of monounsaturated fats like oleic acids (omega-9) from foods like olives and avocados (and their oils); as well as higher proportions of fruits and vegetables, and lower proportions of saturated fats.

High saturated fat diets are also associated with increased obesity, and a number of studies have shown that obesity is directly related to inflammatory diseases—including allergies as we've discussed. High saturated fat diets and diets high in trans fatty acids have also been clearly shown to accompany higher levels of inflammation—illustrated by increases in inflammatory factors such as IL-6 and CRP (Basu *et al.* 2006).

To maximize anti-inflammatory factors, the ideal proportion of omega-6s to omega-3s is recommended at about two to one (2:1). The western diet has been estimated by researchers to up to thirty to one (30:1) of omega-6s to omega-3s. This large imbalance (of too much omega-6s and too little omega-3s) has also been associated with inflammatory diseases, including asthma, arthritis, heart disease, ulcerative colitis, Crohn's disease, and others. When fat consumption is out of balance, the body's metabolism will trend towards inflammation. This is because in the absence of omega-3s and GLA, omega-6 oils convert more easily to arachidonic acid. And remember, ARA is pro-inflammatory (Simopoulos 1999).

Noting the research showing the relationships between the different fatty acids and inflammation, and the condition of the liver (which can be burdened by too much saturated fat), scientists have logically arrived at a model for dietary fat consumption for a person who is either dealing with or wants to prevent inflammation-oriented conditions and toxicity:

Omega-3	20%-25% of dietary fats
Omega-6+Omega-9	40%-50% of dietary fats
Saturated	5%-10% of dietary fats
GLA	10%-20% of dietary fats
Trans fats	0% of dietary fats

Nuts, seeds, grains, beans, olives and avocados can provide the bulk of these healthy fats in balanced combinations. Walnuts, pumpkin seeds, flax, chia, soy, canola and algal-DHA can fill in the omega 3s. Healthy saturated fats can be found in coconuts, palm and dairy products. These foods are typical of the Mediterranean diet.

Traditional Antioxidant Food Recipes

This brings us to some traditional food recipes that provide superior antioxidant power. The science on quercetin, enzymes and antioxidants now gives some of these cleansing remedies significant credibility:

> *Lemon and honey:* This remedy is often blended with an herbal tea such as peppermint or chamomile. The combination of lemon juice and honey provide an alkalizing and cleansing effect.

> *Super salsa:* This Mexican dish provides cilantro, garlic, cayenne peppers and tomatoes to stimulate blood purification and

> *Honion syrup:* Equal parts chopped onions and raw honey provides constituents to stimulate the immune system.

> *Horseradish syrup:* Equal parts grated horseradish and honey will clear the sinuses and open the airways, while providing an alkalizing effect.

> *Garlic syrup:* Garlic and raw honey combine two anti-microbials and immune-system boosters.

> *Super pickles:* Jerusalem Artichokes, celery and carrot, pickled in apple cider vinegar provide a great alkalizer and blood purifier.

> *Raw vegetable juices:* Juiced endive, celery and carrots. These feed us with immediate nutrients that stimulate our immune system and alkalize our blood.

> *Super soup:* Barley, celery, carrots, beets and ginger. These also provide significant blood alkalizing effects, liver cleansing and stimulate the immune system.

> *Super fruits:* Raw apricots, blueberries, blackberries, strawberries. These provide significant levels of antioxidants.

> *Miso soup:* Miso provides a fermented form of soybeans that stimulates immunity. This remedy has been a long-time favorite among Asian countries.

> *Turmeric curry dishes:* Ayurvedic cooking provides many traditional dishes steeped in spices that stimulate the immune system and provide antioxidants. Turmeric is a favorite that has shown to reduce cancer risk. This is only one type of spiced dish that Ayurvedic cooking provides. An Ayurvedic cookbook is suggested.

The Importance of Raw, Fresh Foods

Most nutrients are heat-sensitive. Vitamin C, fat-soluble vitamins A, E and B vitamins are reduced during pasteurization. Many fatty acids are transformed by high heat to unhealthy fats. Important plant nutrients, such as anthocyanins and polyphenols, are also reduced during pasteurization, along with various enzymes. Proteins are denatured or broken down when heated for long. While this can aid in amino acid absorption, it can also form unrecognized peptide combinations. In milk, for example, some of the nutritious whey protein, or lactabumin, will denature into a number of peptide combinations that are not readily absorbed.

A 2008 study on strawberry puree from the University of Applied Sciences in Switzerland showed a 37% reduction in vitamin C and a significant loss in antioxidant potency after pasteurization. A 1998 study from Brazil's Universidade Estadual de Maringa determined that Barbados cherries lost about 14% of their vitamin C content after pasteurization. During heat treatment, vitamin C will also convert to dehydroascorbic acid together with a loss of bioflavonoids.

A 2008 study at Spain's Cardenal Herrera University determined that glutathione peroxidase—an important antioxidant contained in milk—was significantly reduced by pasteurization. In 2006, the University also released a study showing that lysine content was significantly decreased by milk pasteurization. A 2005 study at the Universidade Federal do Rio Grande determined that pasteurizing milk reduced vitamin A (retinol) content from an average of 55 micrograms to an average of 37 micrograms. A study at North Carolina State University in 2003 determined that HTST pasteurization significantly reduced conjugated linoleic acid (CLA) content—an important fatty acid in milk shown to reduce cancer and encourage good fat metabolism.

A 2006 study on bayberries at the Southern Yangtze University determined that plant antioxidants such as anthocyanins and polyphenolics were reduced from 12-32% following UHT pasteurization. Polyphenols, remember, are the primary nutrients in fruits and vegetables that render anticarcinogenic and antioxidant effects.

One of the most important losses from pasteurization is its enzyme content. Diary and plant foods contain a variety of enzymes that aid in the assimilation or catalyzing of nutrients and antioxidants. These include xanthenes, lysozymes, lipases, oxidases, amylases, lactoferrins and many others contained in raw foods. The body uses food enzymes in various ways. Some enzymes, such as papain from papaya and bromelain from pineapples, dissolve artery plaque and reduce inflammation. While the body makes many of its own enzymes, it also absorbs many food enzymes or uses their components to make new ones.

Pasteurization also typically leaves the food or beverage with a residual caramelized flavor due to the conversation of the enzymes, flavonoids and sugars to other compounds. In milk, for example, there is a substantial conversion from lactose to lactulose (and caramelization) after UHT pasteurization. Lactulose can cause intestinal cramping, nausea and vomiting.

In the case of pasteurized juices, pasteurization can leave the beverage in a highly acidic state, which can irritate our mucous membranes and intestines.

As for irradiation, there is little research on the resulting nutrient content outside of a few microwave studies (which showed decreased nutrient content and the formation of undesirable metabolites). There is good reason to believe that irradiation may thus denature some nutrients.

Whole foods in nature's packages are significantly different from pasteurized processed foods. Fresh whole foods produced by plants contain various antioxidants and enzymes that reduce the ability of microorganisms to grow. The Creator also provided whole foods with peels and shells that protect nutrients and keep most microorganisms out. Microorganisms may invade the outer shell or peel somewhat, but the peel's pH, dryness and density—together with the pH of the inner fruit—provide extremely effective barriers to microorganisms and oxidation.

For this reason, most fruits and nuts can be easily stored for days and even weeks without having significant nutrient reduction. Once the peel or shell is removed, the inner fruit, juice or nut must be consumed to prevent oxidation and contamination—depending upon its pH and sugar content.

Whole natural foods also contain polysaccharides and oligosaccharides that combine nutrients and sugar within complex fibers. These combinations also help prevent oxidation and pathogenic bacteria colonization. With heat processing, however, the sugars are broken down into more simplified, refined form, which allows microbial growth and oxidation. Why? Because simple sugars provide convenient energy sources for aggressive bacteria and fungi colonies. By contrast, our probiotics are used to eating the complexed oligosaccharides in fibrous foods. In other words, heat-processing produces the perfect foods for pathogenic microorganism colonization.

As we discussed in the last chapter, pathogenic microorganisms provide the fuel for systemic inflammation. They can infect the body's (and airways') tissues directly, and/or their endotoxins—waste products—stream into our bloodstream to max out our immune system and detoxification processes. This causes systemic inflammation, and toxicity.

Healthy Cooking

While raw whole foods are often more wholesome to the body, some foods must be cooked to make them more digestible. These include most grains, beans, and some vegetables. Our section on Chinese medicine earlier illustrated that some herbs also require cooking to eliminate certain toxins.

The question is: how much cooking and processing do we need to do to our foods? How much cooking is necessary? Yes, cooking some foods often increases their digestibility. This is particularly important with grain-based foods and beans. Cooking these foods will help break down their fibers and complex carbohydrates into more digestible forms.

Also, many vegetables are more assimilable when they are cooked—or even better, steamed. Steaming vegetables in a pot with a covered lid will preserve most nutrients, while softening some of fibers that hold the nutrients. Foods such as beets, asparagus, broccoli, rhubarb, squash and many others are delicious and nutritious after being steamed or lightly boiled in clean water.

Other plant foods are best eaten raw. These include lettuce, cucumbers, avocado, onions and many others. Because the nutrients in these foods are not so tightly bound within the cell walls of the plants, they can be destroyed by the heat and/or easily separated during cooking.

While the cell walls of plants do contain nutrients, they must be broken down during mastication and digestion. Some cell walls are tougher than others are, and require cooking or processing to break their cell walls. Chlorella—a blue-green algae—is a good example. Many nutrients in chlorella are bound within tightly-packed cell walls, so chlorella is more nutritious when the cell walls have been broken prior to ingestion.

A healthy diet strikes a balance between raw and cooked foods. A perfect way to accomplish this is a dinner that includes a salad topped with seeds, yogurt, olive oil and apple cider vinegar; and an entrée of cooked grains and/or beans with a nice sauce spiced with antioxidant herbs. Breakfast and lunch can include fresh fruit, nuts, raw cheese and fermented dairy; with lightly cooked grains such as oats and barley. Snacks can go raw with apples, nuts, raisins and seeds for sustained, slow-digesting energy and essential fats.

A plant-based food diet can be extremely creative and varied. It can also be extremely colorful and exotic. This is because there are so many different foods and spices to choose from. A flip through a Mediterranean diet cookbook will confirm this immediately.

Detoxifying Probiotics

As we've discussed, probiotics are called 'friendly' because they boost our immunity and our body's ability to purge toxins and microorganisms from our systems. They make up the strongest part of our living immune system, making up over 70% of our immunity.

Probiotics also help us digest food and they secrete beneficial nutritional products. Unbelievably, probiotics are a good source of a number of essential nutrients. They can manufacture biotin, thiamin (B1), riboflavin (B2), niacin (B3), pantothenic acid (B5), pyridoxine (B6), cobalamine (B12), folic acid, vitamin A and vitamin K. Their lactic acid secretions also increase the assimilation of minerals that require acid for absorption, such as copper, iron, magnesium, chromium, selenium and manganese among many others.

Probiotics are also critical to nutrient absorption. They break away amino acids from complex proteins, and mid-chain fatty acids from complex fats. They help break down bile acids. They help convert polyphenols from plant materials into assimilable biomolecules. They also aid in soluble fiber fermentation, yielding digestible fatty acids and sugars. Among many other nutritive tasks, they also help increase the bioavailability of calcium.

Nutrients and Probiotics

Biotin	Produced by probiotics
Thiamin (B1)	Produced by probiotics
Riboflavin (B2)	Produced by probiotics
Niacin (B3)	Produced by probiotics
Pantothenic Acid (B5)	Produced by probiotics
Pyridoxine (B6)	Produced by probiotics
Cobalamine (B12)	Produced by probiotics
Folic Acid (B9)	Produced by probiotics
Vitamin A	Produced by probiotics
Vitamin K	Produced by probiotics
Copper	Probiotics increase bioavailability
Calcium	Probiotics increase bioavailability
Magnesium	Probiotics increase bioavailability
Iron	Probiotics increase bioavailability
Manganese	Probiotics increase bioavailability
Selenium	Probiotics increase bioavailability
Chromium	Probiotics increase bioavailability
Potassium	Probiotics increase bioavailability
Zinc	Probiotics increase bioavailability
Proteins	Probiotics break down for digestibility
Fats	Probiotics break down for digestibility
Carbohydrates	Probiotics break down and process
Sugars	Probiotics break down and process
Milk	Probiotics increase digestibility

| Phytonutrients | Probiotics increase digestibility |
| Cholesterol | Probiotics bind to + reduce blood levels |

Many of the nutrients found in vitamin supplements and supplemented foods are in fact produced by probiotics. Most commercial forms of vitamin B12, for example, are derived from the probiotics *Propionibacterium shermanii*, *Pseudomonas denitrificans* or *Streptomyces griseus*.

We should note here that not all probiotics produce the same nutrients. Some, in fact, will consume some nutrients that others manufacture. For example, *Lactobacillus bulgaricus* will produce folic acid in yogurt, and *Lactobacillus acidolphilus* will consume folic acid. At the end of the day, a mixture of probiotics will still have a net increase in nutrients, however. For this reason, most cultured dairy products have significantly higher nutrient contents than the milk or cream they were made with.

Probiotics also assist in peristalsis—the rhythmic motion of the digestive tract—by helping move intestinal contents through the system. They also produce antifungal substances such as acidophillin, bifidin and hydrogen peroxide, which counteract the growth of not-so-friendly yeasts. Probiotic hydrogen peroxide secretions are also oxygenating, providing free radical scavenging. In addition, they can manufacture some essential fatty acids, and are the source of 5-10% of all short-chained fatty acids essential for healthy immune system function.

An example of the extent of probiotics' ability to produce antimicrobials is the antibiotic streptomycin. This antibiotic, produced by the probiotic bacteria, *Streptomyces griseus* was discovered in 1943 by Selman Waksman.

Probiotics directly and indirectly break down toxins utilizing biochemical secretions and colonizing activities. Nutrients produced by probiotics have been found to have antitumor and anticancer effects within the body. Some probiotics can prevent assimilation of toxins like mercury and other heavy metals. Others will directly bind these toxins or will facilitate their binding to other molecules in order to remove them.

Probiotic nutrients are instrumental in slowing cellular degeneration and the diseases associated with it. Through their nutritive mechanisms, probiotics help normalize serum levels of cholesterol and triglycerides. Some probiotics even help break down and rebuild hormones.

Probiotic nutrients can also increase the productivity of the spleen and thymus—the key organs of the immune system.

Probiotics are necessary components to healthy digestion. Their populations dwell along and within the intestinal mucosal lining, providing a protective barrier to assist in the process of filtering and digesting toxins and other matter prior to these toxins encountering the intestinal wall cells. This mechanism helps maintain the brush barrier cells and keep the mucosal lining of our intestines from damage caused by foreign molecules coming from our foods and their metabolites. Damage to the brush cells of the intestinal lining is the prime cause for a number of irritable bowel disorders.

Illustrating probiotic production of one critical nutrient, Italian researchers (Strozzi and Mogna 2008) gave 23 healthy volunteers *Bifidobacterium adolescentis* DSM 18350, *B. adolescentis* DSM 18352, or *Bifidobacterium pseudocatenulatum* DSM 18353. Stool samples taken before and 48 hours after administration showed a significant increase of bioavailable folic acid from each of the probiotic strains.

Probiotics will also compete with pathogenic organisms for nutrients. Assuming good numbers, this strategy can check pathobiotic growth substantially. Nutrients produced by probiotics will also help stimulate the immune cell production, and normalize their activity during inflammatory circumstances.

Let's review some of the most available probiotic foods. These are fermented or cultured foods that are teeming with probiotic bacteria and yeasts. These include yogurt and kefir, but also raw cheeses, traditional cottage cheese, traditional sour cream, traditional buttermilk, traditional sauerkraut, lassi, amasake (Japanese sweet rice drink), traditional miso, traditional tempeh, traditional tamari, traditional soy sauce and traditional kombucha tea and others.

Other foods utilize probiotics in their preparation. Traditional sourdough bread and bauerbrot are good examples. Most bread, in fact, uses some sort of (often probiotic) yeast fermentation process to prepare the flour for baking. In these, however, the probiotics are likely all killed during baking.

Some of the foods mentioned here are preceded by the word "traditional" because sadly, many of today's versions are pasteurized or otherwise acidified enough to kill any viable probiotic colonies. Both cottage cheese and butter were originally probiotic foods, for example, when we used to eat dairy products from our local dairies or own farms. Today, these two foods are produced commercially without probiotics. Ironically, even many commercial yogurts are unbelievably pasteurized prior to shipping—killing off most if not all of their viable colonies.

Another example is tamari and soy sauce. Today, most commercial versions are brewed with solvents. Probiotics are no longer part of these processes, as were the traditional versions.

Some More Research

In case the reader is not yet convinced of the benefit of probiotic foods on the immune system, here are several other studies illustrating this effect (note that the author's book *Probiotics: Protection Against Infection* reviews several hundred studies illustrating similar effects.)

Illustrating this, Japanese scientists (Hirose *et al.* 2006) gave *Lactobacillus plantarum* strain L-137 or placebo to 60 healthy men and women, average age 56, for twelve weeks. Increased Con A-induced proliferation (acquired immunity), increases in IL-4 production by CD4+ T-cells, and a more balanced

Th1:Th2 ratio was seen in the probiotic group. Quality of life criteria were also higher among the probiotic group.

Researchers from Britain's Scarborough Hospital (McNaught *et al.* 2005) gave a placebo or *Lactobacillus plantarum* 299v to 103 critically ill patients along with conventional therapy. On day 15, the probiotic group had significantly lower serum IL-6 levels compared to the control group.

Researchers from the Department of Immunology at Japan's Juntendo University School of Medicine (Takeda *et al.* 2006) gave a placebo or *Lactobacillus casei* Shirota to 9 healthy middle-aged adults and 10 elderly adults daily for three weeks. After three weeks of supplementation, *L. casei* significantly increased natural killer cell activity among the volunteers, especially among those who had low NK-cell activity before probiotic supplementation.

Researchers from the University of Vienna (Meyer *et al.* 2007) gave healthy women yogurt with starters *Lactobacillus bulgaricus* and *Streptococcus thermophilus*, with or without *Lactobacillus casei*. After two weeks, both yogurt groups had significantly increased blood levels of tumor necrosis factor-alpha (TNF-a): by 24% with the regular yogurt and by 63% with the *L. casei* yogurt. They also observed significantly higher levels of cytokines interleukin (IL)-1beta (by 40%) and interferon gamma (by 108%). In addition, IL-10 decreased during *L. casei*-enhanced yogurt treatment, but then significantly increased after the yogurt treatment was stopped (by 129%).

French scientists (Paineau *et al.* 2008) gave 83 healthy volunteers a placebo or seven probiotic strains, and tested their resulting antibody levels and immune response rates. IgG levels increased in the *Bifidobacterium lactis* Bl-04 and *Lactobacillus acidophilus* La-14 groups; and serum immunoglobulin levels increased significantly from six of the seven probiotic strains.

Probiotics will bind to and prevent LDL-cholesterol from being released back into the bloodstream. This effect reduces levels of cholesterol, and more importantly, levels of LDL-cholesterol in the blood. By reducing LDL-c and increasing HDL-c, less oxidation will take place and less artery damage will result.

Scientists from Denmark's The Royal Veterinary and Agricultural University (Agerholm-Larsen *et al.* 2000) gave 70 overweight and obese adult volunteers 1) placebo pills; 2) a placebo yogurt; 3) a yogurt with two strains of *Streptococcus thermophilus* and two strains of *Lactobacillus acidophilus*; 4) a yogurt with two strains of *Streptococcus thermophilus* and one strain of *Lactobacillus rhamnosus*; or 5) a yogurt with one strain of *Enterococcus faecium* and two strains of *Streptococcus thermophilus*. After eight weeks, LDL-cholesterol decreased by 8.4% (0.26) while fibrinogen increased (0.74) in the *Enterococcus faecium-Streptococcus thermophilus* group (#4). Groups #3 and #4 showed significant decreases in blood pressure as well.

Twenty healthy men were given either milk fermented with *Lactobacillus casei* or a placebo for eight weeks in a double-blind, placebo-controlled study from Japan (Kawase *et al.* 2000). Blood samples were taken before, after 4 weeks and after 8 weeks. After 4 and 8 weeks, the high-density lipoprotein cholesterol levels (HDL-c) were significantly higher for the probiotic group while the placebo group showed no change. The probiotic group also had lower triglycerides levels after 4 weeks while the placebo group showed no change.

Researchers from the Tehran University of Medical Sciences (Ataie-Jafari *et al.* 2009) gave 14 healthy subjects with serum total cholesterol levels of 200 to 300 mg/dL 300 grams of ordinary yogurt or yogurt fermented with *Lactobacillus acidophilus* and *Bifidobacterium lactis*. After the six-week period, the probiotic yogurt group showed a significant decrease in total cholesterol levels compared to the ordinary yogurt group.

Forty-three volunteers were given either a placebo or *Enterococcus faecium* M-74 plus 50 micrograms of organically bound selenium in a double-blind, placebo-controlled study (Hlivak *et al.* 2005). After 56 weeks, total cholesterol among the probiotic group reduced from 229 to 201 mg/dL. LDL cholesterol fell from 149 to 119 mg/dL. No significant changes were seen in the placebo group. The researchers concluded that *E. faecium* reduced serum cholesterol by 12% during the test period.

Japanese researchers (Xiao *et al.* 2003) gave yogurt with a combination of *Streptococcus thermophilus* and *Lactobacillus delbrueckii* subsp. bulgaricus (SL), or the same combination with *Bifidobacterium longum* strain BL1 to 32 human subjects with total cholesterol from 220 to 280 mg/dL. After four weeks, the total cholesterol reduced by half in the *B. longum* group, while the cholesterol levels among the normal yogurt group remained nearly unchanged.

In research from Germany's Friedrich Schiller University (Klein *et al.* 2008), 26 healthy volunteers took a yogurt supplement with probiotic strains *L. acidophilus* 74-2 and *B. lactis* 420 or a placebo for five weeks. After the five weeks, they were tested and crossed over. Final test results revealed that the probiotic group's triglyceride levels decreased by 11.6%. Immune system granulocytes and monocytes with phagocytic activity significantly increased in the probiotic group as well.

Researchers from the Department of Neurology and Geriatrics at Japan's Kagoshima University Graduate School of Medical and Dental Sciences (Matsuzaki *et al.* 2005) studied *Lactobacillus casei* Shirota as a treatment of HTLV-1 associated myelopathy/tropical spastic paraparesis. Ten HTLV-1 patients with myelopathy/tropical spastic paraparesis were given either a placebo or *Lactobacillus casei* Shirota fermented in milk for four weeks. NK-cell activity significantly increased. Spasticity—gauged by a modified Ashworth Scale—significantly decreased. Other urinary components indicating enhanced immunity were also seen following the probiotic treatment.

Researchers from Finland's University of Turku (Ouwehand *et al.* 2008) gave a placebo, *Bifidobacterium longum*, or *Bifidobacterium lactis* Bb-12 to 55 institutionalized elderly subjects for 6 months. The probiotic groups had modulated pro-inflammatory cytokine TNF-alpha and cytokine IL-10 levels compared with the placebo group.

Scientists from Spain's University of Navarra (Parra *et al.* 2004) investigated the effects of fermented milk with *Lactobacillus casei* DN114001 on 45 healthy volunteers, ages 51-58. The probiotic group showed increased oxidative burst capacity among monocytes, and increased NK-cell tumor suppression activity. The researchers concluded that *L. casei* can have "a positive effect in modulating the innate immune defense in healthy-middle-age people."

Here are a few probiotic foods (among many others) to consider adding to our diets:

Traditional Yogurt

Because yogurt is usually produced using *L. bulgaricus, S. thermophilus* and sometimes *L. acidophilus*, it is certainly a good source of probiotics. However, we should clarify again that pasteurization kills many probiotics. This means that commercial yogurts that pasteurize the yogurt after it has been cultured will have killed most or all of those colonies used to convert the milk to yogurt. Some producers pasteurize the milk first and then make the yogurt.

The best yogurt is made using raw milk. It is quite simple to make yogurt: After heating a pot of milk to 180 degrees F (82 C) momentarily, we can add a half-cup of starter (active yogurt from a previous batch or an active commercial yogurt) into the milk after it cools to about 105 degrees F (40 C). After stirring thoroughly, we can put the container in a warm, clean, dry place, with a clean towel or loose seal over the container. The mixture will sour and gel in about six to ten hours depending upon temperature. Then we can jar and refrigerate.

The ideal blend of probiotic species for a yogurt starter—one that was developed over the centuries by the Bulgarians—is a ratio of seven parts *S. thermophilus* to one part *L. bulgaricus*. This ratio produces the ideal sourness that is tasty yet tart. It also prevents the *L. bulgaricus* from outgrowing and overwhelming the *S. thermophilus*.

This later point is one of the reasons why yogurt starters that include *L. acidophilus* often fail to supply any *L. acidophilus* in the end product. *L. bulgaricus* is a hardy organism that will easily overtake *L. acidophilus* in a culture. The use of *L. acidophilus* in yogurt is not only wasteful, but possibly can result in an overly acidic flavor, as *L. bulgaricus* colonies swell with the lactic acid produced initially by *L. acidophilus*. In addition, it appears that *L. bulgaricus* produce small amounts of hydrogen peroxide—which knocks out the *L. acidophilus* colonies.

The moral of this also is not to expect much in the way of *L. acidophilus* in a commercial yogurt that blends *L. acidophilus* with *L. bulgaricus*.

Yogurt and other fermented dairy foods have little or no lactose. This is because the probiotics convert the lactose to lactic acid. The lactic acid is healthy for the intestinal tract, because it renders a medium that helps promote our own probiotic colonies. Lactic acid also offers a pleasing tart flavor to yogurt and other fermented dairy.

Traditional Kefir

Kefir is a traditional drink originally developed in the Caucasus region of what is now considered southern Russia, Georgia, Armenia and Azerbaijan. Here Moslem tribe leaders vigorously protected their kefir recipe, as it was considered an esteemed and regal food with healing properties. The secret recipe was eventually ransomed by a young beautiful female Russian emissary who was kidnapped by a local prince. She wrestled a few kefir grains from the secrecy of the prince's family as a settlement for her abduction. She brought kefir into the Moscow market shortly thereafter and it spread as a highly prized healing food all over Russia and Europe. Kefir also became a focus of Soviet research, discovering some of the surprising benefits of probiotics we have outlined in this book.

Kefir uses fermented milk mixed with kefir grains that resemble little chunks of cauliflower. One tablespoon of kefir grains can be mixed with whole milk and sealed in a jar at room temperature. The milk is fermented overnight in a warm location with the starter grains. Depending upon the temperature, milk and kefir grains, it will take 1-3 days to completely ferment. The jar should be opened and swirled one to two times a day. The grains are screened or filtered out and utilized for the next batch. Cow's milk is most used, but sheep's milk, goat's milk or deer milk can also be used.

Buttermilk

Buttermilk is a soured beverage that was originally curdled from cream. Traditional buttermilk utilized the acids that probiotic bacteria produce for curdling. Today, forced curdling is done using commercially available acidic products. Cream of tartar, lemon juice or vinegar is added to heated and stirred whole milk at a rate of one tablespoon per cup of milk, until the curdling starts. After standing for 15 minutes and stirring another 15, it is refrigerated. See the butter section for the traditional method.

Traditional Butter

Today commercial butter contains no probiotics. Traditionally, butter was made with the cow's natural probiotics. The raw milk sits for a half-day or day depending upon temperature, until the cream rises to the top. The cream is taken from the milk to be churned and aged; letting the probiotics convert lactose to lactic acid. This creates a mix of buttermilk and butter. The buttermilk is strained off, leaving the butter. The butter can be further dried of moisture and mixed with salt for taste. Again, the probiotics from the raw milk will have matured the butter and buttermilk naturally.

Traditional Cottage Cheese

Commercial cottage cheese is now made without probiotics. It was a probiotic process before dairy processors began to pasteurize the product and force the curdling with lactic acids. Again, probiotics also produce the lactic acids that were used to curdle the product in traditional cottage cheese making. Skim milk with cream and buttermilk is probably the easiest way to make cottage cheese at home today, using the curds off the cream separation. The probiotics arising from the buttermilk help curdle the thickened milk and cream before separating the curds. Salt is one of the secrets to making a tasty cottage cheese.

Traditional Kimchi

Kimchi is a fermented cabbage with a wonderful history from Korea. Kimchi was considered a ceremonial food served to emperors and ambassadors. It also was highly regarded as a healing and tonic food. There are a variety of different recipes of kimchi, depending upon the region and occasion.

Kimchi can be made by slicing and mixing cabbage with warm water, salt, ginger, garlic, red pepper, green onions, oil and a crushed apple. It is then put into a sealed jar(s) at room temperature for 24 hours, before putting into the refrigerator to continue the fermenting process (*Lactobacillus kimchii* is a typical colonizer). After several weeks of continued fermentation in the fridge, it is ready for eating.

Traditional Miso

Miso is an ancient food from Japan. A well-made miso will contain over 160 strains of aerobic probiotic bacteria. This is because the ingredients are perfect prebiotics for these probiotics.

Miso is produced by fermenting beans and grains. Soybeans are often used, but other types of beans are also used. Equal parts soaked and cooked soybeans and rice are mixed. A fungi spore (koji, or *Aspergillus oryzae*) and salt is added to the rice prior to mixing. The mixture is put into a covered container in a dark, dry, room-temperature location and stirred occasionally. It can take up to a year of aging like this for the fermentation to result in a tasty miso.

When other beans other than soy are used, they will produce different varieties of miso. Shiromiso is white miso, kuromiso is black miso, and akamiso is red miso. They are each made with different beans. There are also various other miso recipies, many of which are highly guarded by their makers.

Traditional Shoyu

Shoyu is a traditional form of soy sauce made by blending a mixture of cooked soybeans and wheat, again with koji, or *Aspergillus oryzae*. The combination is fermented for an extended time. The aging process for shoyu is dependent upon the storage temperature and cooking methods used, and is also guarded.

Traditional Tempeh

Tempeh is an aged and fermented soybean food. It is extremely healthy and contains a combination of probiotics and naturally metabolized soy. Tempeh is made by first soaking dehulled soybeans for 10-12 hours. The beans are then cooked for 20 minutes and strained. The dry, cooked beans are then mixed with a tempeh starter containing *Rhyzopus oryzae, Rhizopus oligosporus* or both. The mixture is shaped and flattened (about a half-inch high) and put into a warm (room temperature) incubation container for a day or two. The cake will be full with white mycelium (fungal roots) when it is ready. It can then be eaten raw, baked, or toasted.

Other beans other than soy are also sometimes used to make tempeh. The trick is in getting good starter colonies.

Traditional Kombucha Tea

Kombucha tea is an ancient beverage from the orient. Its use dates back many centuries; and was used by China and Taiwanese emperors. Its use was later popularized in Russia, and then in Eastern Europe, where its reputation grew. A quality kombucha tea will contain a number of probiotics, including *Acetobacter xylinum, Acetobacter xylinoides, Glucobacter bluconicum, Acetobacter aceti, Saccharomycodes Ludwigii, Schizosaccharomyces pombe,* and *Picha fermentans*—and other yeasts in the *Schizosaromyces* genus. The fermenting of these organisms renders a beverage that is full of nutrients and enzymes as well as healthy biotics. Kombucha has enjoyed a reputation of being detoxifying and revitalizing. Many alternative health experts have described it as a tonic.

Kombucha is made by blending a black or green tea with sugar, kombucha starter culture, and sometimes a bit of vinegar to create a slightly acidic environment. It is critical that a healthy starter be used. The mixture is then fermented in a warm, dry environment. It requires oxygen, yet will suffer from any toxins or bacteria from the air. Following a couple of weeks of fermentation, the product should be refrigerated to slow down growth and acidity.

Care should be taken to make sure the yeasts have adequately fermented the ethanols. Otherwise, the kombucha can be as high as 3-5% alcohol, and not healthy. Also be leery of a funky "mother." A kombucha mother might have been passed around for many years amongst those who have brewed their kombucha in their basements or other locales where molds and pathogenic bacteria could have joined and thus contaminated the mother.

Traditional Lassi

Lassi is a traditional and popular beverage from India—once enjoyed by kings and governors in ancient India. It is quite simple to make, as it is made with yogurt, fruit and spices. Quite simply, it is a blend of diluted yogurt with fruit pulp—often mango is used in the traditional lassi. A little salt, turmeric and sweetener give it a sweet-n-salty taste. Other spices are also sometimes used. Sugar is often added in today's versions, but honey and/or fruit are preferable.

Traditional Sauerkraut

Sauerkraut is a traditional German fermented food. It is made quite simply, by blending shredded cabbage and pickling salt (12:1, or 3 tablespoons of salt per five pounds of cabbage). The mixture is covered with water and put into a covered bowl or container. It is then stored in the dark in this semi-airtight cover for a month to two months at room temperature. Then it should be stored in the refrigerator in an enclosed container for a month or two to complete the fermentation of the cabbage. Probiotic bacteria such as *Lactobacillus plantarum* and *L. brevis* will typically overtake the early-growth bacteria during fermentation. This is a testament to the power of probiotics.

There are a number of other wonderful fermented foods that can be included into a probiotic-rich diet. This sampling illustrates the general techniques of fermentation. As we can see here, bacteria and fungi in our foods are not necessarily bad. To the contrary, if cultured correctly, they can be healthy for us, and may even help prevent infection from their more lethal cousins.

Most of these foods are traditional and even ancient foods that have been passed down through generations over thousands of years. This does not mean that we cannot be creative, however.

For example, there is a lot that can be done with yogurt. We've all heard of frozen yogurt, and certainly that is one. But yogurt in some cultures, such as among Indians, is eaten with every meal. It is eaten with and in salads, and rice dishes. Yogurt is creamy and delicious, and can make for an excellent salad dressing with a little oil and vinegar and dill. It can also be added to nearly every sauce to make the sauce creamy and delicious.

Kefir and lassi cultures can be added to nearly every combination of beverage, including smoothies and shakes.

Just about every vegetable can be pickled. Pickles using brine with probiotics is delicious and healthy. We can pickle peppers, olives and so many other foods.

Fermented beverages are now the rage among healthy foods. There are now many fermented beverages, including kombucha and others.

Raw vs. Pasteurized Milk

This naturally brings us to the topic of milk, since there are many reports that indicate that dairy may not be so healthy—and not conducive to detoxification processes.

To the contrary, numerous experiments have shown that raw milk, and dairy containing probiotics such as yogurt is not only healthy, but stimulates the immune system and fights off disease.

First let's consider a study by researchers at Switzerland's University of Basel (Waser *et al.* 2007). The researchers studied 14,893 children between the ages of five and 13 from five different European countries, including 2,823 children from farms, and 4,606 children attending a Steiner School (known for its farm-based living and instruction). The researchers found that drinking farm milk was associated with decreased incidence of allergies and asthma. Why?

Raw milk from the cow can contain a host of bacteria, including *Lactobacillus acidophilus, L. casei, L. bulgaricus* and many other healthy probiotics. Cows that feed from primarily grasses will have increased levels of these healthy probiotics. This is because a grass diet provides prebiotics that promote the cow's own probiotic colonies. Should the cow be fed primarily dried grass and dried grains, probiotic counts will be reduced, replaced by more pathogenic bacteria. As a result, most non-grass fed herds must be given lots of antibiotics to help keep their bacteria counts low. Probiotics, on the other hand, naturally keep bacteria counts down.

As a result, the non-grass fed cow's milk will have higher pathogenic bacteria counts than grass-fed cows. This means that the milk itself will also have high counts. When the non-grass-fed cow's milk is pasteurized, the heat kills most of these bacteria. The result is a milk containing dead pathogenic bacteria parts. These are primarily proteins and peptides, which get mixed with the milk and are eventually consumed with the milk.

In other words, pasteurization may kill the living pathogenic bacteria, but it does not get rid of the bacteria proteins. This might be compared to cooking an insect: If an insect landed in our soup, we could surely cook it until it died. But the soup would still contain the insect parts—and proteins.

Now the immune system of most people, and especially infants with their hypersensitive immune system, is trained to attack and discard pathogenic bacteria. And how does the body identify pathogenic bacteria? From their proteins.

In the case of pasteurized commercial milk, our immune systems will readily identify heat-killed microorganism cell parts and proteins and launch an immune response against these proteins as if it were being attacked by the microorganisms directly. This was shown in research from the University of Minnesota two decades ago (Takahashi *et al.* 1992).

It is thus not surprising that weak immune systems readily reject pasteurized cow's milk. In comparison, healthy cow raw milk has fewer pathogenic microorganisms and more probiotic organisms. This has been confirmed by tests done by a California organic milk farm, which compared test results of their raw organic milk against standardized state test results from conventional milk farms.

In addition, pasteurization breaks apart or denatures many of the proteins and sugar molecules. This was illustrated by researchers from Japan's Nagasaki International University (Nodake *et al.* 2010), who found that when beta-lactoglobulin is naturally conjugated with dextran-glycylglycine, its allergenicity is decreased. A dextran is a very long chain of glucose molecules—a polysaccharide. The dextran polysaccharide is naturally joined with the amino acid glycine in raw state. When pasteurized, beta-lactoglobulin is separated.

This is not surprising. Natural whole cow's milk also contains special polysaccharides called oligosaccharides. They are largely indigestible polysaccharides that feed our intestinal bacteria. Because of this trait, these indigestible sugars are called prebiotics.

Whole milk contains a number of these oligosaccharides, including oligogalactose, oligolactose, galactooligosaccharides (GOS) and transgalactooligosaccharides (TOS). Galactooligosaccharides are produced by conversion from enzymes in healthy cows and healthy mothers.

These polysaccharides provide a number of benefits. Not only are they some of the more preferred foods for probiotics: Research has also shown that they reduce the ability of pathogenic bacteria like *E. coli* to adhere to our intestinal cells.

These oligosaccharides also provide environments that reduce the availability of separated beta-lactoglobulin. This is accomplished through a combination of probiotic colonization and the availability of the long-chain polysaccharides that keep these complexes stabilized.

This reduced availability of beta-lactoglobulin has been directly observed in humans and animals following consistent supplementation with probiotics (Taylor *et al.* 2006; Adel-Patient *et al.* 2005; Prioult *et al.* 2003).

It is not surprising, given this information, that people with many conditions have benefited from withdrawing from pasteurized milk and cheese. Raw milk, yogurt, kefir, goat's milk and cheese, along with soy and almond milk, are great alternatives.

What About Casein and Beta-lactoglobulin?

In a number of studies, the milk protein casein has been shown to be implicated in a number of conditions, including cancer (Campbell and Campbell 2006).

In addition, beta-lactoglobulin has been implicated in allergies.

For example, Japanese researchers (Nakano *et al.* 2010) found that casein and beta-lactoglobulin were the main allergens in cow's milk—as confirmed by other research. They also found that 97% of 115 milk allergy children had casein-specific IgE antibodies, while 47% had IgE antibodies against beta-lactoglobulin (beta-LG).

However, fermented dairy and probiotic-rich raw dairy presents an altogether different casein and beta-lactoglobulin molecular structure than does pasteurized milk.

When milk is heated to extremely high degrees, the surfaces of casein micelles—minute fat globules about 100 nanometers in diameter—become harder, and more stable. They move within the fluid but remain in a highly rigid state. Other molecules within the milk do not affect these casein micelles. Thus, the consumption of these rigid casein micelles results in a macromolecule—large protein the body does not easily break down.

However, when dairy is fermented, these casein molecules become destabilized by the probiotics. Once a particular acidity is reached in the milk culture, the casein molecules will become sticky, and they will become congealed—observed as "curdling."

As this curdling takes place—driven by the conversion of lactose to lactic acid by probiotic bacteria—an interesting combination occurs. The destabilized casein micelles react with the beta-lactoglobulin whey protein, which produces a *beta-lactoglobulin-kappa-casein complex*. This neutralizes both the effects of separated beta-lactoglobulin molecules and the casein micelles within the body. In other words, both of these proteins—which spawn radicals in the body—become neutralized through the enzymatic processes driven by probiotic bacteria.

As this occurs, another whey protein, called lactoferrin, also undergoes degradation. This process liberates an immune-stimulating derivative called lactoferricin. This lactoferricin released during the degradation of lactoferrins is also produced by probiotic bacteria, most notably *Streptococcus thermophilus* and *Lactobacillus delbrueckii* ssp. *bulgaricus* (Paul and Somkuti 2010).

Thus we find that these whey-casein components and their derivatives create an altogether different combination of elements in raw milk compared to pasteurized milk. They also maintain known antimicrobial components such as lactoferricin and other bacteriocins.

Prebiotic Foods

One of the most important factors in establishing a healthy environment for our probiotic colonies is making sure they have the right mix of nutrients available. The nutrients our probiotic families favor are called prebiotics. In other words, some foods are particularly beneficial for *bifidobacteria, lactobacilli* and other probiotic populations. These are the oligosaccharides, fructooligosaccharides, galactooligosaccharides, and transgalactooligosaccharides—also referred to as inulin, FOS, GOS and TOS. Even two or three grams of one of these prebiotics will dramatically increase probiotic populations assuming healthy colonies. Inulin, FOS, GOS and TOS are also antagonistic to toxic microorganism genera such as *Salmonella, Listeria, Campylobacter, Shigella* and *Vibrio*. These and other pathogenic bacteria tend to thrive from refined sugars as opposed to the complex saccharides of inulin, FOS, GOS and TOS.

Oligosaccharides are short stacks of simple yet mostly indigestible sugars (from the Greek *oligos*, meaning "few"). If the sugar molecule is fructose, the stacked molecule is called a fructooligosaccharide. If the sugar molecule is galactose, the stacked molecule is called a galactooligosaccharide. These molecules are very useful for human cells and probiotics because they can be processed directly for energy as well as be combined with fatty acids to create cell wall structures and cellular communication molecules. These nutrients also provide energy and nourishment to our probiotic colonies.

The oligosaccharides inulin and oligofructose are probably the most recognized prebiotics. Inulin is a naturally occurring carbohydrate used by plants for storage. It has been estimated that more than 36,000 plant species contain inulin in varying degrees (Carpita *et al.* 1989). The roots often contain the greatest amounts of inulin.

Commercial sources of inulin include Jerusalem artichoke, agave cactus and chicory. Chicory, the root of the Belgian endive, is known to contain some of the highest levels of both inulin at 15-20%, and oligofructose at 5-10%. Inulin from agave has been described as highly branched. This gives it a higher solubility and digestibility than inulin derived from Jerusalem artichoke or chicory.

Notable prebiotic FOS-containing foods include beets, leeks, bananas, tree fruits, soybeans, burdock root, asparagus, maple sugar, whole rye and whole wheat among many others. Bananas contain one of the highest levels of FOS. Bananas are thus a favorite food for both humans and probiotics.

GOS and TOS are natural byproducts of milk. They are produced as lactose is enzymatically converted or hydrolyzed within the digestive tract. This process can also be done commercially. Before much of the recent research on prebiotics was performed, nutritionists simply thought of GOS and TOS as indigestible byproducts of milk.

Another element in plant foods providing prebiotic nutrition for probiotics is the polyphenol group. Polyphenols are groups of biochemicals produced in plants such as lignans, tannins, resveratrol, and flavonoids. There is some uncertainty as to which of these are most helpful to probiotic populations.

Some prebiotics have interesting side effects. For example, there seems to be a relationship between oligofructose inulin and calcium absorption. Inulin has been shown to improve calcium absorption by 20%, and yogurt supplemented with TOS has increased calcium absorption by 16% (van den Heuvel *et al.* 2000)

Galactooligosaccharides have another side effect that is important to note. Dr. Kari Shoaf and fellow researchers at the University of Nebraska (Shoaf *et al.* 2006) found in laboratory tests that galactooligosaccharides reduce the ability of *E. coli* to attach to human cells within tissue cultures. This effect was isolated from GOS' ability to nourish probiotics. This means that GOS provides more than nutrition to our probiotic colonies. This once considered useless indigestible nutrient also helps keep *E. coli* and other pathogenic bacteria from attaching to our cells. A nice package deal indeed.

FOS and GOS have been known to cause digestive disturbance in rare cases. Such a digestive disturbance is likely caused by dysbiosis, however.

Conclusively, a preponderance of scientific literature indicates that probiotics thrive from a diet of plant-based natural foods with plenty of phytonutrients, while overly processed, sugary and meat diets tend to promote pathogenic bacteria and their disease-causing endotoxins.

Yeast Foods and Supplements

Baking yeast and brewer's yeast are common yeasts that are primarily derived from an organism called *Saccharomyces cerevisiae*. In most applications, the yeast is not eaten alive, however. It is *heat-killed* prior to eating. This simply means that it is cooked to a temperature that kills off the viable organisms. This doesn't mean that living *S. cerevisiae* organisms are toxic or anything. In reasonable colony sizes, they are perfectly docile, and even healthy to our bodies because they produce nutrients that our bodies use.

For baking, brewing and supplementation, the heat-killed version of this organism can be very healthy, because when it is alive, it produces a variety of nutrients and immune factors that are left behind in whatever food it was used to ferment.

Just before these yeasts die during heating or baking, they will release intense immune factors in an attempt to protect themselves. These immune factors also help protect our bodies, by stimulating our body's detoxification processes and boosting our immune system. In addition, some of their nutrients, such as B-vitamins produced by yeasts, will donate methyl groups to our liver's glutathione radical-neutralizing processes.

Furthermore, because the biofactors that yeasts produce tend to be acidic, they will lend a tart flavor to the food. This of course lends the flavoring that we relish among our traditional probiotic foods such as cottage cheese, pickles, and so many other foods as we discussed above.

This is the case for sourdough bread, for example. Sourdough bread is not only delicious. It is healthy, even if it is made with white flour (for best results, try whole wheat sourdough bread). Fermented brews such as beer and wine Originally, all the fermented brews such as ginger ale and root beer, were all made using probiotic fermentation.

Yeast Supplements

Baking yeast and Brewer's yeast, Nutritional Yeast and EpiCor®, are all derived from an organism called *Saccharomyces cerevisiae*. This organism is used in brewing and baking. It is thus considered a healthy organism, and acts in a territorial manner to repel organisms and toxins that are seen as foreign to their territories.

For this reason, EpiCor®, Brewer's Yeast or Nutritional Yeast come in dehydrated forms. In other words, the yeast colonies are killed by heat. This heat-killing preserves their nutrients, yet prevents their overgrowth in the body. (However, a person who has mold allergies might still have a reaction to heat-killed yeast because those proteins are still present.)

So what is the difference between EpiCor®, Brewer's Yeast and Nutritional Yeast? The answer lies in their unique processes of fermentation.

Brewer's Yeast is a byproduct of the brewing industry, thus it typically does not have the higher levels of nutrients that the other two have. Brewer's yeast still has a variety of nutrients, including many trace elements (such as chromium and selenium), B vitamins (but typically not B12 as many assume), many antioxidants and proteins.

Nutritional Yeast will typically produce more of these same nutrients, because it has been prepared in such a way that both stresses the yeasts more, and preserves more of their nutrients. Nutritional yeast will contain chromium and selenium, as well as thiamin, riboflavin, niacin, vitamin B6, folate, vitamin B12, pantothenic acid, magnesium, zinc, and a number of amino acids. It is a great protein source, with 50% protein by weight.

EpiCor® is another yeast derivative that is produced using a proprietary method. EpiCor®, however, may have even more enhanced levels of certain nutrients, which include those mentioned above, along with nucleotides and possibly additional antioxidants and immune factors. The reason that EpiCor® may have additional immune factors is because during fermentation, the yeast is *stressed*. Like any organism, when it is stressed, it produces immune factors to protect itself.

After EpiCor® has been stressed, it is then heat-killed, dehydrated and powdered, rendering those immune factors and nutrients.

EpiCor® has been the subject of focused research, which has found that it significantly lowers systemic inflammation.

In one study (Robinson *et al.* 2009), 500 milligrams of EpiCor® or a placebo was given to 80 healthy volunteers with seasonal grass allergies during pollen season. After six and twelve weeks, the EpiCor® group experienced a significant reduction of allergy symptoms compared to the placebo group.

Other EpiCor® studies have shown that it increases salivary IgA (mucosal immunity), and reduces serum IgE (pro-allergy sensitivity).

Red Yeast Rice: The yeast *Monascus purpureus,* when fermented with rice, becomes what is known as red yeast rice. Red yeast rice has been shown in research to lower LDL cholesterol (Liu *et al.* 2006). The mechanism renders red yeast the ability to help prevent lipid peroxidation in the body. Red yeast rice has been used in China for over a thousand years. However, red yeast rice use as a supplement has been questioned by the FDA and pharmaceutical industry. This might have something to do with the fact that correctly fermented red yeast rice can be a significant source of the constituent monacolin K, the primary active ingredient of the statin drug lovastatin.

While there are others, these yeast products have been shown to maximize the body's antioxidant capacities, increase tolerance, and stimulate detoxification processes. They also have considerable research backing up these claims.

Raw Vinegars

Vinegars are excellent living foods that stimulate the body's living purification systems. Vinegar made from apples, grapes or other fruits also contain a variety of antioxidants, as well as acetic acid, which helps stimulate a good environment for our body's own probiotics, and one that repels pathogenic microorganisms.

There are a variety of different types of vinegars, depending upon the raw material used. In all cases, the raw material of a healthy vinegar will be a plant source, fermented by a healthy yeast culture. The yeast culture will convert the sugars of the plant source (and added sugars if used) to alcohol. As the alcohol is fermented further, it is oxidized by the zymase enzymes in the yeast, which convert to alcohol to carboxylic acetic acids. These acetic acids are the main constituent of vinegar, and what gives vinegar its tartness.

To speed up the process, alcohols are often used commercially to make vinegars. These include cheaper or turned wines, distilled alcohol (from wood or grain) and other spirits. The conversion of alcohol to vinegar is much quicker because the first step (sugar to alcohol) has already been made.

Fresh vinegar is typically made by crushing whole apples, grapes, potatoes, barley or other fruits or grains - even pears, bananas and others - into a mash. Sugar can be added to speed up the process, typically at a ratio of one-to-four of mash.

Brewer's yeast (*Saccharomyces cerevisiae*) can then be added for fermentation. One-quarter of a yeast cake will typically inoculate a liter of the mash. Alternatively, a "mother" of fresh vinegar that has been retained from a previous vinegar can be used. Such a "mother" will likely contain more yeast species than just the *S. cerevisiae* yeast, and possibly even some probiotic bacteria. The amount needed depends upon the strength of the "mother," but one cup of the mother (from the top center of the previous batch) per liter should probably do it.

The mix is then put aside in a warm place, with the jar covered by a cloth to let in oxygen. The period of fermentation depends upon the sugar content and the temperature stored. The vinegar may be strained or unstrained. Unstrained retains more living yeasts.

Balsamic vinegars will ferment for years in oak barrels, for example. An apple vinegar might take 60 days to nine months. Care should be taken that the alcohol levels are reduced down to well below .5% (legal alcohol limit). Higher acetic acid levels will mean lower alcohol levels. Testing with a round piece of fine marble (5/6 of marble weight reduction equates to acetic acid levels). Look for 30-32 grams reduction per marble piece, after vinegar loses sour taste for a 5% acetic acid vinegar.

Vinegar can be used in salads, for pickling vegetables and other creative recipes. It can also simply be taken by the teaspoon. A traditional raw cider is the Bragg's brand of apple cider vinegars (no financial affiliation).

Alcohol Warning

A key point to remember regarding fermented beverages is that unless the alcohol level is fermented down to a level below .5%, it will be considered an alcoholic beverage. Alcohol is unhealthy for body. Alcohol is ethanol, which is highly toxic to the liver. Alcohol damages the liver. This means that the liver will produce less enzymes and filter the blood poorly. This leaves the body in a state of increased toxicity. Over time this can produce severe liver disease, which can result in death.

Often people consider that because wines and other spirits are made from natural ingredients, they must be healthy. For example, resveratrol from wine is touted as being healthy. Resveratrol, however, comes from the grapes themselves. While red wine certainly will also contain resveratrol, the alcohol content of the wine can do more damage than the resveratrol can help.

As for those reputed to have been drinking a glass or two of wine every day and remain seemingly healthy, yes, the liver can certainly manage a minimal amount of alcohol every day. This doesn't mean that the alcohol is healthy for the liver. There have been a few studies that have indicated the possibility that a drink or two of wine every day may increase longevity. This type of epidemiological research, however, is highly questionable, notably because those who have a glass or two of wine everyday may also well be doing something else—such as socializing while drinking or reducing stress levels—that might also account for their longevity. Other studies have shown that socializing and reducing stress levels also extend life.

The bottom line is that the research showing that the liver is damaged by alcohol consumption is irrefutable. For example, Canadian scientists (Rehm et al. 2010) reviewed seventeen studies that analyzed the relationship between alcohol and cirrhosis of the liver. They found that all of them linked alcohol consumption with liver disease and death from liver disease. They also found that the same amount of alcohol consumption produces a higher incidence of liver disease among women.

Alcohol also damages our probiotic colonies.

Living Nutritional Supplements

As we've discussed, antioxidant nutrition can significantly lighten our body's inflammatory load, and stimulate our detoxification processes. For example, researchers from the Human Nutrition Research Center on Aging at Tufts University (Tucker *et al.* 2004) studied the relationships between homocysteine and B vitamins. They studied 189 healthy volunteers between 50 and 85 years old. They gave the subjects either one cup daily of fortified cereal (with 440 micrograms of folic acid, 1.8 milligrams of vitamin B-6, and 4.8 micrograms of vitamin B-12) or an unfortified cereal (placebo). After twelve weeks, the fortified cereal eaters had significantly less homocysteine levels than did the placebo cereal.

A diet with a variety of plant-based fresh foods of sufficient quantity requires minimum supplementation, assuming organically-grown foods and/or foods grown in healthy soils. This said, there is a great likelihood that our diets are lacking in some nutrients, especially if we suffer from systemic inflammation.

In such a condition, we are likely eating a narrow range of foods and/or exposed to a significant amount of toxins or infections. In other words, because toxins and infections 'burn up' nutrients—as the body requires these to neutralize radicals and produce enzymes—a person with systemic inflammation living in a toxic environment will likely require more nutrients than a healthy person living in a natural environment.

There are a number of isolated nutrients that have been shown to help reduce toxins. A few, like antioxidant vitamins C, A, D, and E and others have been shown to reduce inflammation by modulating inflammatory mediators and balancing Th1 and Th2 (Mainardi *et al.* 2009). Others, such as selenium, directly relate to the liver's glutathione processes for reducing toxins and radicals.

When a person's diet is lacking in an important nutrient, the body sometimes responds with critical weaknesses in immunity and inflammation. This can produce a greater tendency for toxin accumulation, simply because the body's supply of radical-neutralizing nutrients is decreased.

Many people are deficient in some or many nutrients, depending upon their diet. Even people who regularly take multi-vitamins become deficient in some nutrients. Why is this? This is an extremely complicated subject—one that could take an entire book to fully explore. To summarize, there are a number of reasons why people don't get the nutrients their body needs. These range from the more obvious—of poor diet choices—to the less obvious—of not being able to absorb certain nutrients due to enzyme issues, probiotic deficiencies and/or intestinal defects.

As has been shown in a number of studies, especially regarding B vitamins, a person may take a good multivitamin yet still be deficient because they lack the intrinsic factors that help assimilate those nutrients. In other cases, there is a chelation problem, where the nutrient is not absorbed because it doesn't have the right intestinal biofactors available within either the diet or the intestines. In still other cases, a nutrient may not be in a form that the body recognizes. This is often the case with synthetic multivitamins. In some cases, the body might treat the particular nutrient as a foreign molecule, and decide to break it down and expel it!

For those who are deficient in one or more nutrients, a good food-source supplement or change in the diet can immediately help their inflammatory hypersensitivity. Yet for another person, who may not be deficient in that nutrient, the nutrient supplement may not offer a significant change in toxicity and/or inflammation.

If a person is not deficient in the nutrient, taking more of the nutrient may not help them at all. Furthermore, overloading on isolated nutrients that have been shown to help those who are deficient can lead to a worsening of inflammation. This is due to the fact that synthesized, isolated nutrients can overload the liver and detoxification systems, as they have to be broken down. Some vitamins, such as vitamin A, can be toxic if over-supplemented. The bottom line is that for the most part, more is not necessarily better when it comes to nutrients.

So it is essential that we engage in a supplement strategy very logically. First, we need to have a healthy amount of plant-based foods in our diet, with raw, fresh foods with plenty of fiber and phytonutrients. This will create a solid foundation.

Secondly, we can add a food-based multivitamin as a sort of insurance policy to make sure we get enough of the most important nutrients. A food-based multivitamin is one where the nutrients are sourced directly from foods, or grown on food substrates such as spirulina. These sorts of multivitamins are more recognized by the body.

Thirdly, we can pay closer attention to certain nutrients that have been shown in some research to decrease inflammation. For these nutrients, we may decide to take a focused combination or isolated nutrient. But here we need to understand that many isolated nutrients can imbalance our body and create other deficiencies. Therefore, we need to approach isolated nutrient supplementation with caution. Best to err on the side of nature's balance of whole food sources, in other words.

For example, if we are taking more vitamin C, we can use a food-based or mineral ascorbate vitamin C supplement that offers chelated versions, and bioflavonoids that help the body assimilate and utilize the vitamin C.

If we are taking a mineral supplement like magnesium, we can take one that offers a chelated version together with calcium and trace minerals— offered by coral or mined sources, for example. The point here is that taking excess magnesium without the supporting and balancing minerals can exhaust the body of calcium, zinc and other essential, supporting elements.

We can also consult with a nutritionally-oriented health professional who can test our body's nutrient levels. Tests range from urine tests to blood tests and hair analyses—the latter of which may be appropriate to establish cellular mineral levels (Wilson 1998). This can be very helpful when trying to determine if we have a particular nutrient deficiency.

What is a Food-Source Supplement?

A food-source supplement is one where the nutrients have been produced by a living organism. The three key sources of natural nutrients are those produced by plants, those produced by probiotics, those produced by yeasts or those produced by the earth. These are nature's nutrients. Living organisms produce nutrients to protect themselves from the environment or other species. Thus, the nutrients they produce stimulate our immune system.

Our immune system also readily recognizes the nutrients, and our body and liver can readily metabolize these nutrients. They can be easily broken down and utilized, in other words.

Nutrients that are produced in a lab or manufacturing facility using synthesized substrates and catalysts can be recognized as a nutrient by the body, but many may not, especially if the immune system is already subject to inflammation. Such an immune system may not tolerate many synthetic nutrients.

As a result, the best nutrients on the market are:

> Nutrients that have been grown by yeasts or probiotics
> Nutrients that have utilized natural substrates (many use spirulina)
> Nutrients that have been derived directly from plant sources (vitamin C from acerola, for example)
> Nutrients that have been gathered from mines or dead coral (magnesium and calcium carbonate, for example)

Because these types of nutrients are produced by living organisms, they are well-recognized by the body, and well-utilized by the body.

A Few Cleansing Nutrients

With that said, we should know that nearly every nutrient has a role in the body's immune system and/or the liver's detoxification process. Thus we can really list practically every nutrient here. Instead, we'll just list a few "heavy-hitters" that are known to significantly stimulate cleansing. Remember, however, that the body needs a balance of nutrients. Therefore, it is advisable to not focus on isolated nutrients, but rather on living nutrients combined (chelated) within natural supplement substrates.

Quercetin: We also discussed quercetin foods previously. Quercetin supplements may be appropriate if the diet is lacking in plant-based foods. As mentioned earlier, this flavonoid inhibits histamine and leukotrienes— inflammatory mediators—in the body.

Vitamin C is considered by researchers as one of the "first line of defense" antioxidants, because it is readily available to neutralize free radicals at mucosal membranes and tissue fluids. A number of studies have shown that vitamin C can reduce inflammation.

Vitamin C supplement doses aimed at reducing inflammation typically range from one to three grams per day. As mentioned, chelated versions and versions with bioflavonoids help the potency of vitamin C. Some health researchers have also noted that vitamin C and quercetin tend to work well together. This is why apples and onions are so healthy. While fruits and many vegetables offer readily-assimilable doses of vitamin C with bioflavonoids, vitamin C drink powders with chelated ascorbates also provide a good way to supplement extra vitamin C.

Lycopene: This phytonutrient, usually isolated from tomatoes, has been shown in some research to reduce inflammation. Best approach here is to consume tomatoes, which have been found to contain about 10,000 different nutrients.

Beta-carotene and other Carotenoids: These vitamin A precursors are essential antioxidants often lacking in many diets. Some research has shown that carotenoids can reduce radical damage to the eyes and other organs.

Vitamin E: Vitamin E supplementation has been shown to provide significant antioxidant benefits. As a result, studies have shown that vitamin E can help prevent cardiovascular disease, respiratory diseases and cognitive impairment.

A few recent studies on vitamin E have shown inconclusive findings, however. What is going on here?

Most people consider vitamin E a single nutrient. But there are actually at least eight forms of vitamin E. Four of them are tocopherols, which include alpha-tocopherol, beta-tocopherol, gamma-tocopherol, and delta-tocopherol. There are also four tocotrienol forms of vitamin E. This includes alpha-tocotrienol, beta-tocotrienol, gamma-tocotrienol, and delta-tocotrienol. The primary vitamin E form in most supplements is alpha-tocopherol.

Most of the research on vitamin E has utilized only alpha-tocopherols. Ongoing research has established that alpha-tocopherols do provide some benefits, but a mix of tocotrienols provide more benefit—especially with regard to cardiovascular health.

Diets can vary in terms of their vitamin E forms. Western diets are typically restricted to alpha-tocopherols and gamma-tocopherols. However, a mixed plant-based diet that includes coconut and palm foods, whole grain rice and other whole grains will render more of the tocotrienol forms.

The bottom line is that the E vitamins are essential antioxidants that help prevent lipid peroxidation—as discussed earlier.

Vitamin Bs: All the vitamin Bs are important to the body's detoxification systems. They are most known for donating methyl groups, used by the liver and glutathione to scavenge free radicals. We should also note that toxins and pharmaceuticals will reduce our stores of Bs. Also, many people lack the intrinsic factor that allows for B vitamin—especially B12—assimilation. For these people, many doctors have advised B12 shots.

Research has recently illustrated, however, that sublingual (under the tongue) B12 is absorbed just as readily into the blood as a B12 shot. There are several sublingual B vitamin supplements on the market today.

Magnesium, Sulfur, Zinc and Other Minerals

Minerals are critical to our detoxification and cleansing processes because they donate ions that neutralize radicals, and are part of key enzymes. Without enough of these important minerals, the body's metabolic systems slow down, due to the lack of enzymes.

Magnesium deficiency has been found to be at the root of a number of conditions, especially those related to anxiety, spasms and muscle cramping. Not surprisingly, inflammation can be significantly reduced with magnesium supplementation.

Magnesium, along with calcium, is critical for smooth muscle tone and nerve conduction. Magnesium is part of the calcium ion channel system. Magnesium regulates calcium infusion into the nerves, which helps keep them stabilized and balanced. This is why magnesium deficiencies within the calcium ion channel system causes overstrain among muscles. This translates to spasms, cramping and muscle fatigue.

If magnesium levels are low, the ion channels will be unstable, stimulating nerve hyperactivity. This nerve hyperactivity can cause changes in the flow of nutrients into cells and toxins out of cells. In other words, magnesium deficiency can result in toxemia.

Magnesium is also a critical element used by the immune system. A body deficient in magnesium will likely be immunosuppressed. Animal studies have illustrated that magnesium deficiency leads to increased IgE counts, and increased levels of inflammation-specific cytokines. Magnesium deficiency is also associated with increased degranulation among mast/basophil/neutrophil cells, which stimulates the allergic response.

Dr. Jabar from the State University of New York Hospital and Medical Center, notes the blood magnesium levels can help determine if magnesium supplements can help. Magnesium levels among red blood cells indicate whether magnesium will likely have any effects.

It is no surprise that magnesium has also been shown to benefit anxiety, as it helps balance nerve firing. Magnesium has also been shown to have anti-inflammatory effects when combined with dosing with larger (one gram or more) doses of vitamin C.

Foods high in magnesium include soybeans, kidney beans, lima beans, bananas, broccoli, Brussels sprouts, carrots, cauliflower, celery, cherries, corn, dates, bran, blackberries, green beans, pumpkin seeds, spinach, chard, tofu, sunflower seeds, sesame seeds, black beans and navy beans, mineral water and beets.

Calcium, is also critical for the functioning of nerves and muscles. Every cell utilizes calcium, evidenced by calcium ion channels present in every cell membrane. Therefore, calcium is necessary for healthy lungs and airways. Thus, calcium deficiency results in more than bone problems. Muscle cramping and airway constriction are also side effects of calcium deficiency. Low calcium levels also result in deranged nerve firing, which can produce anxiety and depression. Supplementing calcium should also be accompanied by magnesium supplementing. For example, a supplement with 1,000 mg of calcium can be balanced by 600 mg of magnesium along with trace minerals.

Good calcium foods include dairy, bok choy, collards, okra, soy, beans, broccoli, kale, mustard greens and others.

Zinc is another important mineral for toxemia. Researchers from Italy's INRAN National Research Institute on Food and Nutrition (Devirgiliis *et al.* 2007) have investigated the relationship between zinc and chronic diseases. Their research determined that an "imbalance in zinc homeostasis" can impair protein synthesis, cell membrane transport and gene expression. These factors, they explained, stimulate imbalances among hormones and tissue systems, producing inappropriate inflammation.

As zinc ions pass through the cell membrane, they assist the cell in the uptake of nutrients. Zinc transporters interact with genes to regulate the transmission of nutrients within the cell, and the pathways in and out of the cell. Zinc concentration within the cell is balanced by proteins called metallothioneins. These proteins require copper and selenium in addition to zinc. Metallothioneins are critical to the cell's ability to scavenge various radicals and heavy metals that can damage the cells. Deficiencies in metallothioneins have been seen among chronic inflammatory conditions, and even fatal diseases such as cancer.

Not surprisingly, research has also shown that zinc modulates T-cell activities (Hönscheid *et al.* 2009).

Good zinc foods include cowpeas, beans, lima beans, milk, brown rice, yogurt, oats, cottage cheese, bran, lentils, wheat and others.

Selenium: Research has shown that greater levels of lipid peroxidation (due to greater consumption of poor fats and fatty foods) decrease our body's levels of selenium. This is because selenium is a critical component of , glutathione peroxidase—which reduces lipid peroxidation. Those with higher levels of lipid peroxidation tend to require more selenium because they exhaust this nutrient more readily, as we discussed earlier. While selenium supplements might offer generous amounts of selenium, one brazil nut will supply about 120 micrograms of selenium. This is 170% of the recommended daily value.

Sulfur: Research has also confirmed that dietary sulfur can significantly relieve inflammation and hypersensitivity. In a multi-center open label study by researchers from Washington state (Barrager *et al.* 2002), 55 patients with allergic rhinitis were given 2,600 mg of methylsulfonylmethane (MSM)—a significant source of sulfur derived from plants—for 30 days. Weekly reviews of the patients reported significant improvements in allergic respiratory symptoms, along with increased energy. Other research has suggested that sulfur blocks the binding of histamine among receptors.

Another study (Kim *et al.* 2006) of 50 patients with knee osteoarthritis given either 6 grams per day of MSM) or a placebo for 12 weeks found that after 12 weeks, the MSM group had significantly less pain and significantly more mobility than the placebo group.

Supplemental MSM is typically derived from plant sources. Good food sources of sulfur include avocado, asparagus, barley, beans, broccoli, cabbage, carob, carrots, Brussels sprouts, chives, coconuts, corn, garlic, leafy green vegetables, leeks, lentils, onions, parsley, peas, radishes, red peppers, soybeans, shallots, Swiss chard and watercress.

Potassium is lowered by many pharmaceutical medications, toxins and sweating. Low potassium levels will contribute to imbalances in blood pressure and the kidneys. These issues reduce our ability to cleanse toxins.

Good potassium foods include bananas, spinach, sunflower seeds, tomatoes, pomegranates, turnips, lima beans, navy beans, squash, broccoli and others.

Trace minerals: These should not be ignored in this discussion. Trace elements are important to nearly every enzymatic reaction in the body.

While minerals have been shown to provide therapeutic results, we must be careful about mineral supplements, especially those that provide single or a few minerals. Minerals co-exist in the body, and a dramatic increase in one can exhaust others as the body depletes the oversupply. Thus, an isolated macro-mineral supplement can easily produce a mineral imbalance in the body, which can produce a variety of hypersensitivity issues.

Better to utilize natural sources of minerals. These include, first and foremost, mineral-intensive vegetables. Nearly all vegetables contain generous mineral content in the combinations designed by nature. Best to eat a mixed combination of vegetables to achieve a healthy array of trace minerals.

Whole food mineral sources also contain many trace minerals in their more-digestible *chelated* forms. Chelation is when a mineral ion bonds with another nutrient, providing a ready ion as the body needs it.

Most organically-grown plant-based foods provide a rich supply of trace minerals, assuming we are eating enough of them. Other good sources of full spectrum trace minerals include natural mineral water, whole (unprocessed) rock salt, coral calcium, spirulina, AFA, kelp and chlorella. These sources will typically have from 60 to 80 trace elements, all of which are necessary for the body's various enzymatic functions. See the author's book, *Pure Water.*

We should also note that research by David Brownstein, M.D. (2006) has illustrated that whole unprocessed salt does not affect the body—high blood pressure, cardiovascular disease, diabetes and so on—as do refined salts (often called sodium).

These naturally-chelated mineral sources also prevent the side effects known for mineral supplements. For example, magnesium can easily produce diarrhea in the 2,000-5,000 milligram level. While this might be considered a minor side effect, diarrhea can also produce dehydration.

Numerous holistic doctors now prescribe full-spectrum mineral combinations for inflammatory conditions. Many have attested to their clinical successes in recommending minerals to balance the inflammatory response and stimulate healthy mucosal membranes. Full range supplements that have

RDA levels of the macrominerals combined with trace levels of the other minerals can provide a good foundation. Eating more than 5-6 servings a day of fruits and vegetables can provide the rest.

Greenfood/Superfood Supplements

Isolated nutrients in large doses can also throw off the body's balance of other nutrients, as we've discussed. Many nutrients are called cofactors because their effectiveness requires the presence of other nutrients. This sort of cooperative character of nutrients is simply because the body's processes are heavily related to each other. As opposed to a lot of research, very little occurs in the body within a vacuum.

Superfood supplements are quite simply, extremely nutritious foods. Many—such as wheatgrass, spirulina, chlorella, barley grass and others—also typically contain generous levels of chlorophyll—which alkalizes the blood, stimulates more red blood cells, and helps neutralize radicals.

Many of these are available as supplements, as they may be dehydrated and encapsulated or pressed into tablets—or simply taken as a powder. Many superfood supplements—primarily nutritious fruits and vegetables such as noni, mangosteen and wheat grass—may also be eaten raw as we've discussed. We've covered some of these as greenfoods earlier, but we'll summarize some of them again just to underscore their importance to cleansing and reducing inflammation. We'll also cover introduce some new superfoods as well:

Chlorella: A virtually complete food. This microalgae is cultivated in pools or tanks under controlled conditions. Chlorella contains numerous antioxidant nutrients, B vitamins, lots of chlorophyll, beta-carotene, trace minerals, and is an excellent source of protein. It also contains Chlorella Growth Factor, (CGF) which helps stimulate growth and immunity.

Spirulina: This is a microalgae, grown in hot climates; also in pools or tanks. It contains most of the antioxidant vitamins, prebiotics, beta-carotene, every essential amino acid, GLA, phycocyanin, B12 and many other nutrients.

Wheatgrass: This is the young plant of the wheat, picked when it is several inches high. Wheatgrass is a concentrated source of greenfood nutrients, and contains many of the phytonutrients and trace minerals found in vegetables. Wheatgrass is also known to help detoxify the blood and liver due to its high levels of chlorophyll and alkalizing mineral content.

Sprouts: Sprouts from beans and wheats contain numerous enzymes, along with high levels of phytonutrients. Sprouts can be homegrown easily, but can now also be found in powder form.

Aloe: Aloe vera has been used traditionally for inflammation, constipation, wound healing, skin issues, ulcers and intestinal issues for at least five thousand years. Aloe's constituents include anthraquinones and mucopolysaccharides, which help replenish the mucosal membranes.

Mushrooms: We discussed Reishi mushroom and Hoelen mushroom (*Wolfiporia extensas*) in the Chinese herbal medicine section earlier. Other mushrooms, such as Maitake (*Grifola frondosa*), Shiitake (*Lentinula elodes*), Turkey Tails (*Coriolus versicolor or Trametes versicolor*), Agaricus (*Agaricus blazeil*), Cordyceps (*Cordyceps sinensis*) and Lion's Mane (*Hericium erinaceus*) all have the distinction of stimulating the immune system and increasing tolerance. Blends of mushrooms are readily available in encapsulated supplement form.

Lecithin: This is derived primarily from brewer's yeast and soy, and is known to contain choline and inositol—two nutrients beneficial for cell membranes and nerve cells. Lecithin has been shown to relax nerves and help smooth muscle function.

Kelp is a macroalgae that contains a host of nutrients and phytonutrients, including fucoidan—shown to be a significant antioxidant. Kelp is also a good source of iodine—a critical trace element for thyroid health. Kelp powder is salty, and can replace refined salt as a condiment.

Green Papaya: This superfood has been used to help rebuild weakened mucosal membranes. It contains a special enzyme called papain, as well as vitamins A, C, E and Bs. In fact, it contains more vitamin A than carrots and more vitamin C than oranges on a per-content basis.

Bee Pollen has been recommended by traditional practitioners for inflammatory conditions because it contains a variety of antioxidant nutrients, enzymes, and proteins—many of which are derived from pollen. Clinicians have documented observing that bee pollen can increase tolerance and immunity in many of their patients. Bee pollen is best used from hives and honeybees harvesting pollens from the local plants if possible.

Royal Jelly: This superfood, made by the Queen, supplies similar nutrients as bee pollen, along with others. Royal jelly supplies vitamins A, C, D, E, Bs, enzymes, steroid hormones, trace minerals and all the essential amino acids. Royal jelly is also a rare source for natural acetylcholine. Royal jelly has been recommended for inflammatory conditions for many centuries. It is also reputed to stimulate the adrenal and thyroid glands.

Manuka Honey: Raw honey in general has been shown to be antimicrobial and soothing to the mucosal membranes. Thus, it is often used in cough syrups and sore throat remedies as we've described. Manuka honey is a special honey that comes from honeybees that harvest from the flowers of the Manuka bush (*Leptospermum scoparium*). This particular honey is thought to exert stronger health properties than normal raw honey. It is also reputed to be a remedy for ulcers, sinus infections and irritable bowels. Most of the world's supply comes from New Zealand, where the Manuka tree flourishes. This honey is also typically treated very gently to preserve its antioxidant and antimicrobial properties.

Super Vegetables: Extraordinary vegetables include parsley, broccoli, spinach, kale and cabbage. Cabbage is also excellent for rebuilding mucosal membranes, supplying what is now termed vitamin U. See the discussion on mucosal membrane strategies for more information on vitamin U.

Super Brans, Fibers and Seeds: These include psyllium seed, oat bran, rice bran, fennel seed, flax seed, sesame seed, sunflower seeds and others. These supply mucilage, lignans and important plant fibers that stimulate mucosal membrane health and decrease levels of lipid peroxidation-sensitive LDL cholesterol.

Plant Gums: These include guar gum and glucomannan. Most gums derived from plants provide mucilage and glucuronolactone, and other special polysaccharides. These constituents help maintain the health of our mucosal membranes. They also bind to toxins. Glucuronolactone is also a key component in many of the body's flexible connective tissues, which include the lungs.

Probiotic Supplementation Strategies

After reviewing hundreds of human clinical studies—some quoted in this book and many more discussed and referenced in the author's two books, *Probiotics–Protection Against Infection* and *Oral Probiotics*—we have selected the probiotic species shown in research to be useful for reducing systemic inflammation.

Below is a brief discussion of each organism. The references for these benefits can be found in the author's books on probiotics mentioned above.

Lactobacillus acidophilus is by far the most familiar probiotic to most of us, and is also by far the most-studied probiotic species to date. They are key residents in the human gut, although supplemented strains may still be transient. In addition to helping digest lactose, probably the most important benefit of *L. acidophilus* is their ability to inhibit the growth of pathogenic intestinal microorganisms such as *Candida albicans, Escherichia coli, Helicobacter pylori, Salmonella, Shigella* and *Staphylococcus* species.

Research illustrates that *L. acidophilus* can:

➢ Help digest milk
➢ Reduce stress-induced GI problems
➢ Inhibit *E. coli*
➢ Reduce infection from rotavirus
➢ Reduce necrotizing enterocolitis
➢ Reduce intestinal permeability
➢ Control *H. pylori*
➢ Modulate PGE2, IgA and IgG
➢ Reduce dyspepsia
➢ Relieve and inhibit IBS and colitis
➢ Inhibit and control *Clostridium* spp.
➢ Inhibit *Bacteroides* spp.
➢ Inhibit *Candida* spp. Overgrowths
➢ Reduce allergic response
➢ Decrease allergic symptoms
➢ Inhibit upper respiratory infections

Lactobacillus helveticus was made popular by cheese-makers from Switzerland. The Latin word *Helvetia* refers to Switzerland. *L. helveticus* is used to make Swiss cheese and other varietals, as it produces lactic acid but not other probiotic metabolites that can often make cheese taste bitter or sour.

Research illustrates that *L. helveticus* can:

➤ Normalize blood pressure by producing natural ACE inhibitors
➤ Stimulate intestinal mucosal immunity
➤ Promote healthy sleep

Lactobacillus salivarius are residents of most humans. They are found in the mouth, sinuses, larynx, pharynx, airways and small intestines, colon, and vagina. They are hardy bacteria that can live in both oxygen and oxygen-free environments. *L. salivarius* is one of the few bacteria species that can also thrive in salty environments. *L. salivarius* produce prolific amounts of lactic acid, which makes them hardy defenders of the teeth and gums. They also produce a number of antibiotics, and are speedy colonizers.

Research illustrates that *L. salivarius* can:

➤ Inhibit mutans streptococci in the mouth
➤ Reduce dental carries
➤ Reduce gingivitis and periodontal disease
➤ Reduce mastitis
➤ Reduce risk of strep throat caused by *S. pyogenes*
➤ Reduce ulcerative colitis and IBS
➤ Inhibit *E. coli*
➤ Inhibit *Salmonella* spp.
➤ Inhibit *Candida albicans*

Lactobacillus casei are transient bacteria within the human body, but are typical residents of cow intestines. They are readily found in natural raw milk and colostrum. *L. casei* have been reported to reduce allergy symptoms and increase immune response. This is accomplished by their regulating the immune system's CHS, CD8 and T-cell responsiveness—an effect seen among immunosuppressed patients. *L. casei* are also competitive bacteria that will overtake other probiotics in a combined supplement. Hence, it is best to supplement *L. casei* individually.

Research illustrates that *L. casei* can:

➤ Inhibit pathogenic microbial infections
➤ Reduce occurrence, risk and symptoms of IBS
➤ Inhibit severe systemic inflammatory response syndrome
➤ Inhibit respiratory tract infections
➤ Inhibit bronchitis
➤ Maintain remission of diverticular disease
➤ Inhibit *H. pylori* (and ulcers)
➤ Reduce allergy symptoms

➤ Inhibit *Pseudomonas aeruginosa*
➤ Decrease milk intolerance
➤ Increase CD3+ and CD4+
➤ Increase phagocytic activity
➤ Support liver function
➤ Decrease proinflammatory cytokine TNF-alpha
➤ Strengthen the immune system
➤ Inhibit and reduce diarrhea episodes
➤ Stimulate cytokine interleukin-1beta (IL-1b)
➤ Stimulate interferon-gamma
➤ Inhibit *Clostridium difficile*
➤ Reduce inflammation
➤ Reduce constipation
➤ Decrease beta-glucuronidase
➤ Stimulate natural killer cell activity (NK-cells)
➤ Increase IgA levels
➤ Increase lymphocytes
➤ Decrease IL-6 (pro-inflammatory)
➤ Increase IL-12 (stimulates NK-cells)
➤ Reduce lower respiratory infections
➤ Inhibit *Candida* overgrowth
➤ Inhibit vaginosis
➤ Prevent colorectal tumor growth
➤ Restore NK-cell activity in smokers
➤ Stimulate the immune system among the elderly
➤ Increase CD56 lymphocytes
➤ Decrease rotavirus infections
➤ Decrease colds and influenza
➤ Reduce risk of bladder cancer
➤ Increase (good) HDL-cholesterol
➤ Decrease triglycerides
➤ Decrease blood pressure
➤ Inhibit viral infections
➤ Inhibit malignant pleural effusions secondary to lung cancer
➤ Reduce cervix tumors when used in combination radiation therapy
➤ Inhibit tumor growth of carcinomatous peritonitis/stomach cancer
➤ Break down nutrients for bioavailability

Lactobacillus rhamnosus: These bacteria can colonize in the intestines and airways. Much of the research on this species has been done on a particular strain, *L. rhamnosus* GG. *L. rhamnosus* GG have been shown in numerous studies to significantly stimulate the immune system and inhibit allergic inflammatory responses. This is not to say, however, that non-GG strains will not perform similarly. In fact, studies with *L. rhamnosus* GR-1, *L. rhamnosus* 573/L, and *L. rhamnosus* LC705 strains have also showed positive results. The GG strain is trademarked by the Valio Ltd. Company in Finland and patented in 1985 by two scientists, Dr. Sherwood Gorbach and Dr. Barry Goldin, who also led most of the exhaustive research on this strain.

Research illustrates that *L. rhamnosus* can:

➤ Inhibit a number of pathogenic microbial infections
➤ Improve glucose control
➤ Reduce risk of respiratory infections
➤ Decrease beta-glucosidase
➤ Reduce eczema
➤ Reduce colds and flu
➤ Strengthen the immune system
➤ Increase IgA levels in mucosal membrane
➤ Increase IgA levels in mothers breast milk
➤ Inhibit *Pseudomonas aeruginosa* infections in respiratory tract
➤ Inhibit *Clostridium difficile*
➤ Inhibit enterobacteria
➤ Reduce IBS symptoms
➤ Decrease IL-12, IL-2+ and CD69+ T-cells in IBS
➤ Reduce constipation
➤ Reduce the risk of colon cancer
➤ Modulate skin IgE sensitization
➤ Inhibit *H. pylori* (ulcer-causing)
➤ Reduce atopic dermatitis in children
➤ Increase Hib IgG levels in allergy-prone infants
➤ Reduce colic
➤ Stimulate IgM, IgA and IgG levels (modulates IgE)
➤ Stabilize intestinal barrier function (decreased permeability)
➤ Increase INF-gamma
➤ Modulate IL-4
➤ Help prevent atopic eczema
➤ Reduce *Streptococcus mutans*
➤ Stimulate tumor killing activity among NK-cells
➤ Stimulate IL-10 (anti-inflammatory)
➤ Reduce inflammation

Lactobacillus reuteri is a species found residing permanently in humans. As a result, most supplemented strains attach fairly well, though temporarily, and stimulate colony growth for resident *L. reuteri* strains. *L. reuteri* will colonize in the mouth, airways, stomach, duodenum and ileum regions. *L. reuteri* will also significantly modulate the immune response of the gastrointestinal mucosal membranes. This means that *L. reuteri* are useful for many of the same digestive ailments that *L. acidophilus* are also effective for. *L. reuteri* have several other effects, including the restoration of our oral cavity bacteria. They also produce a significant amount of antibiotics.

Research illustrates that *L. reuteri* can:

➤ Inhibit gingivitis
➤ Reduce pro-inflammatory cytokines

➤ Stimulate growth and feeding among preterm infants
➤ Inhibit and suppress *H. pylori*
➤ Decrease dyspepsia
➤ Reduce nausea
➤ Reduce flatulence
➤ Reduce diarrhea (rotavirus and non-rotavirus)
➤ Reduce TGF-beta2 in breastfeeding mothers (reducing eczema)
➤ Reduce salivary *mutans streptococcus*
➤ Strengthen the immune system
➤ Reduce plaque on teeth
➤ Decrease symptoms of IBS
➤ Increase (inflammatory) CD4+ and CD25 T-cells (in IBS)
➤ Decrease (inflammatory) TNF-alpha (in IBS)
➤ Decrease (inflammatory) IL-12 (in IBS)
➤ Reduce eczema-specific IgEs in infants
➤ Reduce infant colic
➤ Reduce colds and influenza
➤ Stabilize intestinal barrier function (intestinal permeability)
➤ Decrease atopic dermatitis

Lactobacillus plantarum has been part of the human diet for thousands of years. They are used in numerous fermented foods, including Sauerkraut, Gherkins, Olive brines, Sourdough bread, Nigerian Ogi and Fufu, Kocha from Ethiopia, Sour Mifen noodles from China, Korean Kimchi and other traditional foods. *L. plantarum* are also found in dairy and cow dung.

L. plantarum is a hardy strain. They will colonize the oral cavity, airways, stomach and intestines. Temperature for optimal growth is 86-95 degrees F. *L. plantarum* are not permanent residents, however. When supplemented, they vigorously attack pathogenic bacteria, and create an environment hospitable for incubated resident strains to expand before departing. *L. plantarum* also produce lysine, and a number of antibiotics, including lactolin. They also strengthen mucosal membranes and reduce intestinal permeability.

Research illustrates that *L. plantarum* can:

➤ Strengthen the immune system
➤ Help restore healthy liver enzymes (and alcohol-induced liver injury)
➤ Reduce frequency and severity of respiratory diseases
➤ Reduce intestinal permeability
➤ Inhibit various intestinal pathobiotics (incl. *Clostridium difficile*)
➤ Reduce Th2 (inflammatory) levels and increase Th1/Th2 ratio
➤ Reduce inflammatory responses
➤ Reduce symptoms of multiple traumas among injured patients
➤ Reduce fungal infections
➤ Reduce IBS symptoms
➤ Reduce pancreatic sepsis (infection)
➤ Reduce (inflammatory) interleukin-6 (IL-6) levels
➤ Decrease flatulence

Lactobacillus bulgaricus: We owe the *bulgaricus* name to Ilya Mechnikov, who named it after the Bulgarians—who used the bacteria to make the fermented milks that produced the original kefirs apparently related to their extreme longevity. In the 1960s and 1970s, Russian researchers, notably Dr. Ivan Bogdanov and others, began focused research on *L. bulgaricus.* Early studies indicated antitumor effects. As the research progressed into Russian clinical research and commercialization, it became obvious that even heat-killed *L. bulgaricus* cell fragments have immune system-stimulating benefits.

L. bulgaricus bacteria are transients that assist in *bifidobacteria* colony growth. They significantly stimulate the immune system and have antitumor effects as mentioned. They also produce antibiotic and antiviral substances such as bulgarican and others. *L. bulgaricus* bacteria have also been reported to reduce IBS symptoms. *L. bulgaricus* require more heat to colonize than many probiotics—at 104-109 degrees F.

Research illustrates that *L. bulgaricus* can:

➤ Reduce intestinal permeability
➤ Decrease IBS symptoms
➤ Help manage HIV symptoms
➤ Stimulate TNF-alpha
➤ Stimulate IL-1beta
➤ Decrease diarrhea (rotavirus and non-rotavirus)
➤ Decrease nausea
➤ Increase phagocytic activity
➤ Increase leukocyte levels
➤ Increase immune response
➤ Increase CD8+ levels
➤ Lower CD4+/CD8+ ratio (reducing inflammation)
➤ Increase IFN-gamma
➤ Lower total cholesterol
➤ Lower LDL levels
➤ Lower triglycerides
➤ Inhibit viruses
➤ Reduce salivary mutans in the mouth
➤ Increase absorption of dairy (lactose)
➤ Increase white blood cell counts after chemotherapy
➤ Increase IgA (immunity) to rotavirus
➤ Reduce intestinal bacteria

Bifidobacterium bifidum are normal residents in the human intestines, and by far the largest residents in terms of colonies. Their greatest populations occur in the colon, but also inhabit the lower small intestines. Breast milk typically contains large populations of *B. bifidum* along with other bifidobacteria. *B. bifidum* are highly competitive with yeasts such as *Candida albicans.* As a result, their populations may be decimated by large yeast overgrowths.

This will also result in a number of endotoxins, including ammonia, being leached out of the colon into the bloodstream. As a result, *B. bifidum* populations are extremely important to the health of the liver, as has been illustrated in the research. They produce an array of antibiotics such as bifidin and various antimicrobial biochemicals such as formic acid. *B. bifidus* populations can also be severely damaged by the use of pharmaceutical antibiotics.

Research illustrates that *B. bifidum* can:

➤ Increase cell regeneration in alcohol-induced liver injury
➤ Stimulate immunity in very low birth weight infants
➤ Increase TGF-beta (anti-inflammatory) levels
➤ Reduce allergies
➤ Reduce *H. pylori* colonization
➤ Increase CD8+ T-cells as needed
➤ Establish infant microflora
➤ Inhibit *E. coli*
➤ Reduce intestinal bacteria infections
➤ Reduce acute diarrhea (rotavirus and non-rotavirus)

Bifidobacterium infantis are also normal residents of the human intestines—particularly among children. As implicated in the name, infants colonize a significant number of *B. infantis* in their early years. They will also colonize in the vagina, leading to the newborn's first exposure to protective probiotic bacteria. For this reason, it is important that pregnant mothers consider probiotic supplementation with *B. infantis*. *B. infantis* are largely anaerobic, and thrive within the darkest regions, where they can produce profuse quantities of acetic acid, lactic acid and formic acid to acidify the mucosal membranes and intestinal tract.

Research illustrates that *B. infantis* can:

➤ Reduce acute diarrhea (rotavirus and non-rotavirus)
➤ Reduce or eliminate symptoms of IBS
➤ Reduce death among very low birth weight infants
➤ Increase immunity among very low birth weight infants
➤ Establish infant microflora
➤ Normalize Th1/Th2 ratio
➤ Reduce inflammatory allergic responses
➤ Normalize IL-10/IL-12 ratio
➤ Improve immune system efficiency

Bifidobacterium longum are also normal inhabitants of the human digestive tract. They dominate the colon but also live in the small intestines. They are one of our top four bifidobacteria inhabitants. Like *B. infantis,* they produce acetic, lactic and formic acid. Like other bifidobacteria, they resist the growth of pathogenic bacteria, and thus reduce the production of harmful nitrites and ammonia. *B. longum* also produce B vitamins. Healthy breast milk contains significant *B. longum* counts.

<u>Research illustrates that *B. longum* can:</u>

➤ Reduce death among very low birth weight infants
➤ Reduce sickness among very low birth weight infants
➤ Reduce acute diarrhea (rotavirus and non-rotavirus)
➤ Reduce vomiting
➤ Reduce nausea
➤ Reduce ulcerative colitis
➤ Reduce or alleviate symptoms of IBS
➤ Stabilize intestinal barrier function (decreased permeability)
➤ Inhibit *H. pylori*
➤ Increase TGF-beta1 (anti-inflammatory) levels
➤ Decrease (inflammatory) TNF-alpha
➤ Decrease (inflammatory) IL-10 cytokines
➤ Reduce lactose-intolerance symptoms
➤ Reduce diarrhea
➤ Increase helper T-cells type2 (Th2)
➤ Increase (anti-inflammatory) IL-6
➤ Reduce (inflammatory) Th1
➤ Reduce pro-inflammatory IL-12 and interferon
➤ Stimulate healing of liver in cirrhosis
➤ Reduce constipation
➤ Reduce hypersensitivity
➤ Reduce IBS symptoms
➤ Inhibit intestinal pathogenic bacteria
➤ Decrease prostate cancer risk
➤ Decrease itching, nasal blockage and rhinitis in allergies
➤ Reduce (inflammatory) NF-kappaB
➤ Reduce (inflammatory) IL-8 levels
➤ Reduce progression of chronic liver disease
➤ Increase absorption of dairy nutrients

   Bifidobacterium animalis/B. lactis was previously thought to be distinct from *B. lactis,* but today they are considered the same species with *B. lactis* being a subspecies of *B. animalis. B. lactis* has also been described as *Streptococcus lactis.* They are transient bacteria typically present in raw milk. They are used as starters for traditional cheeses, cottage cheeses and buttermilks. They are also found among certain plants.

<u>Research illustrates that *B. animalis* can:</u>

➤ Reduce constipation
➤ Improve digestive comfort
➤ Decrease total cholesterol
➤ Increase blood glucose control
➤ Reduce respiratory diseases (severity and frequency)
➤ Strengthen the immune system
➤ Reduce salivary mutans in mouth
➤ Increase body weight among preterm infants

➤ Reduce (inflammatory) CRP levels
➤ Reduce (inflammatory) TNF-alpha levels
➤ Reduce acute diarrhea (rotavirus and non-rotavirus)
➤ Reduce (inflammatory) IL-10 levels
➤ Reduce (inflammatory) TGF-beta1 levels
➤ Reduce (inflammatory) CDE4+CD54(+) cytokines
➤ Stimulate improvement in atopic dermatitis patients
➤ Reduce IBS symptoms
➤ Reduce diarrhea
➤ Normalize bowel movements
➤ Decrease intestinal permeability
➤ Reduce blood levels of interferon-gamma
➤ Stimulate IgA among milk-allergy infants
➤ Improve atopic dermatitis symptoms and sensitivity
➤ Inhibit *H. pylori*
➤ Reduce allergic inflammation
➤ Increase T-cell activity as needed
➤ Increase immunity among the elderly
➤ Increase absorption of dairy

Bifidobacterium breve are also normal inhabitants of the human digestive tract—living mostly within the colon. They produce prolific acids, and also B vitamins. Like the other bifidobacteria, they reduce ammonia-producing bacteria in the colon, aiding the health of the liver. They have been shown to reduce allergies and respiratory condition severity. They also inhibit and control populations of *H. pylori*. Remember that *H. pylori* overgrowths are seen in conditions of GERD and ulcers. Latin *brevis* means short.

Research illustrates that *B. breve* can:

➤ Reduce severe systemic inflammatory response syndrome
➤ Increase resistance to respiratory infection
➤ Reduce (inflammatory) TNF-alpha
➤ Reduce (inflammatory) IL-10
➤ Reduce (inflammatory) TGF-beta1
➤ Reduce IBS symptoms
➤ Decrease (pro-colon cancer) beta-glucoronidase
➤ Inhibit *H. pylori*
➤ Increase antipoliovirus vaccination effectiveness
➤ Reduce acute diarrhea (rotavirus and non-rotavirus)
➤ Reduce allergy symptoms
➤ Increase growth weights among very low birth weight infants

Streptococcus thermophilus are common participants in yogurt making. They are also used in cheese making, and are even sometimes found in pasteurized milk. They will colonize at higher temperatures, from 104-113 degrees F. This is significant because this bacterium readily produces lactase, which breaks down lactose. (This is the only streptococci known to do this.)

Like many other supplemented probiotics, *S. thermophilus* are temporary microorganisms in the human body. Their colonies will typically inhabit the system for a week or two before exiting (unless consistently consumed). During that time, however, they will help set up a healthy environment to support resident colony growth. Like other probiotics, *S. thermophilus* also produce a number of different antibiotic substances, including acids that deter the growth of pathogenic bacteria.

Research illustrates that *S. thermophilus* can:

➢ Reduce acute diarrhea (rotavirus and non-rotavirus)
➢ Reduce intestinal permeability
➢ Inhibit *H. pylori*
➢ Help manage AIDS symptoms
➢ Increase lymphocytes among low-WBC patients
➢ Increase (anti-inflammatory) IL-1beta
➢ Decrease (inflammatory) IL-10
➢ Increase tumor necrosis factor-alpha (TNF-a)
➢ Increase absorption of dairy
➢ Decrease symptoms of IBS
➢ Inhibit *Clostridium difficile*
➢ Increase immune function among the elderly
➢ Restore infant microflora similar to breastfed infants
➢ Increase (anti-inflammatory) CD8+
➢ Increase (anti-inflammatory) IFN-gamma
➢ Reduce acute gastroenteritis (diarrhea)
➢ Reduce baby colic
➢ Reduce symptoms of atopic dermatitis
➢ Reduce nasal cavity infections
➢ Increase HDL-cholesterol
➢ Increase growth in preterm infants
➢ Reduce intestinal bacteria
➢ Reduce upper respiratory tract infections from *Staphylococcus aureus*, *Streptococcus pneumoniae*, beta-hemolytic streptococci, and *Haemophilus influenzae*
➢ Reduce salivary mutans streptococci in the mouth
➢ Reduce flare-ups of chronic pouchitis
➢ Reduce LDL-cholesterol in overweight subjects
➢ Reduce ulcerative colitis

Streptococcus salivarius are vigorous probiotic bacteria that station themselves throughout the upper respiratory tract, but primarily inhabit the oral cavity and pharynx. *S. salivarius* are the primary and most aggressive of our oral cavity probiotic bacteria. They are extremely territorial, and produce a number of antibiotics, including salivaricin A and salivaricin B, along with a host of other antibiotic substances.

They are also permanent residents in the human body, being primarily inherited from mom. *Streptococcus salivarius* are organizers. They produce a number of enzymes and acids that manage the growth of other bacteria. One might conclude that *Streptococcus salivarius* are one of the most important bacteria to maintaining the health of the airways, because they are the principal gatekeepers when it comes to preventing the entry and survival of infective microorganisms.

Research illustrates that *S. salivarius* can:

➤ Reduce dental plaque
➤ Reduce dental caries
➤ Inhibit gingivitis
➤ Inhibit *Streptococcus pyogenes* (strep throat)
➤ Prevent mastitis among breast-feeding mothers
➤ Reduce ulcerative colitis

Saccharomyces boulardii are yeasts (fungi). They render a variety of preventative and therapeutic benefits to the body. Yet should this or another yeast colony grow too large, they can quickly become a burden to the body due to their dietary needs (primarily refined sugars) and waste products. *S. boulardii* are known to enhance IgA—which, as we've discussed, will typically reduce IgE atopic sensitivities. This is likely why this probiotic helps clear skin disorders. *S. boulardii* also help control diarrhea, and have been shown to be helpful in Crohn's disease and irritable bowel issues. *S. boulardii* have also been shown to be useful in combating cholera bacteria (*Vibrio cholerae*).

Research illustrates that *S. boulardii* can:

➤ Decrease infectious *Entameba histolytica* (intestinal)
➤ Inhibit *H. pylori*
➤ Decrease intestinal permeability
➤ Decrease diarrhea infections
➤ Stimulate T-cells as needed
➤ Decrease C-reactive protein
➤ Decrease beta-glucoronidase enzyme (associated with colon cancer)
➤ Inhibit *E. coli*
➤ Reduce ulcerative colitis
➤ Reduce symptoms of Crohn's disease
➤ Reduce *Clostridium difficile*

Supplementing with Probiotics

The main consideration in probiotic supplementation is consuming *live* organisms. These are typically described as "CFU" which stands for *colony forming units*. In other words, live probiotics will produce new colonies once inside the intestines. Heat-killed ones are not as beneficial, although they can also stimulate the immune system. So the key is keeping the probiotics alive while in the capsule and supplement bottle, until we are ready to consume them. Here are a few considerations about probiotic supplements:

Capsules: Vegetable capsules contain less moisture than gelatin or enteric-coated capsules. Even a little moisture in the capsule can increase the possibility of waking up the probiotics while in the bottle. Once woken up, they can starve and die. Enteric coating can minimally protect the probiotics within the stomach, assuming they have survived in the bottle. Some manufactures use oils to help protect the probiotics in the stomach. In all cases, encapsulated freeze-dried probiotics should be refrigerated (no matter what the label says) at all times during shipping, at the store, and at home. Dark containers also better protect the probiotics from light exposure, which can kill them.

Powders of freeze-dried probiotics are subject to deterioration due to increased exposure to oxygen and light. Powders should be refrigerated in dark containers and sealed tightly to be kept viable. They should also be consumed with liquids or food, preferably dairy or fermented dairy. Powders can also be used as starters for homemade yogurt and kefir.

Caplets/Tablets: Some tablet/caplets have special coatings that provide viability through to the intestines without refrigeration. If not, those tablets would likely be in the same category as encapsulated products, requiring refrigeration.

Shells or Beads: These can provide longer shelf viability without refrigeration and better survive the stomach. However, because of the size of the shell, these typically come with less CFU quantity, increasing the cost per therapeutic dose. Another drawback may be that the intestines must dissolve this thick shell. An easy test is to examine the stool to be sure that the beads or shells aren't coming out the other end whole.

Lozenges: These are the newest way to supplement with probiotics, and should be a consideration for sinus infections and respiratory disorders. A correctly formulated chewable or lozenge can inoculate the mouth, nose and throat with beneficial bacteria to compete with and fight off pathogenic bacteria as they enter or reside in our mouth, nose, throat and airways of the lungs.

Probiotic supplements that survive well among the mucous membranes of the airways, sinuses and oral cavity include *L. reuteri, L. rhamnosus, L. plantarum, L. paracasei, and Streptococcus salivarius.* As we discussed in the research, several of these, notably *L. reuteri,* have been shown to increase airway health and decrease lung infections.

However, most of the probiotics in a lozenge will not likely survive the stomach acids and penetrate the intestines. (Therefore, intestinal probiotics in one of the forms above are recommended in addition to probiotic lozenges.)

As the research showed in the last chapter (see topic on oral probiotics), lozenges are an excellent way to help prevent new infections and sore throats during increased exposures. The bacteria in a good lozenge or chewable will allow the probiotics to colonize around our gums and throat, fending off microorganisms that threaten their welfare.

This type of supplement should still be kept sealed, airtight and cool. Refer to the author's book *Oral Probiotics* for detailed information regarding species, strategies and additional research on these probiotics.

Liquid Supplements: There are several probiotic supplements in small liquid form. One brand has a long tradition and a hardy, well-researched strain. A liquid probiotic should be in a light-sealed, refrigerated container. It should also contain some dairy or other probiotic-friendly substrate, giving the probiotics some food while awaiting delivery to the intestines.

Probiotic Hydrotherapy: This method of supplementation is a great way to implant live colonies of probiotics into the lower colon. Colon hydrotherapy (or colonic) is one of the healthiest things we can do for preventative and therapeutic health in general. Colon hydrotherapy is performed by a certified colon hydrotherapist who uses specialized (and sanitary) equipment to flush out the colon with water. This colon flushing usually takes about 30 minutes. Once the process is complete, the hydrotherapist can "insert" a blend of probiotics into the tube and "pump" the probiotics directly into our colon. Colon hydrotherapy is a wonderful treatment recommended for most anyone, especially those with disorders related to systemic inflammation.

Colonic treatments are relatively inexpensive, compared with their benefit. Two to three colonics a year are often recommended for ultimate colon health. Those with sensitive or irritable bowels should consult with their health professional before submitting to a colonic, however.

Probiotic Dosage: A good dosage for intestinal probiotics for prevention and maintenance can be ten to fifteen billion CFU (*colony forming units*) per day. Total intake during an illness or therapeutic period, however, will often double or triple that dosage. Much of the research shown in this text utilized 20 billion to 40 billion CFU per day, about a third of that dose for children and a quarter of that dose for infants. (*B. infantis* is often the supplement of choice for babies.)

Supplemental oral probiotic dosages can be far less (100 million to two billion), especially when the formula contains the hardy *L. reuteri*.

People who must take antibiotics for life-threatening reasons can alternate doses of probiotics between their antibiotic dosing. The probiotic dose can be at least two hours before or after the antibiotic dose. (Always consult with the prescribing doctor.)

Remember that these dosages depend upon delivery to the intestines. Therefore, a product that passes into the stomach with little protection would likely not deliver many colonies to the intestines. Such a supplement would likely require higher dosage to achieve the desired effects.

Alkaline Nutrition

This discussion of nutrients should also include the reflective effects of a healthy diet: The proper acid-alkaline balance among the blood, urine and intercellular tissue regions. The reference to acidic or alkaline body fluids and tissues has been made by numerous natural health experts over the years. Is there any scientific validity to this?

Many nutritionists condemn an acidic metabolism and loosely call appropriate metabolism as a *state of alkalinity*. Strictly speaking, however, an alkaline environment is not healthy. The blood, interstitial fluids, lymph and urine should be *slightly acidic* to maintain the appropriate mineral ion balance. Let's dig into the science.

Acidity or alkalinity is measured using a logarithmic scale called pH. The term pH is derived from the French word *pouvoir hydrogene,* which means 'hydrogen power' or 'hydrogen potential.' pH is quantified by an inverse log base-10 scale. It measures the proton-donor level of a solution by comparing it to a theoretical quantity of hydrogen ions (H+) or H_3O+.

The scale is pH 1 to pH 14, which converts to a range of 10^{-1} (1) to 10^{-14} (.00000000000001) moles of hydrogen ions. This means that a pH of 14 maintains fewer hydrogen ions. It is thus *less acidic* and *more alkaline* (or basic).

The pH scale has been set up around the fact that water's pH is log-7 or simply pH 7—due to water's natural mineral content. Because pure water forms the basis for so many of life's activities, and because water neutralizes and dilutes so many reactions, water was established as the standard reference point or neutral point between what is considered an acid or a base solution. In other words, a substance having greater hydrogen ion potential (but lower pH) than water will be considered acidic, while a substance with less H+ potential (higher pH) than water is considered a base (alkaline).

Now the solution with a certain pH may not specifically maintain that many hydrogen ions. But it has the same *potential* as if it contained those hydrogen ions. That is why pH is hydrogen power or hydrogen potential.

In human blood, a pH level in the range of about 6.4 is considered healthy because this state is slightly more acidic than water, enabling the bodily fluids to maintain and transport minerals. It enables the *potential* for minerals to be carried by the blood, in other words. Minerals are critical to every cell, every organ, every tissue and every enzyme process occurring within the body. Better put, a 6.4 pH offers the appropriate *currency* of the body's fluids: This discourages acidosis and toxemia, maintaining a slight mineralized status.

Acidosis is produced with greater levels of carbonic acids, lactic acids, and/or uric acids among the joints and tissues. These acids are readily oxidizing, which produces free radicals. However, an overly alkaline state can precipitate waste products from cells, which also floods the system with radicals. For this reason, *toxemia* results from either an overly acidic blood-tissue content or an overly alkaline blood-tissue content. In other words, pH *balance* is the key.

Ions from minerals like potassium, calcium, magnesium and others are usually positively oriented—with alkaline potential. But to be carried through a solution, the solution must have the pH potential to carry them.

Besides being critical to enzymatic reactions, these minerals bond with lipids and proteins to form the structures of our cells, organs and tissues—including our airways, nerves and mucosal membranes.

Natural health experts over the past century have observed among their patients and in clinical research that an overly acidic environment within the body is created by a diet abundant in refined sugars, processed foods, chemical toxins and amino acid-heavy animal foods. More recently, research has connected this acidic state to toxemia. The toxemia state is a state of free radical proliferation, which damages cells and tissues. It is also a state that produces systemic inflammation, because the immune system is over-worked as it tries to remove the cell and tissue damage.

As mentioned earlier, animals accumulate toxins within their fat tissues. They are bioaccumulators. Thus, animals exposed to the typical environmental toxins of smog and chemical pollutants in their waters and air—along with pesticides and herbicides from their foods—will accumulate those toxins within their fat cells and livers. And those who eat those animals will inherit (and further accumulate) these accumulated toxins. In addition, animals secrete significant waste matter as they are being slaughtered.

Plants are not bioaccumulators. While they can accumulate some pesticides and herbicide chemicals within their leaves and roots, they do not readily absorb or hold these for long periods within their cells. This is because many environmental toxins are, as mentioned, fat soluble. Because plants have little or no fat, they can more easily systemically rid their tissues of many of these toxins over time.

Further, as the research has shown, a diet heavy in complex proteins—which contain far more amino acids than our bodies require—increases the risk and severity of inflammation. Amino acids are the building blocks of protein. A complex protein can have tens of thousands of amino acids. While proteins and aminos are healthy, a diet too rich in them will produce deposits in our joints and tissues, burdening our immune system.

As we discussed in the last chapter, research also reveals that diets rich in red meats discourage the colonization of our probiotics, and encourage the growth of pathogenic microorganisms that release endotoxins that clog our metabolism and overload our immune system. Diets rich in red meats also produce byproducts such as phytanic acid and beta-glucuronidase that can damage our intestinal cells and mucosal membranes within the intestines. Greater levels of cooked saturated fats also raise cholesterol levels, especially lipid peroxidation-prone low-density lipoproteins (LDL).

The complexities of digesting complex proteins produce increased levels of beta-glucuronidase, nitroreductase, azoreductase, steroid 7-alpha-dehydroxylase, ammonia, urease, cholylglycine hydrolase, phytanic acid and others. These toxic enzymes deter our probiotics and produce systemic inflammation. Not surprisingly, they've been linked to colon cancer.

By contrast, plant-based foods contain many antioxidants, anti-carcinogens and other nutrients that strengthen the immune system and balance the body's pH. Plant-based foods also discourage inflammatory responses. Plant-based foods feed our probiotics with complex polysaccharides called prebiotics. They are also a source of fiber (there is little fiber in red meat)—critical for intestinal health.

The Mediterranean diet does not completely eliminate meat, but it is focused on more plant-based foods, healthier oils and less red meat. However we configure our diet, there are choices we can make at every meal. The research shows that the greater our diet trends toward the Mediterranean diet, the lower our toxic load will be and the stronger our immunity will be. This will allow us to better combat and eventually lower systemic inflammation.

This also not a condemnation of dairy. Milk is a great food, assuming it contains what nature intended: probiotics. Real milk is inseparable from probiotics, and when probiotics are killed off by pasteurization, milk becomes a dubious food.

Chapter Five

Cleansing Herbs

There are numerous herbs that have been utilized in traditional medicine to modulate the immune system and stimulate the body's purification processes. Some of these were in response to serious disease conditions.

In addition, a number of modern companies have developed cleansing formulations that stimulate the body's detoxification processes in a dramatic way. Some of these formulations pile up upwards of 10-15 different herbs, some of which are laxatives, purgatories and emetics.

Some of the herbs within these are quite harsh upon the body, and can result in stressing the body to the point of producing full body toxemia. Examples of these include black walnut hulls, wormwood, cat's claw and others.

Now for diseased conditions of parasites, Lyme disease and other infective situations, some of these intense herbs could be called for. But these would require a careful evaluation by a medical professional, and clear guidelines on dosage, strength and duration.

This text does not advocate the use of such intense medicinal herbs to stimulate the body's own immune and detoxification systems, without a specific prescription by a medical professional and herbalist.

What this text advocates is that incorporation of common culinary spices and herbs that have a gradual and gentle effect upon the body. These effects will be seen by the stimulation of the strength of those organs and tissue systems that drive our body's purification programs. They will:

- ➢ Strengthen the immune system
- ➢ Increase tolerance
- ➢ Stimulate detoxification processes
- ➢ Donate key nutrients
- ➢ Balance and strengthen the adrenal glands
- ➢ Subdue anxious nervous response
- ➢ Strengthen mucous membranes
- ➢ Feed probiotics
- ➢ Reverse systemic inflammation
- ➢ Alkalize the bloodstream
- ➢ Rebuild the airways
- ➢ Relax smooth muscles
- ➢ Neutralize free radicals
- ➢ Strengthen the adrenal glands

Our discussion is far from exhausting. One of the reasons is because just about every medicinal herb can affect and stimulate the body's purification systems in one way or another. We will focus, instead, upon those common herbs that are easily accessible in western society to the public: In other words, they can easily be grown in our gardens, purchased and blended into our food recipes, or mixed and steeped into herbal teas.

These uses are by far the most sustainable means to use these herbs, and they are also the safest. This is because nature provides a full spectrum of nutrients among an herb's active ingredients among the natural parts of the plant. The roots, stems, leaves and flowers of one of these herbal plants typically provide a safe means of consumption—assuming we are selecting one of these herbs and not some poisonous plant we have never seen.

On the contrary, an herbal formulation that has undergone extraction or refining can eliminate some of these natural buffers—such as fibers, polysaccharides and mucilages. Cooking these away can result in side effects and pronounced effects that might not be expected.

This presentation of the science and traditional use of medical herbs is not simply the personal opinion of the author. Rather, this discussion utilizes the medical science and research of numerous researchers, scientists and physicians trained in herbal medicines. Here traditional clinical uses of herbal medicine have been derived from a number of *Materia Medica* texts from various traditions, as well as from documented histories of using these herbs upon significant populations over centuries—some even over thousands of years. Unless otherwise noted in the text, this information utilizes the following reference materials (see reference section for complete citation):

Bensky *et al.* 1986; Bisset 1994; Blumenthal 1998; Blumenthal and Brinckmann 2000; Bruneton 1995; Chevallier 1996; Chopra *et al.* 1956; Christopher 1976; Clement *et al.* 2005; Duke 1989; Ellingwood 1983; Fecka 2009; Foster and Hobbs 2002; Frawley and Lad 1988; Gray-Davidson 2002; Griffith 2000; Gundermann and Müller 2007; Halpern and Miller 2002; Hobbs 2003; 1997; Hoffmann 2002; Hope *et al.* 1993; Jensen 2001; Kokwaro 1976; Lad 1984; LaValle 2001; Lininger *et al.* 1999; Mabey 1988; Mehra 1969; Mindell and Hopkins 1998; Murray and Pizzorno 1998; Nadkarni and Nadkarni 1908/1975; Newall *et al.* 1996; Newmark and Schulick 1997; O'Connor and Bensky 1981; Potterton 1983; Schulick 1996; Schauenberg and Paris 1977; Schulz *et al.* 1998; Shi *et al.* 2008; Shishodia *et al.* 2008; Tierra 1992; Tierra 1990; Tiwari 1995; Tisserand 1979; Tonkal and Morsy 2008; Weiner 1969; Weiss 1988; Williard 1992; Williard and Jones 1990; White and Foster 2000; Wood 1997.

Bupleurum

Bupleurum (*Bupleurum chinense* or *Bupleurum falcatum*) has also been called Hare's Ear, Saiko and Thorowax. Bupleurum belongs in the Umbelliferae family, and thus is related to fennel, dill, cumin, coriander and others—and exerts similar medicinal effects.

The root is typically used, and its constituents include triterpenoid saponins called saikosides, flavonoids such as rutin, and sterols such as bupleurumol, furfurol and stigmasterol. The saikosides in Bupleurum have been known to boost liver function and reduce liver toxicity. In general, Bupleurum appears to also stimulate detoxification.

Bupleurum is used to stimulate the spleen, purify the blood and rejuvenate the liver—and has been used to treat hepatitis. Bupleurum was studied by researchers at the Beijing University of Traditional Chinese Medicine (Chen *et al.* 2005) on 58 patients with spleen deficiency. After one month of treatment, tests showed that levels of epinephrine and dopamine were decreased and beta-endorphin levels had increased substantially among the Bupleurum-treated group. They concluded that Bupleurum significantly *"regulates nervous and endocrine systems."*

Szechwan Pepper

This is the fruit from *Zanthoxylum simulans* which is also sometimes referred to as *Fructus Zanthoxyli Bungeani* or *Pericarpium zanthoxyli bungeani* in traditional Chinese medicine. More precisely, this herb is also referred to as Sichuan pepper. The tree is also called Prickly ash, and is grown around the world. The small peppers that come from the Prickly ash tree can be dried and ground or used fresh.

Chuan Jiao is also referred to as Fagara, Sansho, Nepal pepper or Szechwan pepper.

Because it is very spicy and hot, it is often used in Sichuan dishes—known for their spiciness. Chuan Jiao contains limonene, geraniol and cumic alcohol, among with a number of other medicinal constituents.

In traditional Chinese medicine, Chuan Jiao is known to remove abdominal pain, vomiting, nausea and parasites—especially roundworm. It is also used as a skin wash for eczema, and has a mild diuretic effect.

Dong Quai

This is *Angelica sinensis,* also referred to as *Corpus radix angelicae sinensis* in traditional Chinese medicine. The roots and rhizomes are used. In Western herbology, it is sometimes referred to simply as Angelica. It is also called Dong quai.

This herb contains courmarins and a number of volatile oils. Thus it is known to lower blood pressure, relax tense muscles and improve circulation, as it inhibits platelet aggregation. It is also known as a potent anti-inflammatory, and is known to rejuvenate the adrenal glands.

Dong quai is also considered antispasmodic, which means it reduces hypersensitivity. It stimulates tolerance. It is a very popular herb for balancing the female reproductive system and irregular menstruation. It is considered a tonic in general, and has been used in traditional medicine for colds, fevers, inflammation, arthritis, rheumatic issues and anemia.

Licorice and Gan Cao (Chinese Licorice)

Glycyrrhiza uralensis is also called Chinese Licorice. It is not the common Licorice (*Glycyrrhiza glabra*) known in Western and Ayurvedic herbalism.

However, the two plants have nearly identical uses and constituents. So this discussion also serves *Glycyrrhiza glabra*.

Chinese licorice is known in Chinese medicine as giving moisture and balancing heat to the lungs. It has thus been extensively used to stop coughs and wheezing. It is also known to clear fevers. Taken either internally or topically, it is known to ease carbuncles and skin lesions. It is also soothing to the throat and eases muscle spasms. The root is thus described as antispasmodic.

Researchers from New York's Mount Sinai School of Medicine (Jayaprakasam *et al.* 2009) extensively investigated *Glycyrrhiza uralensis*. They found that *G. uralensis* had five major flavonoids: liquiritin, liquiritigenin, isoliquiritigenin, dihydroxyflavone, and isoononin. Liquiritigenin, isoliquiritigenin, and dihydroxyflavone were found to suppress inflammation via inhibiting eotaxin. Eotaxin stimulates the release of eosinophils during inflammation.

Licorice also contains glactomannan, triterpene saponins, glycerol, glycyrrhisoflavone, glycybenzofuran, cyclolicocoumarone, glycybenzofuran, cyclolicocoumarone, licocoumarone, glisoflavone, cycloglycyrrhisoflavone, isoflavone, apigenin, isokaempferide, glycycoumarin, isoglycycoumarin, glycyrrhizin and glycyrrhetinic acid (Li *et al.* 2010; Huang *et al.* 2010).

One of its main active constituents, isoliquiritigenin, has been shown to be a H2 histamine antagonist (Stahl 2008). Chinese Licorice has been shown to prevent the IgE binding that signals the release of histamine. This essentially disrupts the histamine inflammatory process while modulating immune system responses (Kim *et al.* 2006).

Another important constituent, glycyrrhizin, is a potent anti-inflammatory biochemical. It has also been shown to halt the breakdown of cortisol produced by the body. Let's consider this carefully. Like cortisone, cortisol inhibits the inflammatory process by interrupting interleukin cytokine transmission. If cortisol is prevented from breaking down, more remains available in the bloodstream to keep a lid on inflammation.

This combination of constituents gives Licorice aldosterone-like effects. This means that the root stimulates the production and maintenance of steroidal corticoids. Animal research has confirmed that Licorice is anti-allergic, and decreases anaphylactic response. It also balances electrolytes and inflammatory edema (Lee *et al.* 2010; Gao *et al.* 2009).

Ginger

This is *Zingiberis officinalis*, also called *Rhizoma zingiberis officinalis* in traditional Chinese medicine. It is quite simply common Ginger root.

Ginger is extensively used in both Chinese and Ayurvedic medicine. It is also commonly used in Western herbalism and a number of other traditional medicines around the world.

Ginger is one of the most versatile food-spice-herbs known to humanity. In Ayurveda—the oldest medical practice still in use—Ginger is the most recommended botanical medicine. Ginger is referred to as *vishwabhesaj*—meaning "universal medicine"—by Ayurvedic physicians.

An accumulation of studies and chemical analyses has determined that Ginger has at least 477 active constituents. As in all botanicals, each constituent will stimulate a slightly different mechanism—often moderating the mechanisms of other constituents. Many of Ginger's active constituents have anti-inflammatory and/or pain-reducing effects. These include a number of gingerols and shogaols.

Clinical evaluation has documented that Ginger blocks inflammation by inhibiting lipoxygenase and prostaglandins in a balanced manner. This allows for a gradual reduction of inflammation and pain without the negative GI side effects that accompany NSAIDs. Ginger also stimulates circulation, inhibits various infections, and strengthens the liver.

Properties of Ginger supported by traditional clinical use include being analgesic, anthelmintic, anticathartic, antiemetic, antifungal, antihepatotoxic, antipyretic, antitussive, antiulcer, cardiotonic, gastrointestinal motility, hypotensive, thermoregulatory, analgesic, tonic, expectorant, carminative, antiemetic, stimulant, anti-inflammatory, antimicrobial and more.

Ginger has therefore been used as a traditional treatment for bronchitis, rheumatism, asthma, colic, nervous disorders, colds, coughs, migraines, pneumonia, indigestion, respiratory ailments, fevers, nausea, colds, flu, ulcers, hepatitis, liver disease, colitis, tuberculosis and many digestive ailments to name a few.

Myrrh/Guggulu

Myrrh is from the gum oleoresin taken from the *Commiphora mukul* tree. This tree grows abundantly in India and Asia. In fact, many trees of the genus *Commiphora*—more than 200 species—have been called myrrh and used to treat pain, skin afflictions, inflammatory disorders, diarrhea, and periodontal diseases The frankincense and myrrh trade, along with gold and other spices, was an important commerce between the east, middle east and Africa thousands of years ago. Ayurvedic physicians consider it the most important medicinal resin used. "Guggul" is actually a general term meaning tree resins, but the widespread use of *Commiphora* has taken over the term. Myrrh has been widely used in India and the Middle East for thousands of years for a variety of ailments, including arthritis, rheumatism, gout, gastrointestinal problems, lumbago, nervousness, urinary tract issues, bronchitis, diabetes, asthma, obesity, phthisis, hemorrhoids, skin diseases, ulcers, infected gums, sore throat, intestinal worms, boils, liver disorders, vitiligo, edema, menstrual dysfunction, paralytic seizures and other ailments. It is applied both externally and taken internally. It is calming, considered an all-around tonic for the body, and slightly laxative. More recently, it has been recognized as significantly reducing serum triglycerides and cholesterol. It is considered stimulant, aromatic, expectorant, emmenagogue (stimulates menstruation flow), astringent (externally), antiseptic, antiparasitic, antineoplastic (preventing neoplasms), anesthetic (produces anesthesia), and anticarcinogenic.

A number of studies over the years have confirmed myrrh's immune-stimulating, antimicrobial and antitumor effects (Tonkal and Morsy 2008).

Research done by Banarus Hindu University researchers (Devaraj 1985) showed guggul resin had significant anti-inflammatory and anti-arthritic effects.

In 2008, laboratory testing (Raut *et al.* 2008) confirmed that myrrh oleo-resin was effective at breaking down microcrystals that build up in the joints, kidneys and gallbladder.

Researchers from the University of Kansas (Ding and Staudinger 2005), determined that the plant sterol pregnane X receptor inhibits the expression of the gene cytochrome Cyp2b10. Cyp2b10 apparently plays a role in liver metabolism. This illustrates not only one mechanism of myrrh in terms of its ability to protect the liver. It also shows the capability of botanicals to modulate human gene expression—for the better.

In an *in vivo* study from Glasgow's University of Strathclyde (Duwiejua *et al.* 1993), myrrh significantly reduced joint swelling. The researchers concluded myrrh was an anti-inflammatory agent.

Juniper

Juniper is a round evergreen bush that grows to about ten feet tall. It has short, pointed leaves, small yellow flowers, and produces small green or blue-black berries (actually small cones). Juniper grows throughout Europe, Asia, and the United States—among both plains and alpine regions. Traditional uses have included a variety of inflammatory diseases and infectious diseases including chronic and rheumatic arthritis, edema, gout, bronchitis, colds, fungal infections, hemorrhoids, wounds, gynecological diseases and general inflammation. It is known to purify and balance blood chemistry. It stimulates appetite and digestion. American Indians used juniper for tuberculosis, fevers, colds, coughs, sore throats, liver and kidney infections, and intestinal disorders.

Tinctures from its berries and branches have been used for skin irritations and alopecia (baldness). It has also been used to combat urinary tract infections. In the Middle Ages, herbalists used juniper to prevent the contraction of various contagious diseases. When treating a person during the Black Death epidemic, many herbalists would keep a few juniper berries in the mouth to stave off infection—forming an antiseptic barrier of sorts. North American Indians used juniper berries as a liniment and an infusion for colds, sore throats and tuberculosis. Juniper is considered to be expectorant (detoxifying), analgesic, diuretic, stomach tonic, carminative, rubefacient (irritant when rubbed on), and disinfectant (antimicrobial).

Juniper is also part of the Ayurvedic Indian Materia Medica, as it is quite commonly found in the Himalayan mountains and valleys of India. In Ayurveda, juniper is suggested for urinary issues, digestive ailments, rheumatism,

194

and as an antiseptic. Today herbalists frequently use juniper for cystitis, gout, and rheumatic joints. The German Commission E monograph recommends the dried fruit on a daily basis for rheumatic disorders.

In a study from the Karl-Franzens-University's School of Pharmacognosy, juniper extract inhibited LOX activity—the enzyme conversion process involved in the production of pro-inflammatory leucotrienes (Schneider *et al.* 2004).

Researchers from the University of Zagreb tested juniper essential oil against sixteen different bacterial species, seven different yeast-like fungi, three different yeast species, and four dermatophytes. Juniper illustrated antibacterial properties against both gram-positive and gram-negative bacteria; showed fungicidal activity; and significantly inhibited dermatophytes (Petlevski *et al.* 2008).

The berry extract showed significant antimicrobial ability against gram-positive bacteria. Studies show significant prostaglandin-2 inhibition, producing an anti-inflammatory effect and the blocking of pain (Akkol *et al.* 2009).

A study from Italy's University of Cagliari (Angioni *et al.* 2003) determined that juniper inhibited *Staphylococcus aureus*. Tests have shown juniper's essential oils produce a number of different antifungal effects (Pepeljnjak *et al.* 2005).

Juniper extract exhibited significant antimicrobial effects upon *Candida albicans, Aspergillus niger,* and others (El-Ghorab *et al.* 2008).

In a study from Turkey's Gebze Institute of Technology (Karaman *et al.* 2003), juniper inhibited 57 different strains of bacteria, including those of *Xanthomonas, Staphylococcus, Enterobacter, Cinetobacter, Bacillus, Brevundimonas, Brucella, Escherichia, Micrococcus* and *Pseudomonas.* Eleven *Candida albicans* species were also shown to be inhibited by juniper.

Juniper was shown effective against tumor cells (Moujir *et al.* 2008). This chemoprotective quality seems to relate to the lignans.

In tests against a variety of viruses, juniper essential oils were found to inhibit replication of the SARS-CoV and HSV-1 (herpes simplex) viruses (Loizzo *et al.* 2008; Sassi *et al.* 2008).

Juniper leaves and berries also contain a significant amount of antioxidant potency and free radical scavenging abilities. (Al-Mustafa 2008; Lim *et al.* 2002).

Juniper's safety has been established in a number of reports (Petlevski *et al.* 2008; Wang *et al.* 2002; Schilcher and Leuschner 1997).

Juniper extract also appears to increase the level of phosphorylation in adipose tissue with increased AMP-activated protein kinase—in mice studies this reduced obesity and increased the efficiency of insulin and leptin (Kim *et al.* 2008).

The polysaccharides in juniper stimulated macrophage and mononuclear phagocyte activity in a study by researchers from the Montana State University (Schepetkin *et al.* 2005).

Some of the terpenoids in juniper displayed anti-malarial effects (Oka-saka *et al.* 2006).

Juniper proved to be toxic to cells infected with HIV-1 and HIV-3 at 50% concentration (Salido *et al.* 2002).

Juniper also showed antimicrobial activity against *Fusobacterium necrophorum, Clostridium perfringens, Actinomyces bovis* and *Candida albicans* in research performed at Oregon State University (Johnston *et al.* 2001).

Juniper's diterpenes and sesquiterpene showed activity against *Mycobacterium tuberculosis* (Topcu *et al.* 1999).

In an *in vivo* study, juniper oil resulted in higher levels of TNF (stimulated immune system) and lower levels of PGE2 and cytokines IL-6 and IL-10 (reduced inflammation) compared to controls (Chavali *et al.* 1998).

In another study, juniper oil reduced liver damage and increased liver microcirculation and bile flow, illustrating that juniper was liver-protective (Jones *et al.* 1998).

Cinnamon

This is *Cinnamomum cassia*, also referred to as *Ramulus cinnamomi cassiae* in traditional Chinese medicine. It is commonly called cinnamon—a delicious culinary spice present in most kitchens.

Cinnamon is used in just about every traditional medicine. The bark is often used, although the twigs are also utilized. Its constituents include limonene, camphor, cineole, cinnamic aldehyde, gums, mannitol, safrole, tannins and oils.

According to Western herbalism, Ayurvedic medicine and traditional Chinese medicine, it is useful for colds, sinusitis, bronchitis, dyspepsia, asthma, muscle tension, toothaches, the heart, the kidneys, and digestion. It is also thought to strengthen circulation in general. Its properties are described as expectorant, diuretic, stimulating, analgesic and alterative. In other words, it is an immune-system modulator. It is also thought to dilate the blood vessels and warm the body according to these traditional disciplines.

Astragalus

Astragalus (*Astragalus mongholicus* or *Astragalus membranaceus*) root is a well-known immune system adaptogen. In other words, it strengthens the immune system, allowing it to become more tolerant. Astragalus has also been proven to be calming, anti-inflammatory and anti-microbial.

In Chinese medicine, Astragalus is known to treat *qi* deficiency. Remember, *qi* (or *chi*) is the vigor of the body, expressed in circulation, heat, detoxification and immunity. Thus, Astragalus invigorates the body. Astragalus is often used to treat exhaustion, adrenal deficiency, spleen deficiency and circulation issues. Laboratory and *in vivo* research has shown it can reduce blood pressure and increase circulatory health.

Astragalus contains a number of constituents, such as astragalosides, isoastragalosides, astramembrannin, afrormosin, catycosin, daucosterol, formononetin, ononin, pinitol, sitosterol, and various flavonoids, including methoxyisoflavone. It also contains two polysaccharide glucans, heteroglycans, and calycosin.

Researchers from China's Sichuan University (Wang *et al.* 2010) found that Astragalus reduced IL-4 cytokines and modulated the Th1/Th2 ratio, reducing pro-inflammatory processes—evidenced by changes in genetic signalling.

Researchers from Shanghai's Huashan Hospital of Fudan University (Xie *et al.* 2006) found that Astragalus reduced the production of TNF-alpha and inhibited NF-kappa B activity. This illustrated its adaptogenic properties and ability to inhibit inflammation.

Jujube

The *Ziziphus ziziphus* plant produces a delicious sweet date that tastes very much like a sweet apple. The fruit has many different properties in traditional medicine. It has been used to stimulate the immune system. It has been used to reduce stress, reduce inflammation, sooth indigestion, and repeal GERD.

Jujube contains a variety of constituents, including mucilage, ceanothic acid, alphitolic acid, zizyberanal acid, zizyberanalic acid, zizyberanone, epiceanothic acid, ceanothenic acid, betulinic acid, oleanolic acid, ursolic acid, zizyberenalic acid, maslinic acid, tetracosanoic acid, kaempferol, rutin, quercetin and others.

Panex Ginseng

Panex ginseng is an immune stimulant with thousands of years of use. Panax ginseng will come in white forms and red forms. The color depends upon the aging or drying technique used.

When Ginseng is cultivated and steamed, it is called 'red root' or Hong Shen. Ginseng root will turn red when it is oxidized or processed with steaming. Some feel that red root is better than white, but this really depends upon its intended use, the age of the root, and how it was processed. Soaking Ginseng in rock candy produces a white Ginseng that is called Bai shen. This soaking seems odd, but this has been known to increase some of its constituent levels such as superoxide and nitric oxide. When the root is simply dried, it is called 'dry root' or Sheng shaii shen. Korean Red Ginseng is soaked in a special herbal broth and then dried.

There are a number of species within the *Panax* genus, most of which also contain most of the same adaptogens, referred to as gensenosides. Most notable in the *Panex* genus is American Ginseng, *Panax quinquefolius*.

Ginseng contains camphor, mucilage, panaxosides, resins, saponins, gensenosides, arabinose and polysaccharides, among others.

Eleutherococcus senticosus, often called Siberian Ginseng, is actually not Ginseng. While it also contains adaptogens (eleutherosides), these are not the gensenoside adaptogens within Ginseng that have been observed for their ability to relieve hypersensitivity.

Researchers from Italy's Ambientale Medical Institute (Caruso *et al.* 2008) tested an herbal extract formula consisting of *Capparis spinosa, Olea europaea, Panax ginseng* and *Ribes nigrum* (Pantescal) on allergic patients. They found that allergic biomarkers, including basophil degranulation CD63 and sulphidoleukotriene (SLT) levels were significantly lower after 10 days. They theorized that these biomarkers explain the herbal formulation's *"protective effects."*

Researchers from Japan's Ehime University Graduate School of Medicine (Sumiyoshi *et al.* 2010) tested *Panax ginseng* on mice sensitized to hen's eggs. After the oral feedings, they found that the Ginseng significantly reduced allergen-specific IgG Th2 levels. It also increased IL-12 production, and increased the ratio of Th1 to Th2 among spleen cells. In addition, it enhanced intestinal CD8, IFN-gamma, and IgA-positive counts. The researchers concluded that, *"Red Ginseng roots may be a natural preventative of food allergies."*

Ginseng has been found to stimulate circulation and improve cognition. It is also known to reduce fatigue, and stress. Herbalists also use it to improve appetite, and as a mild stimulant and potent antioxidant.

Black Plum

Prunus mume (Seib et Zucc) is also referred to as *Fructus pruni mume* in Chinese medicine. It is also called *Omae* in Korea, *Ume* or *Umeboshi plum* in Japan, which translates, quite simply, to 'Dark plum' or 'Black plum.' It is also referred to as Mume. It is, quite simply, the fruit of a special variety of plums.

This plum is treasured for its immune-stimulating properties. The Chinese *Materia Medica* describes it as able to alleviate coughing and lung deficiencies. It has a strongly astringent property, and thus helps to cleanse the digestive tract and halt diarrhea. Research documented in the *Medica* has indicated that it stimulates bile production, is anti-microbial, and has been able to relieve fever, nausea, abdominal pain and vomiting.

Gingko

The extracts or powders from the leaves of the *Gingko biloba* plant are now popular all over the world. Ginkgo's standardized extracts are part of many formulas, from brain tonics to blood purification formulations. It also has a long history of use in Chinese medicine for expanding the airways.

Gingko contains numerous flavonoids and terpenoids, including ginkgolide, amentoflavone, biolobetin, bilobalide, ginkgetin, glycosides, ginkgolic acids, quercetin, isorhamnetins, kaempferol and others. Ginkgolide, for example has been shown to inhibit platelet aggregating factor (PAF), which means that it helps prevent clotting events within the arteries.

A study from researchers at Germany's Hannover School of Pharmacy and Medicine (Wilkens *et al.* 1990) found that gingko resulted in an almost immediate reduction in platelet factor 4 (PF4) and beta-thromboglobulin (beta-TBG).

Boswellia (Frankincense)

The medicinal Boswellia species include *Boswellia serratta*, *Boswellia thurifera*, and *Boswellia spp.* (other species). Boswellia contains a variety of active constituents, including a number of boswellic acids, diterpenes, ocimene, caryophyllene, incensole acetate, limonene and lupeolic acids.

The genus of *Boswellia* includes a group of trees known for their fragrant sap resin that grow in Africa and Asia. Frankincense was extensively used in ancient Egypt, India, Arabia and Mesopotamia thousands of years ago, as an elixir that relaxed and healed the body's aches and pains. The gum from the resin was applied as an ointment for rheumatic ailments, urinary tract disorders, and on the chest for bronchitis and general breathing problems. It is classified in Ayurveda as bitter and pungent.

Over the centuries, boswellia has been used as an internal treatment for a wide variety of inflammatory ailments and a variety of infections. Its properties are described as stimulant, diaphoretic, anti-rheumatic, tonic, analgesic, antiseptic, diuretic, demulcent, astringent, expectorant, and antispasmodic.

In two studies, boswellic acids extracted from Boswellia were found to have significant anti-inflammatory action. The trials revealed that Boswellia inhibited the inflammation-stimulating LOX enzyme (5-lipoxygenase) and thus significantly reduced the production of inflammatory leukotrienes (Singh *et al.* 2008; Ammon 2006).

Another study (Takada *et al.* 2006) showed that boswellic acids inhibited cytokines and suppressed cell invasion through NF-kappaB inhibition.

In *in vivo* studies by researchers from the University of Maryland's School of Medicine (Fan *et al.* 2005), Boswellia extract exhibited significant anti-inflammatory effects. The report also concluded that, *"these effects may be mediated via the suppression of pro-inflammatory cytokines."*

In an *in vitro* study also from the University of Maryland's School of Medicine (Chevrier *et al.* 2005), boswellia extract proved to modulate the balance between Th1 and Th2 cytokines. This illustrated Boswellia's ability to strengthen the immune system and increase tolerance.

A similar-acting anti-inflammatory Ayurvedic herb is **Guggul**. Guggul is another gum derived from the resin of a tree—*Commiphora mukul*.

Black Pepper

In Ayurveda, *Piper nigrum* is considered medicinal. Yet it is probably one of the most common spices used in Western foods. In fact, the world probably owes its use of Black pepper in foods to Ayurveda.

Black pepper is used in a variety of Ayurvedic formulations because of its anti-inflammatory action. Ayurvedic doctors describe Black pepper as a stimulant, expectorant, carminative (expulsing gas), anti-inflammatory and analgesic. It has been used traditionally for rheumatism, arthritis, bronchitis, coughs, asthma, sinusitis, gastritis and other histamine-related conditions. It is also thought to stimulate a healthy mucosal membrane among the stomach and intestines.

Black pepper used as a spice to increase taste is certainly not unhealthy, but it takes a significantly greater and consistent dose to produce its anti-inflammatory effects.

A traditional Ayurvedic prescription for gastroesophageal reflux or GERD, for example, is to take Black pepper in a warm glass of water on an empty stomach first thing in the morning over a period of time. This dose of Black pepper, according to Ayurveda, stimulates mucosal secretion, and purifies the mucosal membranes of the stomach and intestines.

Researchers from South Korea's Wonkwang University (Bae *et al.* 2010) found that the *Piper nigrum* extract piperine significantly inhibited inflammatory responses, including leukocytes and TNF-alpha.

Long Pepper

The related Ayurvedic herb, *Piper longum,* has similar properties and constituents as Black pepper. It is often used in Indian recipes. It is used to inhibit the inflammation and histamine activity that results in lung and sinus congestion. Like Black pepper, Long pepper is also known to strengthen digestion by stimulating the secretion of the mucosal membranes within the stomach and intestines. It is also said to stimulate enzyme activity and bile production. One study by researchers from India's Markandeshwar University (Kumar *et al.* 2009) found that the oil of Long pepper fruit significantly reduced inflammation.

Triphala

Triphala means *"three fruits."* Triphala is a combination of three botanicals: *Terminalia chebula, Terminalia bellirica* and *Emblica officinalis.* They are also termed Haritaki, Bihitaki and Amalaki, respectively. This combination has been utilized for thousands of years to rejuvenate the intestines, regulate digestion and create efficiency within the digestive tract.

The 'three fruits' also are said to produce a balance among the three doshas of *vata, pitta* and *kapha.* Each herb, in fact, relates to a particular *dosha:* Haritaki relates to *vata,* Amalaki relates to *pitta* and Bibhitaki relates to *kapha.* The three taken together comprise the most-prescribed herbal formulation given by Ayurvedic doctors for digestive issues.

This use has been justified by preliminary research. For example, in a study by pharmacology researchers from India's Gujarat University (Nariya *et al.* 2003), triphala was found to significantly reverse intestinal damage and intestinal permeability *in vivo.*

The traditional texts and the clinical use of triphala today in Ayurveda have confirmed these types of intestinal effects in humans.

We might want to elaborate a little further on Haritaki in particular. *Terminalia chebula* has been used by Ayurvedic practitioners specifically for conditions related to inflammation, abdominal issues, skin eruptions, itchiness, and epithelial issues. It is also called He-Zi in traditional Chinese medicine.

Research has found that Haritaki contains a large number of polyphenols, including ellagic acids, which have significant antioxidant and anti-inflammatory properties (Pfundstein *et al.* 2010).

Turmeric

Curcuma longa has been extensively used as a medicinal herb for many centuries, and this predicated its use as a curry food spice—as Ayurveda has long incorporated healing herbs with meals. The roots or rhizomes of Turmeric are used. It is a relative of Ginger in the *Zingiberaceae* family.

Just as we might expect from a medicinal botanical, Turmeric has a large number of active constituents. The most well known of those are the curcuminoids, which include curcumin (diferuloylmethane, demethoxycurcumin, and bisdemethoxycurcumin). Others include volatile oils such as tumerone, atlantone, and zingiberene; as well as polysaccharides and a number of resins.

As stated in a recent review of research from the Cytokine Research Laboratory at the University of Texas (Anand 2008), multiple studies have linked Turmeric with *"suppression of inflammation; angiogenesis; tumor genesis; diabetes; diseases of the cardiovascular, pulmonary, and neurological systems, of skin, and of liver; loss of bone and muscle; depression; chronic fatigue; and neuropathic pain."*

Indeed, Turmeric has been used for centuries for arthritis, asthma, inflammation, gallbladder problems, diabetes, wound-healing, liver issues, hepatitis, respiratory disease, menstrual pain, anemia, and gout. It is described as alterative, antibacterial, carminative and stimulating. It is also known for its wound-healing, blood-purifying and circulatory powers. Studies have illustrated that curcumin has about 50% of the effectiveness of cortisone, without its damaging side effects (Jurenka 2009).

A number of studies have proved over the past decade that Turmeric and/or its key constituents such as curcumin halt or inhibit both inflammatory COX and LOX enzymes. Curcumin has specifically been shown to inhibit IgE signaling processes, and slow mast cell activation (Aggarwal and Sung 2009; Thampithak *et al.* 2009; Sompamit *et al.* 2009; Kulka 2009).

Coriander/Cilantro/Parsley

Coriandrum sativum has documented throughout traditional medicines as an anti-allergy and antioxidant herb. The seeds are called Coriander, and the leaves are called Cilantro. Cilantro has been popularly used throughout Central America, Italy, and also Asia—where it is sometimes called Chinese parsley. Cilantro is the backbone ingredient—together with tomatoes and garlic—of salsa. It is related to Italian parsley, with many of the same constituents. Coriander is taken as fresh or juiced fresh, and it has been used by Ayurvedic practitioners primarily for allergic skin rashes and hay fever.

Fresh Italian parsley can readily be found in supermarkets and farmers' markets. While often used as a garnish (for looks and/or to clean the breath), a therapeutic quantity of parsley is about a *bunch*. A bunch of parsley is about two ounces or about ten stalks together with their branches and leaves. A *bunch* can be added to a salad or put into a soup. Parsley can be delicious with tomatoes, vinegar and olive oil. And of course, it can also freshen the breath.

Cumin Seed

Cuminum cyminum has a long history of use among European and Asian herbalists. It is described as antispasmodic and carminative, so it tends to soothe inflammatory responses. Like Fennel, Cumin has been used traditionally to ease abdominal cramping and gas.

Cumin seed contains mucilage, gums and resins. Traditional herbalists consider these constituents primarily responsible for Cumin's ability to help strengthen the mucosal membranes. This makes Cumin part of a strategy to rebuild the mucosal membranes of the airways.

Dandelion

Dandelion species include *Taraxum officinale, Taraxum mongolicum,* and *Taraxum spp.* Dandelion's role is not directly pulmonary, but rather, a strong supporting herb to purify the blood, restore the liver and reduce inflammation and hypersensitivity.

Dandelion contains hundreds of active constituents, which include beta-carboline alkaloids, beta-sitosterol, boron, caffeic acid, calcium, coumaric acid, coumarin, four steroids, furulic acid, gallic acid, hesperetin, hesperidin, indole alkaloids, inulin, iron, lupenol, lutein, luteolin, magnesium, mannans, monoterpenoids, myristic acid, palmitic acid, potassium, quercetins, rufescidride, sesquiterpenes, silicon, steroid complexes, stigmasterol, syringic acid, syringin, tannins, taraxacin, taraxacoside, taraxafolide, taraxafolin-B, taraxasterol, taraxasteryl acetate, taraxerol, taraxinic acid beta-glucopyranosyl, benzenoids, triterpenoids, violaxanthin, vitamin A, Bs, C, D, K and zinc among others (Hu and Kitts 2003; Hu and Kitts 2004; Seo *et al.* 2005; Trojanová *et al.* 2004; Leu *et al.* 2005; Kisiel and Michalska 2005; Leu *et al.* 2003; Michalska and Kisiel 2003; Kisiel and Barszcz 2000).

Taraxum is derived from the Greek words *taraxos* meaning 'disorder' and *akos* meaning 'remedy.' Dandelion is a common weed with a characteristic beautiful yellow flower that assumes a globe of seeds to spread its humble yet incredible medicinal virtues. Its hollow stem is full of milky juice, with a long, hardy root; and leaves that taste good in a spring salad. Dandelion is one of the most well known traditional herbs for all sorts of ailments that involve toxicity within the blood, liver, kidneys, lymphatic system and urinary tract. Dandelion has been listed in a variety of herbal formularies around the world for many centuries.

Dandelion's use was expounded by many cultures from the Greeks to the Northern American Indians—who used it for stomach ailments and infections. It is also used for the treatment of viral and bacterial infections as well as cancer.

The latex or milky sap that comes from the stem has a mixture of polysaccharides, proteins, lipids, rubber, and metabolites such as polyphenoloxidase. The latex has been used to heal skin wounds and protect those wounds from infection—also the sap's function when the plant is injured. For this reason, Dandelion can significantly increase mucosal membrane health.

Dandelion is known to stimulate the elimination of toxins and clear obstructions from the blood and liver. This is thought to be why Dandelion helps clear stones and scarring from kidneys, gallbladder and bladder. It has also been used to treat stomach problems, and has been used to reduce blood pressure.

In ancient Chinese medicine, it has been recommended for issues related to the imbalance between liver enzymes and pancreatic enzymes. It has been used in traditional treatments for hypoglycemia, hypertension, urinary tract infection, skin eruptions, breast cancer, appetite loss, flatulence, dyspepsia, constipation, gallstones, circulation problems, skin issues, spleen and liver complaints, hepatitis and anorexia.

Probably the best indication of Dandelion's purifying benefits is its ability to reduce leukotrienes—the inflammatory mediators that indicate a situation of toxicity. Laboratory testing has showed that leukotriene production is significantly decreased with an extract of Dandelion (Kashiwada *et al.* 2001).

Dandelion also inhibits other inflammatory mediators. A study by researchers at Canada's University of British Columbia (Hu and Kitts 2004) found that Dandelion extract suppressed the inflammatory mediator prostaglandin E2 (PGE2) without causing cell death. Further tests indicated that COX-2 was inhibited by the luteolin and luteolin-glucosides in Dandelion.

In another study by Hu and Kitts (2005), inflammatory nitric oxide levels were inhibited. Reactive oxygen species—free radicals—were also significantly reduced by Dandelion—attributed to the plant's phenolic acid content. This in turn prevented lipid peroxidation—one of the mechanisms in heightened LDL (bad cholesterol) levels and artery inflammation.

In a 2007 study from researchers at the College of Pharmacy at the Sookmyung Women's University in Korea (Jeon *et al.* 2008), Dandelion was found to reduce inflammation, leukocytes, vascular permeability, abdominal cramping, pain and COX levels among exudates.

Dandelion also supports probiotic survival. Dandelion was found to stimulate fourteen different strains of bifidobacteria—important components of the intestinal immune system (Trojanová *et al.* 2004).

Another study found that Dandelion extract significantly prevented cell death in Hep G2 (liver) cells, while stimulating TNF and IL-1 levels—illustrating its ability to boost immunity and liver health (Koo *et al.* 2004).

This was also illustrated in research showing that Dandelion increases the liver's production of superoxide dismutase and catalase, increasing the liver's ability to purify the blood of toxins and allergens (Cho *et al.* 2001).

Other studies have illustrated that Dandelion inhibits both interleukin IL-6 and TNF-alpha—both inflammatory cytokines (Seo *et al.* 2005).

Dandelion has also illustrated the ability to inhibit inflammatory IL-1 cytokines (Kim *et al.* 2000; Takasaki *et al.* 1999), and the ability to stimulate the liver's production of glutathione (GST)—an important antioxidant needed to clear the system of mucous and toxins (Petlevski *et al.* 2003).

Evening Primrose

Another herb known by traditional herbalists to be beneficial for allergic skin responses is Evening primrose, or *Oenothera spp.* The seeds are rich in gamma-linolenic acid (GLA)—a fatty acid known to slow inflammatory responses of prostaglandins, especially those relating to skin hypersensitivity. The oil from Evening primrose can be applied directly onto the skin and/or taken internally. Evening primrose oil has thus been used successfully in cases of allergic eczema, for example.

Fennel

Foeniculum vulgare contains anetholes, caffeoyl quinic acids, carotenoids, vitamin C, iron, B vitamins, and rutins. Ayurvedic and traditional herbalists from many cultures have used Fennel to relieve digestive discomfort, gas, abdominal cramping, bloating and irritable bowels; and to treat inflammation. Fennel stimulates bile production. Bile digests fats and other nutrients, increasing their bioavailability.

One of Fennel's constituents, called anethole, is known to suppress pro-inflammatory tumor necrosis factor alpha (TNF-a). This inhibition slows excessive immune response. The combination of anethole and antioxidant nutrients such as rutin and carotenoids in Fennel also strengthen immune response while increasing tolerance.

Fennel is not appropriate for pregnant moms, because it has been known to promote uterine contractions. As with any herbal supplement, Fennel should be used under the supervision of a health professional. Those with birch allergies should also be aware that they may also be sensitive to Fennel. (The same goes for Cumin, Caraway, Carrot seed and a few others).

Mallow

Malva silvestris is a close relative of the *Malva verticillata* herb used in the Chinese Ravas Napas remedy mentioned earlier.

Mallow grows throughout Europe and has had an extensive and popular reputation among Western and Middle Eastern traditional medicines as a demulcent herb: It soothes irritated tissues. Mallow contains polysaccharides, asparagine and mucilage—which stimulates a balance among the body's mucosal membranes. The leaves are typically used.

The mucilage is primarily composed by polysaccharides. These include beta-D-galactosyl, beta-D-glucose, and beta-D-galactoses.

Mallow has been used for sore throats, heartburn, dry sinuses, and irritable bowels.

This herb has also been used in decoctions by European herbalists for allergic skin responses and eczema. For this reason, Swiss doctors during the

World Wars would apply mallow compresses onto skin rashes with good success.

Mallow's leaves, flowers and roots are all used. It is an emollient and demulcent, rendering the ability to soften and coat, while stimulating healthy mucous membranes around the body.

Marsh Mallow

Althaea officinalis, has similar properties and constituents as the *Malva verticillata* L (Mallow). It belongs in the same family, Malvaceaea, and has similar constituents.

Marsh mallow has also enjoyed an extensive and popular reputation among traditional medicines around the world. This is because it contains mucilage, which supports and stimulates a healthy mucosal membrane.

For this reason, Marsh mallow is considered a demulcent: it's leaves soothe irritated sore throats, heartburn, dry sinuses, and irritable bowels.

The leaves, flowers and roots are all used in healing. Marsh mallow is known to be emollient, which gives it properties that soften and coat practically any membrane within the body, including the sinuses, throat, stomach, intestines, urinary tract and of course, the airways.

The root of the Marsh mallow will contain up to 35% mucilage. It also contains a variety of long-chain polysaccharides. Extracts use cold water, so they dissolve the mucilage without the starches. For this reason, tea infusions for drinking and gargling using Marsh mallow often use cold water overnight, although it can also be steeped for 15-20 minutes using hot water.

Mullein

The leaves, flowers and herbs of *Verbascum theapsiforme* and *V. philomoides olanum* have been part of the traditional herbalist repertory for thousands of years. It is classified as a demulcent and expectorant, because it is known to soothe irritated airways and help clear thickened mucous.

Mullein's soothing and demulcent properties are due primarily to its mucilage content, which can be as high as 3%. Other constituents include saponins, which are believed to produce the expectorant properties of this herb.

Mullein has thus been used for centuries for inflammation including respiratory conditions, skin irritations and ear infections. In all these cases, its effects have been considered soothing to epithelial cells.

Pine Bark Extract

Traditional herbalists have used pine bark extracts for respiratory conditions for centuries. The process of extraction is complex, however. Pine bark contains numerous constituents that yield health benefits, but also contains a high-density tannin complex requiring careful purification.

Today's standard for pine bark extracts is an extract of French Maritime Pine (*Pinus pinaster*) called Pycnogenol®. This extract is produced using a process patented by the Swiss company Horphag Research, Ltd. The process renders a number of bioavailable procyanidolic oligomers (PCOs), including catechin and taxifolin, as well as several phenolic acids.

Pycnogenol® has undergone extensive clinical study and laboratory research. Today, Pycnogenol® has been the subject of nearly 100 human clinical studies, testing over 7,000 patients with a variety of conditions. This extract's unique layered proanthocyanidin content has been shown, among other things, to significantly reduce systemic inflammation.

For example, in a German study (Belcaro *et al.* 2008), Pycnogenol® lowered C-reactive protein levels—known to increase during systemic inflammation and allergies—after 156 patients were given 100 milligrams of Pycnogenol® or placebo for three months. The average CRP decrease went from 3.9 to 1.1 following the treatment period. This is a 354% reduction in this important systemic inflammation marker after only three months of use.

In a study from the National Research Institute for Food and Nutrition in Rome, Italy (Canali *et al.* 2009), 150 milligrams of Pycnogenol® were given to six healthy adults for five days. After the five days, blood tests showed that Pycnogenol® interrupted the genetic expression of 5-lipoxygenase (5-LOX) and cyclooxygenase-2 (COX-2). It also inhibited phospholipase A2 (PLA2) activity. The Pycnogenol® supplementation program also reduced leukotriene production and altered prostaglandin levels. As discussed earlier, COX-2 and 5-LOX production is tied to inflammation processes.

Pycnogenol® also reduces histamine, another critical systemic inflammatory mediator as we've discussed. Researchers from Ireland's Trinity College (Sharma *et al.* 2003) found that Pycnogenol® inhibited the release of histamine from mast cells. The researchers commented that this effect appeared to be the result of the significant bioflavonoid content of Pycnogenol®.

Pycnogenol® has also been shown to reduce and inhibit NF-kB by an average of 15%. NF-kB is involved in the expression of inflammatory leukotrienes, as well as adhesion molecules. The matrix metalloproteinase 9 (MMP-9) enzymes known as conducive to inflamatory responses, is also reduced by Pycnogenol® (Grimm *et al.* 2006).

The bottom line is that Pycnogenol®, an extract bark of the French maritime pine tree, has been shown not only to reduce systemic inflammation in general through the radical scavenging abilities of procyanidolic oligomers.

Red Algae

Red algae—from the *Rhodophyta* family—have been used for thousands of years for inflammation-oriented conditions.

Researchers from the National Taiwan Ocean University (Kazłowska *et al.* 2010) studied the ability of the red seaweed *Porphyra dentata*, to halt allergic responses. The researchers found that a *Porphyra dentata* phenolic extract suppressed nitric oxide production among macrophages using a NF-kappa-Beta gene transcription process. This modulated the hypersensitivity immune response on a systemic level. The phenolic compounds within the Red algae have been identified as catechol, rutin and hesperidin.

Mucilage Seeds

A number of seeds are helpful for calming inflammation and increasing the body's gentle purification systems. These include Flax, Safflower, Rapeseed, Caraway, Anise, Fennel, Licorice seed, Black seed and others. Seeds contain basic compounds that offer mucilage, saponins and other polysaccharides that contribute to the health of the mucous membranes.

Not surprisingly, combinations or single versions of these seeds have been used in traditional medicine for centuries.

Herbal Ointments and Inhalants

Certain herbal oils of these compounds can clear congestion and increase respiratory purification when rubbed on the chest and neck. Herb-derived ointments that are applied to the skin of the neck and chest have been traditional treatments for chest congestion due to colds and bronchitis for thousands of years among traditional medicine cultures.

In the nineteenth and early twentieth centuries, these traditions were developed into commercial products, primarily as ointments containing menthol and camphor. They were eventually applied to vaporizers, chest rubs and in inhalants.

Camphor

Camphor oil is derived from the camphor tree, which is native to Asia and Japan. The tree will grow from 50 to 100 feet tall, and will live for many decades. The oil has been used for thousands of years throughout Asia and the Middle East for anointing, healing and embalming.

Camphor oil is steam-extracted from the tree's wood and roots. Its central constituents include camphene, eugenol, cineole, pinene, phellandrene, limonene, terpinene, cymene, terpinolene, sabinene, furfural, safrole, linalool, terpinen, caryophyllene, borneol, piperitone, geraniol and cinnamaldehyde, among others.

This extensive list of components illustrates the complexity of camphor. It thus has many properties. It is considered anti-inflammatory, antiseptic, analgesic, carminative, diuretic, rubefacient and stimulating.

Camphor has been used traditionally for coughs, bronchial infections, colds, muscle pain and arthritis. It is either rubbed onto the skin, put into a compress or vaporized with steam. It is not consumed internally. Some consumed herbal formulations have utilized camphor oil, but these have only very tiny portions of camphor. Care must be taken by breastfeeding mothers applying camphor on the chest not to allow the baby to consume any.

Camphor research has typically concentrated on ointments formulated with camphor and menthol.

Eucalyptus

Eucalyptus is a large fragrant genus of trees that have primarily come from Australia, although they have been migrating to different regions over the past few hundred years. Today, California and many Pacific Rim countries are now home to eucalyptus species, as is the Mediterranean, Africa and many parts of Asia. The tree's bark and leaves are a source of a medicinal sap known for its decongestant and anti-inflammatory properties.

Eucalyptus oil is derived from this sap, and it is the 1.8-cineol called eucalyptol—a monoterpene—that is the key constituent of eucalyptus oil. Eucalyptol has been shown to suppress arachidonic acid metabolism as well as inhibit cytokine release from monocytes.

Mints and Menthol

The plants of the mint family include Peppermint (*Mentha piperita*), Watermint (*Mentha aquatica*), Spearmint (*Mentha spicata*), Pennyroyal (*Mentha pulegium*) and several others. They have a variety of common constituents, of which menthol is the most applicable to respiratory issues. Other active constituents of many mints will include menthylacetate, menthone, mentofuran, limonene, cineole, isomenthol, neomenthol, azulenes and rosmarinic acid.

Mint is well-known for its ability to settle digestion and ease flatulence. These effects are due to azulene's ability to relax the smooth muscles around the intestines. Azulene also relaxes the smooth muscles around the airways as well. Note that Chamomile also contains azulene.

Menthol is most known for its ability to clear congestion and expand the airways. It is the expectorant property of menthol that produces this effect. Menthol reduced coughing in a study from Britain's Leicester University Hospitals (Kenia *et al.* 2008) of 42 children.

It should be mentioned that all the mints make delicious herbal teas, a great addition to any breakfast or after-dinner beverage.

Anti-inflammatory Herbal Spices

A number of other herbs also contain anti-inflammatory properties. These work in different ways, and while they may or may not specifically modulate food sensitivities, they can help strengthen the immune system and stimulate our purification processes. Here is a quick overview of some of the most well-known (and most available) of these anti-inflammatory herbs:

Basil (*Osimum basilicum*) contains ursolic acid and oleanolic acid, both shown in laboratory studies to inhibit inflammatory COX-2 enzymes.

Garlic (*Allium sativum*) probably deserves a larger section, but that information could easily encompass a book in itself—as was well documented by Paul Bergner: *The Healing Power of Garlic* (1996). Garlic is an ancient medicinal plant with a wealth of characteristics and constituents that stimulate the immune system, protect the liver, purify the bloodstream, reduce oxidative species, reduce LDL lipid peroxidation, reduce inflammation, and stimulate detoxification systems throughout the body. This is supported by a substantial amount of rigorous scientific research.

Garlic is also one of the most powerful antimicrobial plants known. A fresh garlic bulb has at least five different constituents known to inhibit bacteria, fungi and viruses. Much of this antimicrobial capability, however, is destroyed by heat and oxygen. Therefore, eating freshly peeled bulbs are the most assured way to retain these antimicrobial potencies.

Cooked, aged or dehydrated garlic powder also has a variety of powerful antioxidants, but little of its raw antibiotic abilities. Garlic is also a tremendous sulfur donor as well. The combination of garlic's antibiotic, antioxidant, anti-inflammatory and immune-building characteristics make it a *must* spice-herb-food for any inflammatory condition.

Oregano (*Origanum vulgare*) contains at least thirty-one anti-inflammatory constituents, twenty-eight antioxidants, and four significant COX-2 inhibitors (apigenin, kaempherol, ursolic acid and oleanolic acid).

Rosemary (*Rosmarinus officinalis*) contains ursolic acid, oleanolic acid and apigenin—a few of the many constituents in this important botanical—shown to inhibit inflammatory enzymes in laboratory studies. Research has also shown that rosemary's volatile oils can halt airway constriction by inhibiting mast cell degranulation.

Adding Anti-inflammatory Spices to Our Meals

It should be noted that there is a great difference between a spice dose and a therapeutic dose. A therapeutic dose of one or more of these spices will typically be larger than a spice dose. The sign of a therapeutic dose of these spices within a dish is when the spice can be readily tasted. That is, the pungent flavor of the spice stands out in the food. If the amount of spice simply flavors the food a little, then it will probably not be enough to stimulate any immune response. If the spice can be specifically tasted (for example, *"that dish tastes garlicy"* or *"tastes peppery"*) then the spice will likely be enough to stimulate a therapeutic response.

That said, if multiple spices are used, the dose of each spice can be smaller. After all, the meal should also taste good. This, however, is why traditional Chinese and Indian food is so spicy. The recipes come from therapeutic traditions.

Another element of the therapeutic dose is consistency. It is not enough to have one or more of these spices once a week with a particular dish. The spice(s) should be added to at least one meal every day.

In addition, care must be taken to protect therapeutic spices from degradation. This can occur when spices are left in the light or sun for an extended period, or when spices are left open to oxygen. Often spices are left in kitchen racks exposed to the lights of the kitchen and window, or left in unsealed containers or shakers. Oxygen and light degrade the biochemical constituents that give these spices their therapeutic properties.

This latter point is likely one of the main reasons our culinary spices cannot be considered therapeutic. Leaving the spice exposed can take place during processing, packaging and shipping; as well as in the kitchen. Therefore, we should consider purchasing our therapeutic spices from a bulk herb store, or from suppliers or brands that respect their therapeutic nature.

By far the best way to consume or add these foods to our diet is in their fresh form. Many of these herbs can be grown in our garden or purchased from a local farmers' market or grocery store as fresh. As discussed earlier, fresh foods maintain more bioactive nutrients. This is because their beneficial constituents are naturally sealed within the food's peel, shell or cell walls.

Note also that these anti-inflammatory herbal spices (and most of the other natural products contained in this chapter) will typically not stimulate a therapeutic response immediately. Depending upon the status of our immune system, it may take weeks or months before the daily dosing of these natural elements is seen in the form of strengthening our immunity and reducing our toxin levels.

Other Anti-Inflammatory Herbs

The list does not end here. Still other herbs have been used among traditional medicines throughout the world to reverse the toxic, inflammatory metabolism. Many of these are not direct pulmonary herbs, but rather, serve to purify the blood, strengthen the liver, strengthen the adrenals, strengthen the immune system and inhibit inflammation.

Comfrey, Aloe and **Slippery elm,** for example, aid the health of the mucosal membrane with their high mucilage and mucopolysaccharide content—while **Cayenne, Nutmeg** and **Goldenseal** stimulate the body's detoxification processes to clear catarrh.

In addition to these bronchial herbs, there are herbs that relax the muscles and support the nervous system in general. This is a common formulation strategy used by herbalists. These types of herbs are called nervines, and they include **Chamomile, Tulsi, Hops, Wild lettuce** and **Skullcap.**

Here are more common anti-inflammatory herbs that are readily available in spice form, herbal tea form or in our garden:

- **Aloe (***Aloe vera***)**
- **Anise (***Pimpinella anisum***)**
- **Cayenne (***Capsicum* **spp.)**
- **Chamomile (***Matricaria chamomilla***)**
- **Comfrey (***Symphytum officinale***)**
- **Green Tea (***Camellia sinensis***)**
- **Guggul (***Commiphora mukul***)**
- **Lemongrass (***Cymbopogon citratus***)**
- **Nutmeg (***Myristica fragrans***)**
- **Slippery elm (***Ulmus fulva***)**
- **Stinging Nettle (***Urtica dioica***)**
- **Thyme (***Thymus serphyllum***)**
- **Tulsi (***Ocimum gratissimum***)**
- **Wild onion (***Hymenocallis tubiflora***)**

There are certainly many more gentle herbs we can to this collection. But these are certainly good candidates to consider for one's garden, tea or spice cupboard.

Dosage and Usage Considerations

As mentioned, most of the herbs mentioned here, with the exception of essential oils, are safest when used as *infusions*. An infusion is simply the steeping of the fresh or dried root, bark, leaf, seed, stem or fruit in water. In the case of most herb leaves and stems, the water is brought to a boil, and the herb can be steeped for 5-10 minutes using a strainer or tea-ball. In the case of most roots, seeds and barks, the root can be steeped a little longer, for 10-20 minutes, depending on the herb. In some cases a seed, root or bark is better when it is soaked overnight in room temperature water.

It is suggested that any herb not readily known be taken as a tea or as a spice in a food following some consultation with an herbalist or medical professional. This is especially the case if we are under the care of a doctor for any reason—in such a case, the doctor should be consulted that we are trying some new spices or herbal teas.

Chapter Six

Other Cleansing Strategies

Mucosal Membrane Strategies

As we've illustrated in this text, our ability to cleanse and avoid new toxins is dependent upon the health of our mucosal membranes. Here is why:

> ➤ Toxins and microorganisms come into closer contact with epithelia that have damaged mucosal membrane layers. This allows those toxins more access to our tissues and bloodstream.
> ➤ The cilia within the airways do not have the right basement fluid to operate effectively. Either they are overwhelmed by too much mucous or don't have enough basement membrane to effectively 'sweep' out toxins, cell parts and mucous.
> ➤ Defects in the mucosal membranes stimulate inflammation due to the decreased protection they offer those parts of the body they normally protect.

Foods and Beverages that Deplete Our Mucosal Membranes

The foods and beverages that deplete our mucosal membranes also increase systemic inflammation because they contribute free radicals and other toxins, stimulating systemic inflammation.

These include:

> ➤ Alcohol
> ➤ Foods/beverages high in refined sugars
> ➤ Highly processed foods/beverages
> ➤ Foods/beverages high in refined salt
> ➤ Foods high in saturated fats
> ➤ Fried foods and fast foods
> ➤ Foods that are burnt or overcooked
> ➤ Foods containing chemical additives

These foods and beverages serve to irritate the mucous membranes. This is because they either directly contribute free radicals to the body, or the oxidation occurs as they make contact with the mucosal membranes and body cells.

Other Things that Deplete Our Mucosal Membranes

A number of activities also reduce our mucosal health. These include:

> ➤ Stress
> ➤ Anxiety
> ➤ Anger
> ➤ Pharmaceuticals
> ➤ Illicit drugs
> ➤ Tobacco smoke (primary and secondary)
> ➤ Air pollution

- ➢ Lack of sunshine
- ➢ Infections (fungal, bacterial, viral)
- ➢ Lack of hydration

As for anger and stress, when our body is stressed, our body switches to fight-or-flight metabolic mechanisms that pull energy away from the processes of the sub-mucosal glands and gastric glands—which produce our mucosal membrane fluids. This is why a person who is nervous or anxious will also often have dry mouth and an upset stomach. They are not producing enough mucosal secretions to protect those epithelial cells.

The others on the list are either toxins that directly alter the pH of our mucosal membranes, or simply infect them.

Most pharmaceuticals are toxic to the mucosal membranes. This is why a significant side effect of most medications is dry mouth and an upset stomach. These chemicals can deplete our mucosal membranes and/or block mucosal secretions by virtue of inhibiting the COX-2 process. This also goes for other drugs, chemicals, pollutants, and so on.

Methylmethionine and Cabbage

Nature also provides nutrients from whole foods that can help rebuild our mucosal membranes. One of the more productive whole foods applicable to rebuilding our body's mucosal membranes is cabbage. Cabbage contains a unique constituent, s-methylmethionine, also referred to as vitamin U. Through a pathway utilizing one of the body's natural enzymes, called Bhmt2, s-methylmethionine is converted to methionine and then to glutathione in several steps.

In this form, glutathione has been shown to stimulate the repair of the mucosal membranes within the stomach, intestines and airways. Glutathione has also been shown to increase the health and productivity of the liver.

Raw cabbage or cabbage juice has been used as a healing agent for ulcers and intestinal issues for thousands of years among traditional medicines, including those of Egyptian, Ayurvedic and Greek systems. The Western world became aware of raw cabbage juice in the 1950s, when Garnett Cheney, M.D. conducted several studies showing that methylmethionine-rich cabbage juice concentrate was able to reduce the pain and bleeding associated with ulcers.

In one of Dr. Cheney's studies, 37 ulcer patients were treated with either cabbage juice concentrate or a placebo. Of the 26-patient cabbage juice group, 24 patients were considered "successes"—achieving an astounding 92% success rate.

Medical researchers from Iraq's University Department of Surgery (Salim 1993) conducted a double-blind study of 172 patients who suffered from gastric bleeding caused by nonsteroidal anti-inflammatory drugs (NSAIDs). They gave the patients either cysteine, methylmethionine sulfonium chloride (MMSC) or a placebo. Those receiving either the cysteine or the MMSC stopped bleeding. Their conditions became *"stable"* as compared with many in the control group, who continued to bleed.

Plants use s-methylmethionine to help heal cell membrane damage among their leaves and stems. This is reminiscent of antioxidants: Plants produce antioxidants to help to protect them from damage from the sun, insects and diseases. In other words, the very same biochemicals that protect plants also help heal our bodies.

Note that MMSC or cabbage juice does not inhibit the flow of gastric juices in the stomach to produce these effects as do acid blocking medications. Rather, they stimulate the body's natural production of mucous, which serves to protect the stomach's cells from the effects of acids.

Herbs that Stimulate Mucosal Health

A number of the herbs help revitalize the mucous membranes. Some of these, such as Aloe, Slippery elm, Marsh mallow and Mallow, specifically contribute mucopolysaccharides in the form of mucilage. These constituents supplement the mucosal membranes, providing protection. At the same time, they contain nutrients that stimulate submucosal gland secretions, which include the glycoproteins and mucopolysaccharides that form the foundation for our mucous membranes.

Most will also exert antioxidant effects and, in the case of aloe, will exert an antimicrobial effect upon the mucosal membranes. This of course, helps remove infective microorganisms, which in turn helps lighten the burden on our immune system.

Other gentle herbs that can help stimulate our mucosal membrane health include:

> Triphala (*Terminalia chebula, Terminalia bellirica* and *Emblica officinalis*)
> Black Pepper (*Piper nigrum*)
> Mallow (*Malva sylvestris*)
> Marsh Mallow (*Althaea officinalis*)
> Cumin Seed (*Cuminum cyminum*)
> Aloe (*Aloe vera*)
> Comfrey (*Symphytum officinale*)
> Chamomile (*Matricaria chamomilla*)
> Slippery elm (*Ulmus fulva*)
> Flaxseed (*Linum usitatissimum*)

All of these contain constituents that specifically help stimulate mucosal membrane health.

There are several ways to incorporate these herbs into our daily regimen. We can add more freshly ground Black pepper to our foods. We can add a teaspoon of Aloe to a smoothie or juice. We can spice our foods with fresh Cumin seed (also a spice used in many curries). We can make teas (infusions) from one of the Mallows, some Comfrey and Chamomile. Flaxseeds may be steeped into tea, eaten raw, baked into breads, or sprinkled directly on foods.

We can also take a teaspoon of Triphala in a glass of warm water each day or every few days. Reputable Triphala formulations are available at health food stores and online. A teaspoon can be stirred into a glass of water or a healthy fruit smoothie.

Oral Cleansing Strategies

Our oral cavities are a critical element of our body's ability to not only product the body from toxins and invaders, but to cleanse itself.

Oral Probiotics

Research documented in the last chapter shows that our probiotics are critical elements in the health of our mucosal membranes. This is because they inhabit and police our mucosal membranes. They are defenders and facilitators for the recycling of mucous, and they help break down toxins and pathogens.

They also secrete very important biochemicals—which contribute to the ionic and nutrient makeup of the mucosal membranes. Without healthy probiotic colonies, our mucosal membranes are subject to pathogen attack and inflammatory alteration.

For the health of our mouth, throat and airway mucosal membranes, we can take oral probiotics. These are particular species of probiotic bacteria, such as *Lactobacillus reuteri* and *L. salivarius,* which (among others) line the mucosal membranes of our mouths, sinuses, pharynx, larynx and bronchial airways. Research has illustrated—as we showed earlier—that oral probiotics help clean, prevent infection and maintain the strength and flexibility of our mucosal passages.

General Oral Cleansing

Most of us who have visited with a dental hygienist know how to brush properly. While brushing the enamel is certainly important and should not be overlooked, brushing too harshly and in the wrong direction can harm the gums over time. Best to keep a more circular motion over the enamel and lightly massage the gums.

Our gums require more care than do our teeth. The gums provide the foundation for healthy root systems. Healthy gums deliver nutrients, blood, oxygen and immune cells to our teeth; helping the dental pulp, dentin, roots, and enamel remain strong and better able to prevent infection within.

When the gums are beat up by harsh brushing and flossing, they will recede over time. As they recede, the roots and nerves become exposed to the environment of the mouth, which includes pathogenic bacteria and their acids, which will eat away into the roots, tooth enamel and dentin. This can cause a severe type of decay, which requires serious dental repair.

Receding gums also produce more pockets between the teeth and the gums. Aggressive bacteria will set up shop in these pockets, and grow to outrageous colony sizes. They will produce acids and endotoxins such as leukotoxin, which can leak into the bloodstream. Once in the bloodstream, these toxins will damage arteries and tissues. There is also evidence of some of these bacteria translocating around the body through the bloodstream.

While they are sometimes necessary to repair damage from tooth decay, root canals should be avoided if there is any alterna-tive offered by the dentist. This is because root canal surgery kills the tooth by removing the nerves and blood supply to the nerve root. This prevents the body from defending this region.

This lack of innervation and circulation combined with the possibility of future cracking opens us up to an infection of the dead root canals. Often the bacteria that end up infecting a dead root canal are spirochetes, which, as we described earlier, can be extremely dangerous when they set up shop.

Oil Pulling and Tongue Cleaning

While we are on the topic of the oral cavity let's discuss keeping the oral cavity cleansed. Most of us brush and hopefully floss. The water pik is another useful strategy that can decrease our

The Ayurvedic practice of oil pulling has been shown to reduce pathogenic oral bacteria (Asokan et al. 2011) and stimulate cleansing of the oral cavity. To oil-pull, simply lightly swish (don't gargle or swallow) a teaspoon of virgin sesame seed oil or coconut oil between the teeth and gums.

A tongue cleaner is also useful for decreasing oral pathogens. A tongue cleaner made of silver will help purify our tongue as it pulls saliva and toxins from the back of the tongue out of the mouth. This is an ancient healing tradition that can help relieve our oral cavity of many toxins.

Strategies to Reduce Increased Intestinal Permeability

As discussed earlier, the scientific evidence points to the fact that systemic inflammation can be caused by and worsened by the weakening and breakdown of the intestinal mucosal membrane and intestinal barrier. Once the barrier has broken down, toxins, endotoxins and food macromolecules can come into contact with intestinal tissues and the bloodstream. As this takes place, the immune system launches an attack, producing systemic inflammation.

Now the question is: How can we rebuild our intestinal barrier?

In reality, the intestinal barrier is primarily a mucosal membrane, with the addition of cellular components (villi, microvilli, desmosomes and so on), and the various digestive enzymes and probiotic species. The mucous portion of the intestinal barrier is thus metabolically similar to most other mucosal membranes around the body—excepting its functions of nutrient absorption. Therefore, those same things that damage our other mucosal membranes also damage the intestinal barrier, and those things that increase mucosal health also increase our intestinal barrier health.

The intestinal barrier mucosal membranes are also a part of the body's immune system. They are the body's most important first line of defense against invading microorganisms and toxins—preventing them or their by-products from penetrating the body's tissues to produce inflammation.

We have thoroughly investigated not only the causes of the breakdown of the mucosal membrane and intestinal barrier, but also laid out a variety of strategies to stabilize mucosal health. These have ranged from dietary strategies to herbs, probiotics and water. While some of these may not directly heal the barrier, most will at least strengthen the immune system to help detoxify the body of some of the elements that weaken the brush barrier mucosal membranes.

Decreasing the body's toxic load combined with a healthy, predominantly plant-based diet will also help our gastric and intestinal cells regenerate a healthy mucosal membrane. This will help reduce the toxic burden upon the cells of the intestinal wall, which again will help the intestines regenerate a healthy brush barrier.

As we illustrated in the section on s-methylmethionine, many plants—especially leafy green vegetables—produce substances that will directly stimulate the rebuilding of the mucosal membrane within the stomach and intestines. In the case of s-methylmethionine (vitamin U), research has confirmed its ability to heal ulcers, colitis and gastritis. To this we add that plant-based foods stimulate enzyme activity and provide many other nutrients that help maintain a healthy mucosal membrane.

We must remember that the body's epithelial cells and sub-mucosal cells supporting the mucosal membranes have some of the fastest turnover rates of all the body's cells. Most of these cells will divide and be replaced by new cells within a month. While this doesn't necessarily mean we can heal the mucosal membranes within that short a period of time, it does mean that gradually, over several generations of new, healthier epithelial cells, our mucous membranes can gradually be rebuilt.

Hydration Strategies

The fact that dehydration (lack of sufficient fluid intake) can contribute to systemic inflammation and toxicity has been confirmed by research.

The mucosal membranes are made primarily of water. In a dehydrated state, our mucosal membranes thin. It is for this reason that other research has found that many ulcerated conditions can be cured simply by drinking adequate water (Batmanghelidj 1997).

Water is directly involved in inflammatory metabolism. Research has revealed that increased levels of inflammatory mediators such as histamine are released during periods of dehydration in order to help balance fluid levels within the bloodstream, tissues, kidneys and other organs.

Inadequate water intake will dehydrate the mucosal membranes. This produces irritation and hypersensitivity. Research by Dr. Batmanghelidj (1987; 1990) led to the realization that the blood becomes more concentrated during dehydration. As this concentrated blood enters the capillaries of the respiratory system, histamine is released in an attempt to balance the blood dilution.

The immune system is also irrevocably aligned with the body's water availability. The immune system utilizes water to produce lymph fluid. Lymph fluid circulates immune cells throughout the body, enabling them to target specific intruders. The lymph is also used to escort toxins out of the body.

Intracellular and intercellular fluids are necessary for the removal of nearly all toxins—and pretty much every metabolic function of every cell, every organ and every tissue system.

Water also increases the availability of oxygen to cells. Water balances the level of free radicals. Water flushes and replenishes the digestive tract. Thus, water is necessary for the proper digestion of food, as well as nutrition utilization. The gastric cells of the stomach and the intestinal wall cells require water for proper digestive function. The health of every cell depends upon water.

There is certainly reason to believe that dehydration is a key factor for toxicity and inflammation.

As Dr. Jethro Kloss pointed out decades ago (1939), the average person loses about 550 cubic centimeters of water through the skin, 440 cc through the lungs, 1550 cc through the urine, and another 150 cc through the stool. This adds up to 2650 cc per day, equivalent to a little over 2-½ quarts (about 85 fluid ounces).

Meanwhile many have suggested drinking eight 8-oz glasses per day. This 64 ounces would result in a state of dehydration. In 2004, the National Academy of Sciences released a study indicating that women typically meet their hydration needs with approximately 91 ounces of water per day, while men meet their needs with about 125 ounces per day. This study also indicated that approximately 80% of water intake comes from water/beverages and 20% comes from food. Therefore, we can assume a minimum of 73 ounces of fresh water for the average adult woman and 100 ounces of fresh water for the average adult man should cover our hydration needs. That is significantly more water than the standard eight glasses per day—especially for men.

The data suggests that 50-75% of Americans have chronic dehydration. Fereydoon Batmanghelidj, M.D., probably the world's foremost researcher on water, suggests a ½ ounce of water per pound of body weight. Drinking an additional 16-32 ounces for each 45 minutes to an hour of strenuous activity is also a good idea, with some before and some after exercising. More water should accompany temperature and elevation extremes, and extra sweating or fevers. Note also that alcohol is dehydrating.

A glass of room-temperature water first thing in the morning on an empty stomach can significantly help our mucosal membranes. Then we should be drinking water throughout the day. Our evening should accompany reduced water consumption, so our sleep is not disrupted by urination.

There are easy ways to tell whether we are dehydrated. A sensation of being thirsty indicates that we are already dehydrated. A person with toxicity and/or inflammation should thus be drinking enough water to not ever feel thirsty. Dark yellow urine also indicates dehydration. Our urine color should be either clear, or bright yellow if after taking multivitamins.

Drinking just any water is not advised. Municipal water and even bottled water can contain many contaminants that can burden the immune system, and trigger inflammation. Care must be taken to drink water that has been filtered of most toxins yet is naturally mineralized. Research has confirmed that distilled water and soft water are not advisable. Natural mineral water is best. Please refer to the author's book, *Pure Water* for more information on water content, filters and water treatment options.

Hydrotherapy

The ancient physician Hippocrates was a proponent of hydrotherapy for respiratory conditions, and there have been many treatment successes among the many hydrotherapy treatment centers all over Europe, Asia and the U.S. over the centuries. Early nineteenth century physician Vincent Priessnitz from Austria popularized many types of modern water treatments, as did Father Sebastian Kneipp—a 19th century German monk. These included water compresses, cold-water therapy, contrast baths, hot baths, and warm baths.

Dr. Wilhelm Winternitz, an Austrian neurologist, observed one of Priessnitz's treatment centers and became one of the most celebrated proponents of water treatment in modern times. Dr. Winternitz designed a number of different water treatments and influenced American physicians such as Dr. John Harvey Kellogg, Dr. Jethro Kloss and Dr. Simon Baruch. Dr. Kellogg operated the famous Michigan Battle Creek Health Center for many years until it burnt down in 1902. The center utilized hydrotherapy as a key healing agent. Dr. Kloss ran his own clinic and also worked closely with the Battle Creek Center.

Despite its history of success, opposition to hydrotherapy came from pharmaceutical medicine circles in the decades that followed. Water cures became targeted by the new medical establishment, and many hydrotherapy treatment centers were shut down between 1920 and 1950. Hydrotherapy experienced a resurgence in the U.S. following World War II, when physical therapists found success in whirlpool treatment. Today hydrotherapy is widely used in various modalities, treatments, and physical therapy centers. Many hot springs and wellness spas are unmistakably similar to the hydrotherapy centers of years past. Today these centers draw millions of people seeking therapy and relaxation.

Hot and Cold Water Techniques

Hot and warm water therapy increases circulation, relaxation and detoxification efforts. Let's review some of the techniques recommended:

Cold water showers or a quick cold water rinse off after a warm water shower is invigorating and stimulating to the immune system and nervous system. It also helps balance the body's thermoregulation systems, cool the body in hot weather, as well as heat the body (through muscle contraction) in cold weather.

These actions are produced by our blood vessels' response to cold water. Cold water constricts the blood vessels and leads to involuntary muscle contraction. This type of muscle contraction increases the body's immune function by pumping the lymphatic vessels. In other words, lymph flow is circulated by movement and muscle contraction.

The mechanism works like this: As cold water hits the skin, internal muscles autonomically contract. This effectively pumps or squeezes lymphatic vessels. When the lymph vessels are pumped, the lymphatic fluid speed is increased—much like our heart's pumping increases blood circulation.

Lymph circulation distributes macrophages, T-cells, B-cells and other immune factors throughout the body, enabling them to break down invading bacteria, viruses, and chemical toxins. This effectively speeds up our immune response. As our immune system is responding faster, our toxic load is decreased and our infective burden lightens.

Blood vessel constriction from cold water also stimulates the health of our blood vessels. This serves to increase blood vessel wall elasticity, especially when the cold shower follows a warm or hot shower.

German researchers (Goedsche *et al.* 2007) studied the treatments used of Dr. Kneipp on twenty patients with chronic obstructive pulmonary disease. Cold-water hydrotherapy was tested for immunostimulation, maximal expiratory flow, quality of life, and respiratory function. After ten weeks of three cold effusions and two cold washings on the upper body per day, IFN-gamma lymphocytes increased, quality of life increased, lung function improved and the frequency of respiratory infections decreased.

Many traditional healers have used cold water therapy with great success for many inflammatory conditions. Additional cold water strategies include walking in a few inches to a few feet of cold water by a lake, river or ocean for at least a few minutes, building to up to 30 minutes a day.

Contrast baths reference a therapy of alternating hot water and cold water bathing. This therapy has been used with great success, and can be easily practiced at home by simply following a hot shower with a short cold one before toweling off.

Besides constricting blood vessels and stimulating lymph flow, a cold rinse at the end of a shower causes the skin pores to close. This leaves the body prepared to step out of the shower or bath. A cold rinse also reduces the potential of a basal cell chilling, which can stress the body. In other words, a cold rinse will better prepare the body for the temperature change.

Wet Sock hydrotherapy has been used for respiratory issues for centuries. The feet are soaked in hot water for 10-30 minutes while a pair of thin socks are soaked in cold, icy water. The feet are taken out of the hot water and the cold socks are wrung out and put on, with a pair of thick wool socks over top. This is followed by lying down or sitting with the feet up for an hour or two while relaxing.

Finnish sauna and plunge system: The Fins are famous for their wooden saunas, often built outside near a cold-water plunge. A vigorous sweat in the sauna immediately followed by the cold plunge stimulates the immune system dramatically. This ritual has also been a part of other cultures, including many North American Indian tribes, who used *sweat lodges* with great success. These cultures are known for their long lives and strengthened immunity. Infrared saunas are great modern devices for this purpose. Infrared saunas have the added benefit of quickly and safely dilating blood vessels.

Hot baths also have a great tradition of success among those with respiratory ailments. Hippocrates, known to western medicine as the father of medicine, stated that the hot bath *"...promotes expectoration, improves the respiration, and allays lassitude; for it soothes the joints and the outer skin, and is diuretic, removes heaviness of the heat and moistens the nose."*

Hot water calms the body and slows the heart rate, as the body's blood vessels relax and dilate in response to thermal radiation. A hot bath will open skin pores, allowing a detoxification and exfoliation of skin cells and their contents. For sore or damaged muscle tissues, the dilation of capillaries and micro-capillaries speeds up the process of cleansing the muscle cells of lactic and carbonic acids—the byproducts of inadequate respiration.

Recovery times from strenuous activity are typically reduced by the use of hot water therapy. Hot water is also *hydrostatic*—it gently massages the dermal layers. Hot water also slows internal organ activity, and relaxes the airway smooth muscles. This provides a soothing effect upon the innervations to these areas. The result is reduced stress and widened airways. This effect is increased when hot water is in motion—for example a hot tub.

Hot baths can also be medicated with a variety of anti-inflammatory herbs, as listed earlier. Simply make an infusion tea and pour it into the bath.

It should be noted that too much hot water for too long of a period can lead to cardiovascular stress. Hot water can also lead to heat exhaustion. For best results, hot water applications or saunas should be limited to about 10-15 minutes at the hotter levels.

Also, care should be taken to prevent chlorine and chlorine byproduct overload. The byproducts of chlorine breakdown are trihalomethanes (TTHM) and haloacetic acids (TAA5). Over-exposure to these can increase our toxin burden. Today there are healthier alternatives to chlorine, including bromine and salt water blends.

Hot Mineral Springs: From deep within the earth's surface come special waters of a thermal nature. Geothermal heat from volcanic magma creates a rich environment for charging aquifers with high temperatures and a variety of minerals. Many hot springs have a wholesome mixture of bicarbonates, iron, boron, silica, magnesium, copper, lithium, and many trace elements. Some contain exotic elements such as arsenic—believed to help heal skin issues and digestive issues. In other words, not all hot springs are alike.

Due to the earth's sulfur conveyor system, many of these hot spring waters are rich in sulfur in the form of hydrogen sulfide or sulfate. These can loosen phlegm and relax the airways.

Other mineral ions in hot springs have beneficial effects. Magnesium baths have been shown in studies to relax muscles and ease tension. Magnesium also strengthens arteries and relaxes the airway smooth muscles. Iron in hot springs has been associated with strengthening the immune system. Bicarbonates in hot springs—also called "soda springs"—have been associated with easing tension and aiding digestion.

Epson Salt Bath: For those without a nearby hot springs, a simple bath can be easily turned into therapeutic waters. At home, we can duplicate a magnesium and sulfur mineral springs bath by adding natural mineral salts such as Epson salts to our bath water. Epson salts—originally named after the magnesium-rich waters of Epson, England—are primarily magnesium sulfate, which will ionize in the water into magnesium ions and sulfur ions. As mentioned, ionic magnesium is beneficial to body tissues—relaxing the skin, reducing muscle tension, and lowering stress. Sulfur was also discussed above.

The Epson salt bath can be supplemented with the addition of rock salt. Natural rock salt contains upwards of 80 minerals and trace elements, which can make the bath a nourishing soak for the entire body.

A drop or two of an essential oil such as lavender or rose oil into the bath will further support relaxation. Lavender oil in particular can significantly calm the nerves.

The skin is said to be the largest organ of the body and absorbs water quite readily. The skin is similar to a mucous membrane. Ancient seamen understood this fact well. When out to sea and dehydrated, seamen would soak their garments in seawater for survival.

For this same reason, our bath waters should not contain toxic chemical bubble baths, chemical-laden perfumed soaps, or heavily chlorinated water. The skin will readily absorb these toxins, putting an extra burden upon the liver and detoxification systems. Best to use clean water and only natural additives.

Steam baths are especially helpful for most inflammatory conditions. The steam bath can be accomplished with a formal steam room, by the use of a humidifier, or simply with a hot bath in an enclosed room. A cool or cold-water rinse after is helpful for immune stimulation and temperature adjustment. Eucalyptus can be added to increase the expectoration effect. With this and all hot baths, water intake should be increased dramatically, depending upon duration.

Steams can also be done with a pan of boiled water steeped with anti-inflammatory herbs, or boiled potatoes. Just put a towel over the head and over the pan to breathe in the steam.

Sweating to Cleanse

The adult body has about 2.6 million sweat glands located throughout the body's skin cells. This makes the skin the body's greatest outlet for the elimination of toxins. As exposure to chemicals has increased, our need for regular sweat is even greater. Our ancestors worked and sweated daily in order to survive. Today, many of us sit in our heat-controlled environments all day without ever breaking a sweat. This trend has suspiciously increased with the prevalence of inflammatory and autoimmune diseases. University of Alberta researchers (2010) concluded in a study published in the *Archives of Environmental Contamination and Toxicology* that, *"induced sweating appears to be a potential method for elimination of many toxic elements from the human body."*

Typical methods of sweating include exercise, saunas and steam rooms. However, most people overlook the fact that outdoor work, walking or manual labor can produce a healthy sweat. Most people crank on the air conditioning at the slightest sign of heat. Sweating to cool off is a better strategy, as this will stimulate the turnover of toxins that burden our immune system.

Sweating outdoors in the summer heat also makes our body more heat tolerant, which allows us to live in warmer conditions in general. This means we can use the air conditioner less, which is better for our lungs and sinuses in the long run.

Gentle Fasting

Fasting can quickly reduce our toxic burden and systemic inflammation, because it allows the body's liver, kidneys and immune system to clear waste with a lower dietary workload.

However, fasting must be done cautiously. Fasting too aggressively may stimulate too much detoxification too fast, which can overload the bloodstream with toxin byproducts as the tissues clear waste. For this reason, it may be safer to do short, one-day fasts once or twice a week, or fast with soups, juices or fruits.

Fasting with healthy but limited food selections also allows the liver, kidneys and immune system to do a deep cleanse, yet adds some energy nutrients to sustain blood sugar levels.

A systematic approach to fasting is recommended. Here are a few optional approaches to consider:
> ➤ Fast for one afternoon with lemon juice.
> ➤ Water fast from morning until dinner time once or twice a week
> ➤ Fast for one day with only vegetable soups and fresh juices of carrot and celery.

Any of these fasts should be accompanied by the following:
> ➤ Increased water consumption: 3/4-ounce per pound of weight.
> ➤ Increased relaxation and rest (days off work are suggested).
> ➤ Only light exercise, such as walking or swimming.
> ➤ Peaceful environments (no parties or shouting matches).

This formula will guarantee that the fast is productive and thoroughly detoxifying.

Colonics and Enemas

The colon of practically every adult on a western diet is significantly putrefied. This means there is a thick crusty layer of putrefied pathogenic bacteria lining the colon. For some colons, only a small opening allows waste to move out. The rest of the colon is clogged with crusted old waste products. These waste products include histamines, ketones, ammonia, microorganism endotoxins and various other toxic materials that leak back into our bloodstream. Research has shown these contribute to systemic inflammation, as they produce radical oxygen species (free radicals).

The best strategy for anyone with systemic inflammation and/or toxicity is to periodically cleanse the colon. This can be done with periodic enemas, or more deeply and effectively, with a colonic.

Enemas can be done quite easily in the privacy of ones bathroom:

> ➢ The enema bag can be filled with warm water or herbal tea— anti-inflammatory herbs listed earlier can be used.
> ➢ Hang the bag up, with the tubing clamped.
> ➢ Insert the tubing nozzle into the rectum about 3-4 inches. A small amount of castor bean oil or vegetable oil can be put on the nozzle to help its entry.
> ➢ Unclamp the tubing.
> ➢ The water/herbal tea should begin moving up into the colon, slightly extending the lower abdomen. Maintain the filling until the colon begins to feel full.
> ➢ Reclamp the tubing and remove from the rectum.
> ➢ There will soon be a tremendous urge for a bowel movement. Try to resist this urge for two or three minutes.
> ➢ Lightly massage the lower abdomen before bowel movement.
> ➢ The bowel movement will flush the water and waste out.

An enema can be done fairly regularly, but it is important not to overdo enemas, because they can lead to undisciplined bowel movements. After doing one per day for two or three days, once a week is probably sufficient. Consultation with a health professional is suggested.

Colonics are performed by professionals who graduate from schools that teach and certify what is called *colon hydrotherapy*. The colonic is typically done with a sanitary machine that flushes water through the colon, while vacuuming out the waste. A colonic is significantly better and cleanses more deeply than an enema—or even many enemas.

Hydrotherapists typically recommend a colonic at least twice a year if not more. For someone with toxicity and/or inflammation, three colonics per year is probably minimal. Consult a colon hydrotherapist for more information.

Skin Brushing

Brushing the skin lightly with a natural fiber brush can also stimulate detoxification by stimulating the lymphatic system and opening skin pores. This can also stimulate circulation in general, which increases detoxification.

Skin brushing is best accomplished by brushing toward our heart, along the lymphatic vessels and blood vessels. Light but steady pressure is best. It should stimulate circulation and stimulate the skin. This will be readily felt and even seen by more skin color. We likely will not feel an increase in lymph flow, but our immune system will.

A great time to skin brush is after a bath or shower.

Sun Exposure/Vitamin D

Multiple studies have found that inflammatory diseases are significantly greater among regions further from the equator and those with less sunlight exposure. In both Europe and the U.S.—with the exception of urban areas with greater air pollution—those living in Southern regions have shown significantly lower incidence of many degenerative diseases, along with fewer hospital visits.

Vitamin D induces cathelicidin production (Grant 2008). Cathelicidins are proteins found within the lysosomes of macrophages and polymorphonuclear cells (PMNs). These immune cells are intensely antiviral and antibacterial in nature. They are also stimulated and regulated by vitamin D within the body.

Many conditions have been shown to be improved or prevented by therapeutic sunlight and/or vitamin D. These include, lupus vulgaris, small pox, Pick's disease, tuberculosis, asthma, nervous diseases, adrenal insufficiency, hormone imbalances, congestive heart failure, cardiovascular disease, multiple sclerosis, rheumatoid arthritis, Crohn's disease, irritable bowel syndrome, acne, psoriasis, jaundice, depression, eczema, high blood pressure, heart disease, diabetes, hypothyroidism, angina, prostate cancer, lung cancer, colon cancer, ovary cancer, kidney disease, hyperparathyroidism, uterine cancer, stomach cancer, kidney cancer, lymphoma, pancreatic cancer, ovarian cancer, tooth loss, bone loss, obesity, joint inflammation, insomnia, Parkinson's disease, fibromyalgia and a variety of immune- and autoimmune-related diseases.

In all, research over the past ten years has found that sunlight and/or vitamin D deficiency is implicated in over 70 disease conditions.

The sun's ultraviolet-B rays stimulate our bodies to synthesize vitamin D_3. Vitamin D is more of a hormone than a vitamin. It is a critical biochemical for the body. The cholesterol derivative *7-dehydrocholesterol* undergoes a *conrotatory electrocyclic reaction* to produce a pre-vitamin D. The pre-vitamin D molecule undergoes hydroxylation in the liver and kidneys to convert to the final D_3 structure— 1,25 dihydroxyvitamin D (or 25-OHD).

Within a 7-dehydrocholesterol-saturated biomolecular environment of the epidermis, specialized cells called *melanocytes* produce a protective biochemical called *melanin*. Skin melanocytes are primarily located at the lower strata of the epidermis. Other melanocytes located around the body produce specialized forms of melanin. Melanocytes within the uvea, which contains the iris, produce the melanin that gives the color to our irises. Melanocytes around our hair follicles give color to our hair. Melanocytes within the leptomeninges residing within our brain and spinal cord produce a type of melanin thought to support cerebrospinal fluid circulation.

Once produced in skin melanocytes, melanin is transferred to the keratinocytes, which lie on the external skin barrier. Melanin is the biochemical pigment that makes the skin turn brown. Melanin also provides a natural sunscreen for the skin: The greater the melanin level, the fewer ultraviolet-B rays reach the 7-dehydrocholesterol molecules, and the less vitamin D_3 is produced. Vitamin D is used in thousands of metabolic processes around the body. What is not used is stored within fat cells for later use.

Vitamin D is considered a cell membrane antioxidant. It specifically inhibits the lipid peroxidation process. Research has found that vitamin D inhibits lipid peroxidation better than cholesterol—a typical inhibitor. One study found its lipid peroxidation properties have anti-cancer benefits (Wiseman 1993).

Additional effects and mechanisms of sunlight and vitamin D are discussed in the author's book, *Healthy Sun*.

Sleep Strategies

Sleep is critical to our immune system and our ability to purge toxins. This is especially true when it comes to deep sleep and REM-stage cycles.

When we sleep, our immune system moves into overdrive. Like microscopic elves, our probiotics become more active, taking out pathogenic microorganisms and breaking down toxins. Our T- and B-cells help coordinate the process, and participate in breaking down pathogens and toxins. Our liver will produce more antioxidant enzymes during sleep. The body's purification systems all move into overdrive. When we sleep deeply, we also breathe deeper, which removes more toxins from the lungs and the airway mucosal membranes. Our intestinal probiotics switch into high gear, and our cells dump more toxins into intercellular fluids.

This was illustrated by researchers from Chicago's Rush University Medical Center (Ranjbaran *et al.* 2007), who studied sleep abnormalities and their association with *"chronic inflammatory conditions (CIC)."* They found that changes in the *"sleep-wake cycle"* stimulate an increased systemic inflammation response. Their research also showed that slow wave (deep) sleep can curb inflammation and strengthen immunity.

They also found that sleep disturbances can cause greater levels of inflammatory pain and fatigue, while reducing quality of life. This scenario is often seen amongst those with toxemia. The researchers commented that the underlying mechanism causing a lack of sleep to spurn systemic inflammation relates to the *"dysregulation of the immune system."*

A key strategy for deep sleep is to spend time outside everyday. This helps regulate our light-dark cycles. This means getting outside early in the daytime to stimulate the pineal gland and the SCN cells. Then as the night proceeds towards bedtime, we should turn the lights low and then off. This will regulate the circulation of melatonin and cortisol, allowing us to fall asleep at the right time of the cortisol-melatonin cycle—allowing us to sleep deeper through the night.

If we are consistently tired during the day, we can have someone watch us sleep, looking for irregular breathing, stopping breathing for a short period and/or partial wakening while sleeping. These may be signs of sleep apnea. If someone close says that they see some of these symptoms, we should see a sleep specialist.

Before retiring to bed, we might consider clearing our nose and throat. Going to bed with a stuffy nose and phlegm can inhibit our breathing, and disturb sleep. See the discussion on nasal lavages to clear the sinuses. Deep gargling with slightly salty water can help clear the throat. To gargle deeply, we can try humming while gargling.

We can keep the bedroom clear of dust, mold and other possible allergens. We can consider the bedroom a "safe room" as discussed in the chapter on triggers. Inflammatory symptoms during or following sleeping may indicate toxic exposures from the bedroom or bedroom air.

We can avoid eating late. Food may back up into the esophagus if the sphincter is weak and we are lying down. If the mucous membranes are weak, this may cause acid reflux, which can prevent a good night's sleep. If experiencing some reflux at night, we can raise the head of the bed to help keep stomach contents down, at least while working on mucosal membrane strategies outlined earlier.

For more information on sleep, including many lifestyle, dietary and herbal strategies that promote deep sleep, please refer to the author's book, *Natural Sleep - Insomnia Solutions.*

Exercise Strategies

A plethora of research has shown that sedentary lifestyles dramatically increase the risk of systemic inflammation.

This is based on the fact that exercise increases circulation and detoxification, stimulates the immune system, pumps the lymphatic system and increases lung capacity. Exercise is one of the most assured ways to strengthen the immune system and thus increase tolerance. When we exercise, we contract muscles. Again, muscle contraction is what circulates (or pumps) lymph around the body through the lymph vessels. This is because the lymphatic system does not have a heart like the circulatory system has. The lymphatic system relies on muscle contraction for circulation—as we've discussed.

Lymph circulation is critical for systemic inflammation because immune cells circulating through the blood and lymph break down and carry out of the body those broken-down toxins and cell parts.

And of course, exercise also circulates oxygen and nutrients throughout the body. Exercise also stimulates the thymus gland, and speeds up healing of the intestinal cell walls. In all, exercise is one of the best and cheapest therapies available to boost immunity and tolerance.

All of these effects and more are produced by daily exercise and activity.

Choosing the Routine

Choosing the right type of exercise depends greatly upon the individual and situation. Good forms of exercise include swimming, walking, running, tennis, golf, baseball, basketball, softball, volleyball, surfing, racquetball and squash.

Working out in a warmer, slightly humid environment is probably best for detoxification, but exercising in any weather is better than no exercise. If running or working out outside during the winter, we can wear a ski mask or scarf over the nose and mouth to reduce the cold air, for example. Breathing in through the nose will also help warm the air before it hits the lungs. This will allow our lungs to empty more and work more effectively.

The morning also typically contains less air pollutants because the night usually clears out the air a bit. So early morning exercise is worth considering.

Warming up before exercising is also important. A routine of stretching, jumping jacks, push-ups, knee bends and so on will increase circulation and prepare the body for rigorous exercise.

Days with longer exercise activity can be alternated with shorter-burst activity. Shorter-burst activity increases lung function and increases tolerance. Longer, slower exercise produces more detoxification because there are fewer waste products being produced. For example, a person might alternate between walking, taking a hike in the woods, or slow swimming on one day, and play some basketball, soccer or do wind sprints the next. This can further be supplemented with abdominal and even weight (or isometric) training—both of which can increase immunity and detoxification.

The bottom line that the type of exercise depends upon the individual. If a person enjoys a particular sport, they ought to pursue that sport. They will be better for it because they will more likely to continue that sport.

Manual Activity

Manual labor is shunned in modern western society, yet it is one of the best means to stay healthy. Manual labor works many muscle groups and stimulates detoxification. For most of us, there is always the choice of doing it ourselves or otherwise. A good example is weeding. While pulling weeds by hand or using the hoe to remove them requires virtually no expense or special skill, most westerners elect to spray the weeds with toxic chemicals. The election to spray not only eliminates the potential for exercise: It also exposes us to chemicals that add to our body's toxin load.

Active choices can also be as easy as taking the stairs instead of the elevator; walking to the next store rather than driving the car to the next parking lot; biking to work instead of driving; raking the leaves instead of using a leafblower—and so many other choices.

Breathing and Airway Strategies

Relearning to Breathe

Deep breathing is one of the best ways to purify the blood and strengthen the immune system. It can also increase lung capacity and respiration efficiency. Deep breathing will strengthen and enlarge the diaphragm, strengthen the supporting abdominal muscles, relaxes the smooth muscles of the airways, and helps reduce stress.

We will discuss a number of methods here, but we focus on two established techniques for healthy deep breathing:

Deep core breathing:
➤ Slowly push out the abdomen around the belly button. As the lungs fill, push out the upper abdomen. If lying down, a book may be placed on the abdomen to feel and see it rise.
➤ Continue pushing out until the lungs are full and the abdomen is fully pushed out.
➤ Top it off by expanding the rib cage to completely fill the lungs.
➤ Hold in position and relax for 3-7 seconds.
➤ Then push the air out by slowly contracting the upper abdominal muscles followed by contracting the lower abdomen as the lungs are completely emptied. This last step is called *flooring.*

Deep diaphragm breathing:
➤ Slowly push out at the top of the abdomen, enlarging the diaphragm to its capacity as the lungs fill.
➤ Follow by expanding the rib cage to fill out the lungs. Hold for 2-5 seconds.
➤ Then begin contracting the upper abdominal muscles to contract the diaphragm. This will begin pushing the air out.
➤ Slowly contract the diaphragm completely to force out as much air as possible.

Diaphragm breathing does not as completely fill or empty the lungs as deep core breathing does, but it is often more practical while sitting, walking or exercising. Core breathing can result in sleepiness, so it is best used at home in bed or on a comfortable sofa. Either method, if practiced daily for at least 15 minutes, can significantly increase our lung cavity capacity. We may begin to breathe deeper without trying. Placing a hand on the abdomen to feel its rise and fall can also help us center ourselves on our breathing.

In both methods, good breathing posture can be maintained. If sitting, the lower back can be arched slightly with the upper spine fairly straight and relaxed, and the back of the head in line with our lower spine. We can sit on the front of our 'sit bones' at the base of the pelvis, rather than the backside of our sit bones where the lower spine tends to curve outward. When we are sitting on the right part of our sit bones, our lower back will naturally arch.

If lying down on our back, a large pillow can be put under the knees, with the spine straight and a comfortable neck pillow that keeps the crown of the head aligned with the lower spine. Most *hatha-yoga* postures are also conducive to deep breathing exercises.

Keeping the Lungs Clear

Remember that the sinus cavity, pharynx, larynx, trachea and bronchi are all lined with epithelial cells covered with a thin fluid of mucous membrane and tiny hairs called cilia. Cilia trap foreign particles in the sticky, immune cell-rich mucous before they can enter the lungs. This should clear out most soot, debris, bacteria and viruses before they proceed further.

When toxic air (air pollution) or bacteria sneak past these defenses, the bronchial tree, alveoli and pleural cavity will swell with inflammation. The pleural cavity will also often leak fluids into the lung. These fluids, together with the swollen airways, effectively decrease lung capacity and air clearance.

For many, swollen and irritated air passages and pleura is constant, due to an overloading of air pollution, airborne chemicals, dust and microorganisms. Strategies to increase lung capacity and maintain healthy mucosal membranes are thus tantamount to reducing the impact of modern toxins.

Keeping the Sinuses Clear

This brings us to the logical conclusion that we need to keep the nasal passages clear. Obviously, keeping the sinuses and nasal passages clear is the key to breathing comfortably if we plan to breathe in through the nose. When the sinuses are clogged, our mucous membranes are not draining properly. Mucous needs to be swept out, and if the mucous is too thick or crustified with waste matter, it will narrow our available airways.

So how do we accomplish keeping the sinuses clear? Well, besides breathing in through the nose and general hygiene to help keep them clean—we might consider periodic nasal irrigation.

Nasal lavage is the first consideration. This can utilize a special Ayurvedic lavage device called the neti pot. Neti has been in practice for thousands of years. The pot is simply filled with warm weakly-salty water, and poured through each nostril. A small teapot can also be used.

The technique is to first mix about a quarter-teaspoon of non-iodized, re-fined salt to about a cup of lukewarm water. A pinch of baking soda may also be added, especially if the salt is iodized or otherwise burns in any way.

Lean forward, over the sink. With the chin level with the nose, turn the head sideways so the nose on a plane parallel with the ground as much as possible.

The water is lightly poured into one nostril, traveling around the septum and out the other nostril. There is no force or pressure involved. There is no snuffing in or pulling in. The solution is simply poured into one nostril, and out through the other. Just hold the head still while it pours out.

Nasal Irrigation: This can also be accomplished by gently pushing warm saline (water and salt) into each nostril using a soft squeeze bottle. Soft squeeze bottles designed for cleaning the nostrils are often available at most drug stores. After using the saline in the bottle, the bottle can be refilled. Care must be taken not to forcefully squirt the water through, which can get water into the upper sinuses.

Another technique is to sniff the water up the nose and back down through to the pharynx and throat, where it is spit out into the sink. This can provide a more complete cleansing of the pharynx and sinuses, but should not be overdone, and only if the sinuses are at least partially clear.

Nasal irrigation has been proven in research to aid in allergic conditions and sinusitis. For example, researchers from Taiwan's Chung Shan Medical University Hospital (Wang *et al.* 2009) gave nasal irrigation or not to 69 chil-dren with acute sinusitis. The saline irrigation group improved significantly better than the other group with regard to symptoms and quality of life.

Nasal irrigation was also effective in reducing sinus congestion, rhinor-rhea, sneezing and nasal itching in a study by medical researchers from Italy's University of Milano (Garavello *et al.* 2010). In this study, 23 pregnant women with seasonal allergic rhinitis underwent either nasal irrigation or not for six weeks.

In another study, presented at the 50th Scientific Assembly of the American Academy of Family Physicians, Dr. Richard Ravizza and Dr. John Fornadley of Pennsylvania State University divided 294 students into three groups, one of which did nasal irrigation with salt water and the other two groups either took a placebo pill or did nothing. The nasal irrigation group experienced fewer colds during the treatment period compared to the other two groups.

To be fair, some have questioned whether daily regular nasal irrigation for long periods is necessarily good. In a study presented at a the American College of Allergy, Asthma and Immunology (Nsouli 2009), researchers tested 68 patients with a history of sinusitis, who had been using nasal irriga-tion daily. Of the total, 44 patients discontinued the irrigation while 24 con-tinued the daily treatment. After a year, those who had discontinued the irrigation had 62% less sinusitis infections than the group who continued to use nasal irrigation daily. Dr. Tamal Nsouli commented that daily irrigation may deplete healthy mucous from the sinuses. As we've discussed, healthy mucous membranes also cover the sinuses, helping protect us from infection. Dr. Nsouli also commented that he is not opposed to irrigation for three or four times a week, but suggested avoiding daily irrigation for long periods.

We should note that the study details and protocol have yet to be published, and was only presented in abstract form at the conference. Diane Heatley, M.D., a Professor at the University of Wisconsin School of Medicine, questioned the report, stating, *"nasal irrigation has previously been proven safe and effective for treatment of sinus symptoms in both adults and children in a number of studies already published in peer-reviewed journals."*

An appropriate conclusion here is that regular nasal irrigation should still include some moderation. Using it during periods of congestion and sensitivity is certainly appropriate. Use after or during environmental conditions where there is an increased level of pollution and/or infectious agents is also appropriate. But we can remember that our mucous membranes also house important immune cells and probiotics, which help protect us. We don't want to flush those away needlessly.

Liver Cleansing Strategies

The liver is the primary organ involved in removing toxins that burden the immune system—and contribute to systemic inflammation. In other words, liver health is crucial. The liver produces a number of enzymes that help break down toxins and endotoxins (waste material from microorganisms). The liver also filters blood through its hepatocytes to remove toxins, while breaking apart pathogens using its kuppfer cells.

There are several strategies we can utilize to increase the liver's health. Here are a few:

> ➤ Reducing or eliminating our intake of chemical preservatives, food dyes and synthetic sweeteners. All of these require the liver's resources to break them down.
> ➤ Reducing or eliminating our exposure to formaldehydes, cleaning chemicals, pesticides, herbicides, benzenes, VOCs and other harsh chemicals that the liver must work hard to break down once absorbed into the skin or lungs.
> ➤ Drinking enough water (as outlined earlier). Water nourishes and helps the liver flush and detoxify the blood and lymph.
> ➤ Eliminating unnecessary pharmaceuticals, as pharmaceuticals are typically rough on the liver—as is alcohol. This requires that we work closely with those doctors who have prescribed our pharmaceuticals, while asking the doctor a clear question: *"Do I really need to continue taking this pharmaceutical?"* Most pharmaceuticals are intended and tested for short-term use. Most were never intended for long-term use, and many studies have shown that

long-term use of medications can severely damage the liver. Note also that some pharmaceuticals are worse than others. Acetaminophen is particularly harsh on the liver, for example. For a more complete list of pharmaceuticals that aggravate or cause toxemia, see the list in Chapter Two.

➢ Correcting the fatty acid balance in our diet to comply more closely to that outlined earlier. The liver must work hard to accommodate our fats. High levels of the wrong fats can put a strain on the liver.

➢ Keeping our cholesterol levels in balance through wise dietary choices. Foods that produce high levels of low-density lipoproteins (such as fried foods, saturated fats, grilled meats and so on) will strain the liver as it seeks to balance cholesterol and reduce lipid peroxidation.

➢ Liver strengthening foods include beets, carrots, turnips, radishes, onions, leafy-green vegetables, spirulina, chlorella, squash, celery and other plant-based foods.

➢ Liver restoring herbs include Milk Thistle, Turmeric, Garlic, Dandelion, Goldenseal, Ginger, Bupleurum and Guduchi.

➢ Healthy probiotic colonies are critical for liver health. Consider these studies:

Researchers from Russia's Northern State Medical University (Kirpich *et al.* 2008) studied 66 adult Russian males admitted to a psychiatric hospital with a diagnosis of alcoholic psychosis. They gave the patients standard therapy (abstinence plus vitamins) with *Bifidobacterium bifidum* and *Lactobacillus plantarum* 8PA3 or standard therapy alone without probiotics for five days. Stool cultures and liver enzymes were examined and compared with 24 healthy, matched non-drinker controls. The alcoholic patients had significantly fewer bifidobacteria, lactobacilli, and enterococci than did the healthy non-drinkers. The average starting levels of liver enzymes alanine aminotransferase (ALT), aspartate aminotransferase (AST), and gamma-glutamyl transpeptidase (GGT) were significantly greater in the alcoholic group compared to the healthy non-drinkers.

After 5 days of daily probiotics, alcoholic patients had significantly more bifidobacteria and lactobacilli populations compared to the control group. The probiotic group also had significantly lower AST and ALT levels at the end of treatment than the standard therapy control group. Of the 26 patients with mild alcoholic hepatitis, probiotic therapy significantly reduced liver enzymes ALT, AST, GGT, lactate dehydrogenase and total bilirubin. The researchers concluded that, "Short-term oral supplementation with *B. bifidum* and *L. plantarum* 8PA3 was associated with restoration of the bowel flora and greater improvement in alcohol-induced liver injury than standard therapy alone."

Scientists from Italy's University of Catania (Malaguarnera *et al.* 2007) gave 60 cirrhotic patients *Bifidobacterium longum* plus fructo-oligosaccharides (FOS) or placebo. After 90 days, fasting NH(4) serum levels significantly decreased among the probiotic patients. Other liver tests, including MMSE, Trail Making Test-A and Test-B also significantly improved among the probiotic group as compared with the placebo group.

Researchers from the Liver Failure Group and The Institute of Hepatology at the University College London's Medical School (Stadlbauer *et al.* 2008) studied neutrophil function and cytokine responses in alcoholic cirrhosis patients in an open-label study. Twenty patients with alcoholic cirrhosis were treated with a placebo or *Lactobacillus casei* Shirota for 4 weeks. The data were also compared to 13 healthy control subjects who did not receive probiotics. The cirrhosis patients' starting neutrophil phagocytic capacity was significantly lower than healthy controls (73% versus 98%) before probiotic treatment. Neutrophil phagocytic capacities after the probiotic treatments were equal among the cirrhosis patients and healthy volunteers at the end of the study—while the placebo group's neutrophil capacity did not change. In addition, endotoxin-stimulated TNF-receptor-1, TNFR-2 and interleukin IL10 levels were significantly lower among the probiotic group. The researchers concluded that, "Our data provide a proof-of-concept that probiotics restore neutrophil phagocytic capacity in cirrhosis, possibly by changing IL10 secretion and TLR4 expression."

China's Capital University of Medical Sciences and the Beijing Friendship Hospital (Zhao *et al.* 2004) studied fifty patients with liver cirrhosis. They tested and graded the entire group for intestinal probiotic content and severity of liver disease. The researchers found that the cirrhosis was directly associated with intestinal probiotic content. The more severe the cirrhosis, the more imbalanced the intestinal probiotic content was. The patients were randomized and given *Bifidobacterium, Lactobacillus acidophilus* and *Enterococcus faecium;* or *Bacillus subtilis* and *Enterococcus faecium* for 14 days. Fecal flora, pH and ammonia content, and plasma endotoxin levels were tested before and after. All levels improved after both probiotic treatments. In addition, those given *B. subtilis* and *E. faecium* showed a reduction in endotoxin levels among endotoxemia cirrhosis cases.

Researchers from the Department of Surgery at Japan's Nagoya University Graduate School of Medicine (Kanazawa *et al.* 2005) investigated the effects of *L. casei* with 54 patients following hepatectomy. Infection complications were 19% in the probiotic group and 52% in the placebo group.

Forty cirrhosis patients with hepatic encephalopathy were studied by researchers from the University of Naples (Loguercio, *et al.* 1987). They were given either *Enterococcus* probiotic strain SF68 or lactulose (standard treatment) for 10 days. The probiotics were as effective as lactulose in lowering blood ammonia and improving mental state. The beneficial effects of the probiotics persisted significantly longer after treatment was discontinued

Adrenal Strategies

The adrenal glands respond to stress by way of biochemical signals from the hypothalamus and pituitary gland. These biochemical signals come in the form of adrenocorticotropic hormone (or ACTH). This master hormone signals nerve centers, and stimulates the adrenal glands to produce cortisol and other glucocorticoids. This is called the *hypothalamic-pituitary-adrenal axis stress response.*

Remember that the adrenals are critical to the production of cortisol, and it is cortisol and other glucocorticoids that control inflammation. Therefore, the adrenals are necessary to balance inflammation and detoxification. This is why cortisone is used for inflammation: It blocks and controls the inflammatory response by interrupting the interleukin-1 and IL-2 cytokine communications.

However, cortisone medications over longer periods also depress adrenal function. Because they provide corticoids directly, the adrenal gland begins to switch off its corticoid production. This adrenal switching off has been linked to adrenal insufficiency and systemic inflammation (Polito *et al.* 2007).

For this very reason, withdrawing from or reducing cortisone medications after their long-term use can result in a dramatic rise in uninhibited inflammation throughout the body. This is because inflammatory cytokines such as the interleukins are allowed to act without adequate corticoid control.

This can be compounded by a situation called adrenal exhaustion. Under stressful situations, the healthy adrenal gland is stimulated to produce cortisol. This trigger effect is natural and supports our ability to respond to dire circumstances. However, should we become stressed too often, this automatic adrenal response begins the wear out the adrenals. They become exhausted because they have been over-stimulated.

In other words, healthy adrenals should be balancing inflammatory responses by supplying natural corticoids. In the case of adrenal exhaustion and in the absence of sufficient natural corticoids (and/or inflammatory episodes that have gone way out of control) physicians prescribe synthetic cortisone to achieve what our body's adrenal glands should have: Shutting down inflammation before it got out of control.

Relaxation is critical to the adrenal glands. As the system relaxes more, the adrenal glands are allowed some time to refresh, enabling them to better respond to small inflammatory episodes—before they get out of control.

But what about adrenal glands that are already exhausted? Can we do anything to rebuild and strengthen them? Absolutely.

In fact, many of the strategies we have outlined in this chapter, including many of the herbs, foods, detoxification and exercises will directly or indirectly strengthen the adrenal glands. This is accomplished because they can:

> ➢ Reduce inflammation—unburdening the adrenal glands.
> ➢ Stimulate relaxation—allowing the adrenals to recuperate.
> ➢ Directly stimulate healthy adrenal activity.

> Supply adrenals with the raw materials to produce corticoids and androgens.

With regard to the latter point, the adrenal glands do more than simply produce cortisol. They also produce androgens, glucocorticoids and many other hormones that stabilize and balance the body's metabolism. Without a strong and active adrenal complex, the body's hormone and steroid system becomes unbalanced and out of whack. This encourages inflammatory responses to become uncontrolled, producing a number of possible symptoms.

What are some of the more immediate ways to increase adrenal capacity? Here are a few of the many that either unburden or strengthen the adrenals:

> Decreased toxin consumption, and detoxification efforts.
> Greenfoods, fruits and vegetables that provide antioxidants.
> Plenty of water, as defined earlier.
> Relaxation: Letting things roll off the back, so to speak. Not sweating inconsequential things. This is particularly important for those who drive everyday. Driving is highly stressful. It can help, therefore, to listen to soothing music while driving. Or take public transportation.
> Deep breathing: This is important for relaxation, as we discussed above. Breathing not only nourishes the adrenals with oxygen and alkalinity: It also stimulates the VNO nerves.
> Visual imagery: Looking at scenes of nature, or imagining natural settings.
> Higher sounds: Consider what we hear. Are we hearing a lot of chatter about what other people are stressed about? (This includes television.) Hearing stressful language can stimulate our adrenals. In fact, a dramatic movie or TV program has been shown to stimulate the adrenals and increase cortisol levels. This may be okay periodically, but not constantly. For those with already over-stimulated adrenals, being around uplifting sounds and discussions is a better strategy.
> Foods particularly good for the adrenals include onions, garlic, peppers, papaya, mango, apricots, squash and broccoli.
> Herbs that help strengthen and revitalize the adrenals include Shizandra, Tylophora, Astragalus, Dandelion and Licorice.

We might add that the Licorice mentioned here should not be deglycyrrhized licorice, as in the DGL used primarily for stomach ulcers. This is because glycyrrhizin and its triterpenoid, glycyrrhizinic acid, are considered primary adrenal-restorative constituents. This said, a 2003 European Commission suggested that a person should not consume more than 100 milligrams of glycyrrhizinic acid per day. Note, however, that even concentrated extracts of licorice herb will contain only 4-25% glycyrrhizinic acid. This means that 400-500 mg a day of *raw, unconcentrated* licorice root will contain far less than the maximum levels documented by the European Commission.

Natural licorice root, in fact, has been used safely by Western and Eastern traditional herbalists for many centuries.

The Living Conclusion

When most people think of cleansing the body, the approach is not much different than cleaning out a drain. The problem with this strategy is that our bodies are not sinks and pipes. Our bodies are living organisms.

Our bodies are not only alive: They are also packed with smaller living organisms, and billions of living cells. Each of these living structures must 'come along' with any sort of cleansing protocol. We cannot force our 'drain-cleaning' plan down their throats.

Therefore, a better strategy is to know what those living structures need to operate better and more efficiently remove the toxins that are burdening them.

So we give our living ecology what they need. We give them the foods that nourish them. We give them the prebiotics, the fiber, the polysaccharides, nutrient complexes, chelated minerals, tocopherols and tocotrienols, chelated ascorbates and so on. We also stimulate them with fermented proteins, yeast complexes, probiotic foods and supplements, antioxidants and blood-purifying herbs.

Then we support these efforts with lifestyle activities such as exercise, deep breathing, healthy sweating, light fasting, a colonic now and again, some skin brushing, healthy sun exposure, enough pure water, and some hydrotherapy as we have time and energy.

Now each of these strategies has been shown in the research to benefit the immune system when conducted on an isolated basis. But what will we get if we *combine* these strategies into a healthy, sustainable lifestyle?

We will get a well-balanced and sustainable method of cleansing the body of past toxins, fending off many possible toxins, and efficiently cleansing our body of what toxins do make it through.

Now we're not talking about a one- or two-week cleanse. We're not talking about flushing out the toxins like we flush a toilet. We are talking about gently and safely stimulating the body's own purification systems. This means that it is best to incorporate these strategies gradually. While we can incorporate multiple strategies at once, it is best not to dive into each one too deeply.

In other words, we can begin changing our diet while incorporating supplements all together, but by easing into the change. We can start by adding a few elements the first week, and then adding more each successive week.

In the same way, we can add hydrotherapy into our day first by following each shower with a cold shower. Then later we can consider the wet sock therapy on the weekend, a sauna at the gym, or a mineral hot springs during our next three-day weekend.

As for herbs, we can buy a nice herbal tea mix with some of the herbs mentioned, and add a cup of tea to our morning with some raw honey for sweetness.

To our meals we can add more purifying spices, together with delicious fermented and cultured foods. To these meals we can add more whole grains and vegetables, and more fresh fruits and whole nuts to our deserts and snacks.

By doing these, we will start adding more fiber every day, which in turn binds to toxins, lowers lipid peroxidation, and stimulates healthy elimination.

More and more, we can incorporate the programs outlined here, as we are comfortable. If we feel any loss of energy after any particular change, we can draw back and more slowly add that element, or try something else. In other words, we want to work with our body, not against it.

This is a well-rounded, logical and safe approach to cleansing and revitalizing the body. There is no escaping the fact that our body is alive. We simply have to feed the body what will stimulate it: Living elements.

References and Bibliography

Abdureyim S, Amat N, Umar A, Upur H, Berke B, Moore N. Anti-inflammatory, immunomodulatory, and heme oxygenase-1 inhibitory activities of ravan napas, a formulation of uighur traditional medicine, in a rat model of allergic asthma. *Evid Based Complement Alternat Med.* 2011;2011. pii: 725926.

Aberg N, Hesselmar B, Aberg B, Eriksson B. Increase of asthma, allergic rhinitis and eczema in Swedish schoolchildren between 1979 and 1991. *Clin Exp Allergy.* 1995;25:815-819.

Adel-Patient K, Ah-Leung S, Creminon C, Nouaille S, Chatel JM, Langella P, Wal JM. Oral administration of recombinant Lactococcus lactis expressing bovine beta-lactoglobulin partially prevents mice from sensitization. *Clin Exp Allergy.* 2005 Apr;35(4):539-46.

Adoga AS, Otene AA, Yiltok SJ, Adekwu A, Nwaorgu OG. Cervical necrotizing fasciitis: case series and review of literature. *Niger J Med.* 2009 Apr-Jun;18(2):203-7.

Agache I, Ciobanu C. Risk factors and asthma phenotypes in children and adults with seasonal allergic rhinitis. *Phys Sportsmed.* 2010 Dec;38(4):81-6.

Agarwal KN, Bhasin SK, Faridi MM, Mathur M, Gupta S. *Lactobacillus casei* in the control of acute diarrhea—a pilot study. *Indian Pediatr.* 2001 Aug;38(8):905-10.

Agarwal SK, Singh SS, Verma S. Antifungal principle of sesquiterpene lactones from Anamirta cocculus. *Indian Drugs.* 1999;36:754-5.

Agerholm-Larsen L, Raben A, Haulrik N, Hansen AS, Manders M, Astrup A. Effect of 8 week intake of probiotic milk products on risk factors for cardiovascular diseases. *Eur J Clin Nutr.* 2000 Apr;54(4):288-97.

Aggarwal BB, Harikumar KB. Potential therapeutic effects of curcumin, the anti-inflammatory agent, against neurodegenerative, cardiovascular, pulmonary, metabolic, autoimmune and neoplastic diseases. *Int J Biochem Cell Biol.* 2009 Jan;41(1):40-59.

Aggarwal BB, Sung B. Pharmacological basis for the role of curcumin in chronic diseases: an age-old spice with modern targets. *Trends Pharmacol Sci.* 2009 Feb;30(2):85-94.

Agostoni C, Fiocchi A, Riva E, Terracciano L, Sarratud T, Martelli A, Lodi F, D'Auria E, Zuccotti G, Giovannini M. Growth of infants with IgE-mediated cow's milk allergy fed different formulas in the complementary feeding period. *Pediatr Allergy Immunol.* 2007 Nov;18(7):599-606.

Agustina R, Lukito W, Firmansyah A, Suhardjo HN, Murniati D, Bindels J. The effect of early nutritional supplementation with a mixture of probiotic, prebiotic, fiber and micronutrients in infants with acute diarrhea in Indonesia. *Asia Pac J Clin Nutr.* 2007;16(3):435-42.

Ahmed M, Prasad J, Gill H, Stevenson L, Gopal P. Impact of consumption of different levels of *Bifidobacterium lactis* HN019 on the intestinal microflora of elderly human subjects. *J Nutr Health Aging.* 2007 Jan-Feb;11(1):26-31.

Ahmed, AA, McCarthy RD, Porter GA. Effect of milk constituents on hepatic cholesterogenesis. *Atherosclerosis.* 1979;32:347-57.

Aho K, Koskenvuo M, Tuominen J, Kaprio J. Occurrence of rheumatoid arthritis in a nationwide series of twins. *J Rheumatol.* 1986 Oct;13(5):899-902.

Ahola AJ, Yli-Knuuttila H, Suomalainen T, Poussa T, Ahlström A, Meurman JH, Korpela R. Short-term consumption of probiotic-containing cheese and its effect on dental caries risk factors. *Arch Oral Biol.* 2002 Nov;47(11):799-804.

Aihara K, Kajimoto O, Hirata H, Takahashi R, Nakamura Y. Effect of powdered fermented milk with *Lactobacillus helveticus* on subjects with high-normal blood pressure or mild hypertension. *J Am Coll Nutr.* 2005 Aug;24(4):257-65.

Akil I, Yilmaz O, Kurutepe S, Degerli K, Kavukcu S. Influence of oral intake of *Saccharomyces boulardii* on *Escherichia coli* in enteric flora. *Pediatr Nephrol.* 2006 Jun;21(6):807-10.

Akinbami LJ, Moorman JE, Garbe PL, Sondik EJ. Status of childhood asthma in the United States, 1980-2007. *Pediatrics.* 2009;123:S131-45.

Aldinucci C, Bellussi L, Monciatti G, Passàli GC, Salerni L, Passàli D, Bocci V. Effects of dietary yoghurt on immunological and clinical parameters of rhinopathic patients. *Eur J Clin Nutr.* 2002 Dec;56(12):1155-61.

Alemán A, Sastre J, Quirce S, de las Heras M, Carnés J, Fernández-Caldas E, Pastor C, Blázquez AB, Vivanco F, Cuesta-Herranz J. Allergy to kiwi: a double-blind, placebo-controlled food challenge study in patients from a birch-free area. *J Allergy Clin Immunol.* 2004 Mar;113(3):543-50.

Alexander DD, Cabana MD. Partially hydrolyzed 100% whey protein infant formula and reduced risk of atopic dermatitis: a meta-analysis. *J Pediatr Gastroenterol Nutr.* 2010 Apr;50(4):422-30.

Alexandrakis M, Letourneau R, Kempuraj D, Kandere-Grzybowska K, Huang M, Christodoulou S, Boucher W, Seretakis D, Theoharides TC. Flavones inhibit proliferation and increase mediator content in human leukemic mast cells (HMC-1). *Eur J Haematol.* 2003 Dec;71(6):448-54.

Alfvén T, Braun-Fahrländer C, Brunekreef B, von Mutius E, Riedler J, Scheynius A, van Hage M, Wickman M, Benz MR, Budde J, Michels KB, Schram D, Ublagger E, Waser M, Pershagen G; PARSIFAL study group. Allergic diseases and atopic sensitization in children related to farming and anthroposophic life-style—the PARSIFAL study. *Allergy*. 2006 Apr;61(4):414-21. PubMed PMID: 16512802.

Al-Harrasi A, Al-Saidi S. Phytochemical analysis of the essential oil from botanically certified oleogum resin of Boswellia sacra (Omani Luban). *Molecules*. 2008 Sep 16;13(9):2181-9.

Allen SJ, Okoko B, Martinez E, Gregorio G, Dans LF. Probiotics for treating infectious diarrhea. *The Cochrane Library*. 2004;3. Chichester, UK: John Wiley & Sons, Ltd.

Alleva R, Tomasetti M, Bompadre S, Littarru GP. Oxidation of LDL and their subfractions: kinetic aspects and CoQ10 content. *Mol Aspects Med*. 1997;18 Suppl:S105-12.

Almqvist C, Garden F, Xuan W, Mihrshahi S, Leeder SR, Oddy W, Webb K, Marks GB; CAPS team. Omega-3 and omega-6 fatty acid exposure from early life does not affect atopy and asthma at age 5 years. *J Allergy Clin Immunol*. 2007 Jun;119(6):1438-44.

Amato R, Pinelli M, Monticelli A, Miele G, Cocozza S. Schizophrenia and Vitamin D Related Genes Could Have Been Subject to Latitude-driven Adaptation. *BMC Evol Biol*. 2010 Nov 11;10(1):351.

Amenta M, Cascio MT, Di Fiore P, Venturini I. Diet and chronic constipation. Benefits of oral supplementation with symbiotic zir fos (*Bifidobacterium longum* W11 + FOS Actilight). *Acta Biomed*. 2006 Dec;77(3):157-62.

American Conference of Governmental Industrial Hygienists. *Threshold limit values for chemical substances and physical agents in the work environment*. Cincinnati, OH: ACGIH, 1986.

American Dietetic Association; Dietitians of Canada. Position of the American Dietetic Association and Dietitians of Canada: vegetarian diets. *Can J Diet Pract Res*. 2003 Summer;64(2):62-81.

Ammon HP. Boswellic acids (components of frankincense) as the active principle in treatment of chronic inflammatory diseases. *Wien Med Wochenschr*. 2002;152(15-16):373-8.

Ammon HP. Boswellic acids in chronic inflammatory diseases. *Planta Med*. 2006 Oct;72(12):1100-16.

Anand P, Thomas SG, Kunnumakkara AB, Sundaram C, Harikumar KB, Sung B, Tharakan ST, Misra K, Priyadarsini IK, Rajasekharan KN, Aggarwal BB. Biological activities of curcumin and its analogues (Congeners) made by man and Mother Nature. *Biochem Pharmacol*. 2008 Dec 1;76(11):1590-611.

Anderson JL, May HT, Horne BD, Bair TL, Hall NL, Carlquist JF, Lappé DL, Muhlestein JB; Intermountain Heart Collaborative (IHC) Study Group. Relation of vitamin D deficiency to cardiovascular risk factors, disease status, and incident events in a general healthcare population. *Am J Cardiol*. 2010 Oct 1;106(7):963-8.

Anderson JW, Gilliland SE. Effect of fermented milk (yogurt) containing *Lactobacillus acidophilus* L1 on serum cholesterol in hypercholesterolemic humans. *J Am Coll Nutr*. 1999 Feb;18(1):43-50.

Anderson M., Grissom C. Increasing the Heavy Atom Effect of Xenon by Adsorption to Zeolites: Photolysis of 2,3-Diazabicyclo[2.2.2]oct-2-ene. *J. Am. Chem. Soc*. 1996;118:9552-9556.

Anderson RC, Anderson JH. Acute respiratory effects of diaper emissions. *Arch Environ Health*. 1999 Sep-Oct;54(5):353-8.

Anderson RC, Anderson JH. Acute toxic effects of fragrance products. *Arch Environ Health*. 1998 Mar-Apr;53(2):138-46.

Anderson RC, Anderson JH. Respiratory toxicity in mice exposed to mattress covers. *Arch Environ Health*. 1999 May-Jun;54(3):202-9.

Anderson RC, Anderson JH. Respiratory toxicity of fabric softener emissions. *J Toxicol Environ Health*. 2000 May 26;60(2):121-36.

Anderson RC, Anderson JH. Respiratory toxicity of mattress emissions in mice. *Arch Environ Health*. 2000 Jan-Feb;55(1):38-43.

Anderson RC, Anderson JH. Sensory irritation and multiple chemical sensitivity. *Toxicol Ind Health*. 1999 Apr-Jun;15(3-4):339-45.

Anderson RC, Anderson JH. Toxic effects of air freshener emissions. *Arch Environ Health*. 1997 Nov-Dec;52(6):433-41.

Anderson SD, Charlton B, Weiler JM, Nichols S, Spector SL, Pearlman DS; A305 Study Group. Comparison of mannitol and methacholine to predict exercise-induced bronchoconstriction and a clinical diagnosis of asthma. *Respir Res*. 2009 Jan 23;10:4.

Andoh T, Zhang Q, Yamamoto T, Tayama M, Hattori M, Tanaka K, Kuraishi Y. Inhibitory Effects of the Methanol Extract of Ganoderma lucidum on Mosquito Allergy-Induced Itch-Associated Responses in Mice. *J Pharmacol Sci*. 2010 Oct 8.

André C, André F, Colin L. Effect of allergen ingestion challenge with and without cromoglycate cover on intestinal permeability in atopic dermatitis, urticaria and other symptoms of food allergy. *Allergy*. 1989;44 Suppl 9:47-51.

André C. Food allergy. Objective diagnosis and test of therapeutic efficacy by measuring intestinal permeability. *Presse Med*. 1986 Jan 25;15(3):105-8.

Andre F, Andre C, Feknous M, Colin L, Cavagna S. Digestive permeability to different-sized molecules and to sodium cromoglycate in food allergy. *Allergy Proc*. 1991 Sep-Oct;12(5):293-8.

Anim-Nyame N, Sooranna SR, Johnson MR, Gamble J, Steer PJ. Garlic supplementation increases peripheral blood flow: a role for interleukin-6? *J Nutr Biochem.* 2004 Jan;15(1):30-6.

Annweiler C, Schott AM, Berrut G, Chauviré V, Le Gall D, Inzitari M, Beauchet O. Vitamin D and ageing: neurological issues. *Neuropsychobiology.* 2010 Aug;62(3):139-50.

Antczak A, Nowak D, Shariati B, Król M, Piasecka G, Kurmanowska Z. Increased hydrogen peroxide and thiobarbituric acid-reactive products in expired breath condensate of asthmatic patients. *Eur Respir J.* 1997 Jun;10(6):1235-41.

Anukam K, Osazuwa E, Ahonkhai I, Ngwu M, Osemene G, Bruce AW, Reid G. Augmentation of antimicrobial metronidazole therapy of bacterial vaginosis with oral probiotic *Lactobacillus rhamnosus* GR-1 and *Lactobacillus reuteri* RC-14: randomized, double-blind, placebo controlled trial. *Microbes Infect.* 2006 May;8(6):1450-4.

Anukam KC, Osazuwa E, Osemene GI, Ehigiagbe F, Bruce AW, Reid G. Clinical study comparing probiotic Lactobacillus GR-1 and RC-14 with metronidazole vaginal gel to treat symptomatic bacterial vaginosis. *Microbes Infect.* 2006 Oct;8(12-13):2772-6.

Anukam KC, Osazuwa EO, Osadolor HB, Bruce AW, Reid G. Yogurt containing probiotic *Lactobacillus rhamnosus* GR-1 and *L. reuteri* RC-14 helps resolve moderate diarrhea and increases CD4 count in HIV/AIDS patients. *J Clin Gastroenterol.* 2008 Mar;42(3):239-43.

Aoki T, Usuda Y, Miyakoshi H, Tamura K, Herberman RB. Low natural killer syndrome: clinical and immunologic features. *Nat Immun Cell Growth Regul.* 1987;6(3):116-28.

Apáti P, Houghton PJ, Kite G, Steventon GB, Kéry A. In-vitro effect of flavonoids from Solidago canadensis extract on glutathione S-transferase. *J Pharm Pharmacol.* 2006 Feb;58(2):251-6.

APHA (American Public Health Association). Opposition to the Use of Hormone Growth Promoters in Beef and Dairy Cattle Production. Policy Date: 11/10/2009. Policy Number: 20098. http://www.apha.org/advocacy/policy/id=1379. Accessed Nov. 24, 2010.

Araki K, Shinozaki T, Irie Y, Miyazawa Y. Trial of oral administration of *Bifidobacterium breve* for the prevention of rotavirus infections. *Kansenshogaku Zasshi.* 1999 Apr;73(4):305-10.

Araujo AC, Aprile LR, Dantas RO, Terra-Filho J, Vianna EO. Bronchial responsiveness during esophageal acid infusion. Lung. 2008 Mar-Apr;186(2):123-8. 2008 Feb 23.

Arbes SJ Jr, Gergen PJ, Vaughn B, Zeldin DC. Asthma cases attributable to atopy: results from the Third National Health and Nutrition Examination Survey. *J Allergy Clin Immunol.* 2007 Nov;120(5):1139-45. 2007 Sep 24.

Argento A, Tiraferri E, Marzaloni M. Oral anticoagulants and medicinal plants. An emerging interaction. *Ann Ital Med Int.* 2000 Apr-Jun;15(2):139-43.

Arif AA, Delclos GL, Colmer-Hamood J. Association between asthma, asthma symptoms and C-reactive protein in US adults: data from the National Health and Nutrition Examination Survey, 1999-2002. *Respirology.* 2007 Sep;12(5):675-82. .

Arif AA, Shah SM. Association between personal exposure to volatile organic compounds and asthma among US adult population. *Int Arch Occup Environ Health.* 2007 Aug;80(8):711-9.

Armstrong BK. Absorption of vitamin B12 from the human colon. *Am J Clin Nutr.* 1968;21:298-9.

Armuzzi A, Cremonini F, Bartolozzi F, Canducci F, Candelli M, Ojetti V, Cammarota G, Anti M, De Lorenzo A, Pola P, Gasbarrini G, Gasbarrini A. The effect of oral administration of Lactobacillus GG on antibiotic-associated gastrointestinal side-effects during Helicobacter pylori eradication therapy. *Aliment Pharmacol Ther.* 2001 Feb;15(2):163-9.

Arrigo G, D'Angelo A. Achromycin and anaphylactic shock. *Riv Patol Clin.* 1959 Oct;14:719-22.

Arshad SH, Bateman B, Sadeghnejad A, Gant C, Matthews SM. Prevention of allergic disease during childhood by allergen avoidance: the Isle of Wight prevention study. *J Allergy Clin Immunol.* 2007 Feb;119(2):307-13.

Arslanoglu S, Moro GE, Schmitt J, Tandoi L, Rizzardi S, Boehm G. Early dietary intervention with a mixture of prebiotic oligosaccharides reduces the incidence of allergic manifestations and infections during the first two years of life. *J Nutr.* 2008 Jun;138(6):1091-5.

Arterburn LM, Oken HA, Bailey Hall E, Hamersley J, Kuratko CN, Hoffman JP. Algal-oil capsules and cooked salmon: nutritionally equivalent sources of docosahexaenoic acid. *J Am Diet Assoc.* 2008 Jul;108(7):1204-9.

Arterburn LM, Oken HA, Hoffman JP, Bailey-Hall E, Chung G, Rom D, Hamersley J, McCarthy D. Bioequivalence of Docosahexaenoic acid from different algal oils in capsules and in a DHA-fortified food. *Lipids.* 2007 Nov;42(11):1011-24.

Arunachalam K, Gill HS, Chandra RK. Enhancement of natural immune function by dietary consumption of *Bifidobacterium lactis* (HN019). *Eur J Clin Nutr.* 2000 Mar;54(3):263-7.

Arvaniti F, Priftis KN, Panagiotakos DB. Dietary habits and asthma: a review. *Allergy Asthma Proc.* 2010 Mar;31(2):e1-10.

Arvola T, Laiho K, Torkkeli S, Mykkänen H, Salminen S, Maunula L, Isolauri E. Prophylactic Lactobacillus GG reduces antibiotic-associated diarrhea in children with respiratory infections: a randomized study. *Pediatrics.* 1999 Nov;104(5):e64.

Asero R, Antonicelli L, Arena A, Bommarito L, Caruso B, Colombo G, Crivellaro M, De Carli M, Della Torre E, Della Torre F, Heffler E, Lodi Rizzini F, Longo R, Manzotti G, Marcotulli M, Melchiorre A, Minale P, Morandi P, Moreni B, Moschella A, Murzilli F, Nebiolo F, Poppa M, Randazzo S, Rossi G, Senna GE. Causes of food-induced anaphylaxis in Italian adults: a multi-centre study. *Int Arch Allergy Immunol.* 2009;150(3):271-7.

Asero R, Mistrello G, Roncarolo D, Amato S, Caldironi G, Barocci F, van Ree R. Immunological cross-reactivity between lipid transfer proteins from botanically unrelated plant-derived foods: a clinical study. *Allergy.* 2002 Oct;57(10):900-6.

Ashrafi K, Chang FY, Watts JL, Fraser AG, Kamath RS, Ahringer J, Ruvkun G. Genome-wide RNAi analysis of Caenorhabditis elegans fat regulatory genes. *Nature.* 2003 Jan 16;421(6920):268-72.

Aso Y, Akaza H, Kotake T, Tsukamoto T, Imai K, Naito S. Preventive effect of a *Lactobacillus casei* preparation on the recurrence of superficial bladder cancer in a double-blind trial. The BLP Study Group. *Eur Urol.* 1995;27(2):104-9.

Aso Y, Akazan H. Prophylactic effect of a *Lactobacillus casei* preparation on the recurrence of superficial bladder cancer. BLP Study Group. *Urol Int.* 1992;49(3):125-9.

Ataie-Jafari A, Larijani B, Alavi Majd H, Tahbaz F. Cholesterol-lowering effect of probiotic yogurt in comparison with ordinary yogurt in mildly to moderately hypercholesterolemic subjects. *Ann Nutr Metab.* 2009;54(1):22-7.

Atkinson W, Harris J, Mills P, Moffat S, White C, Lynch O, Jones M, Cullinan P, Newman Taylor AJ. Domestic aeroallergen exposures among infants in an English town. *Eur Respir J.* 1999 Mar;13(3):583-9.

Atsumi T, Tonosaki K. Smelling lavender and rosemary increases free radical scavenging activity and decreases cortisol level in saliva. *Psychiatry Res.* 2007 Feb 28;150(1):89-96.

Backster C. *Primary Perception: Biocommunication with Plants, Living Foods, and Human Cells.* Anza, CA: White Rose Millennium Press, 2003.

Bacopoulou F, Veltsista A, Vassi I, Gika A, Lekea V, Priftis K, Bakoula C. Can we be optimistic about asthma in childhood? A Greek cohort study. *J Asthma.* 2009 Mar;46(2):171-4.

Badar VA, Thawani VR, Wakode PT, Shrivastava MP, Gharpure KJ, Hingorani LL, Khiyani RM. Efficacy of Tinospora cordifolia in allergic rhinitis. *J Ethnopharmacol.* 2005 Jan 15;96(3):445-9.

Bae GS, Kim MS, Jung WS, Seo SW, Yun SW, Kim SG, Park RK, Kim EC, Song HJ, Park SJ. Inhibition of lipopolysaccharide-induced inflammatory responses by piperine. *Eur J Pharmacol.* 2010 Sep 10;642(1-3):154-62.

Bafadhel M, Singapuri A, Terry S, Hargadon B, Monteiro W, Green RH, Bradding PH, Wardlaw AJ, Pavord ID, Brightling CE. Body mass and fat mass in refractory asthma: an observational 1 year follow-up study. *J Allergy.* 2010;2010:251758. 2010 Dec 1.

Bai AP, Ouyang Q, Xiao XR, Li SF. Probiotics modulate inflammatory cytokine secretion from inflamed mucosa in active ulcerative colitis. *Int J Clin Pract.* 2006 Mar;60(3):284-8.

Baik HW. Nutritional therapy in gastrointestinal disease. *Korean J Gastroenterol.* 2004 Jun;43(6):331-40.

Baker SM. *Detoxification and Healing.* Chicago: Contemporary Books, 2004.

Bakkeheim E, Mowinckel P, Carlsen KH, Håland G, Carlsen KC. Paracetamol in early infancy: the risk of childhood allergy and asthma. Acta Paediatr. 2011 Jan;100(1):90-6.

Balch P, Balch J. *Prescription for Nutritional Healing.* New York: Avery, 2000.

Balimane P, Yong-Haen H, Chong S. Current Industrial Practices of Assessing Permeability and P-Glycoprotein Interaction. *J AAPS* 2006; 8(1).

Ballentine R. *Diet & Nutrition: A holistic approach.* Honesdale, PA: Himalayan Int., 1978.

Ballentine RM. *Radical Healing.* New York: Harmony Books, 1999.

Balli F, Bertolani P, Giberti G, Amarri S. High-dose oral bacteria-therapy for chronic non-specific diarrhea of infancy. *Pediatr Med Chir.* 1992 Jan-Feb;14(1):13-5.

Ballmer-Weber BK, Holzhauser T, Scibilia J, Mittag D, Zisa G, Ortolani C, Oesterballe M, Poulsen LK, Vieths S, Bindslev-Jensen C. Clinical characteristics of soybean allergy in Europe: a double-blind, placebo-controlled food challenge study. *J Allergy Clin Immunol.* 2007 Jun;119(6):1489-96.

Ballmer-Weber BK, Vieths S, Lüttkopf D, Heuschmann P, Wüthrich B. Celery allergy confirmed by double-blind, placebo-controlled food challenge: a clinical study in 32 subjects with a history of adverse reactions to celery root. *J Allergy Clin Immunol.* 2000 Aug;106(2):373-8.

Banno N, Akihisa T, Yasukawa K, Tokuda H, Tabata K, Nakamura Y, Nishimura R, Kimura Y, Suzuki T. Anti-inflammatory activities of the triterpene acids from the resin of Boswellia carteri. *J Ethnopharmacol.* 2006 Sep 19;107(2):249-53.

Bant A, Kruszewski J. Increased sensitization prevalence to common inhalant and food allergens in young adult Polish males. *Ann Agric Environ Med.* 2008 Jun;15(1):21-7.

REFERENCES AND BIBLIOGRAPHY

Barnes M, Cullinan P, Athanasaki P, MacNeill S, Hole AM, Harris J, Kalogeraki S, Chatzinikolaou M, Drakonakis N, Bibaki-Liakou V, Newman Taylor AJ, Bibakis I. Crete: does farming explain urban and rural differences in atopy? *Clin Exp Allergy.* 2001 Dec;31(12):1822-8.

Barnetson RS, Drummond H, Ferguson A. Precipitins to dietary proteins in atopic eczema. *Br J Dermatol.* 1983 Dec;109(6):653-5.

Barnett AG, Williams GM, Schwartz J, Neller AH, Best TL, Petroeschevsky AL, Simpson RW. Air pollution and child respiratory health: a case-crossover study in Australia and New Zealand. *Am J Respir Crit Care Med.* 2005 Jun 1;171(11):1272-8.

Baron M. A patented strain of Bacillus coagulans increased immune response to viral challenge. *Postgrad Med.* 2009 Mar;121(2):114-8.

Barrager E, Veltmann JR Jr, Schauss AG, Schiller RN. A multicentered, open-label trial on the safety and efficacy of methylsulfonylmethane in the treatment of seasonal allergic rhinitis. *J Altern Complement Med.* 2002 Apr;8(2):167-73.

Barros R, Moreira A, Fonseca J, de Oliveira JF, Delgado L, Castel-Branco MG, Haahtela T, Lopes C, Moreira P. Adherence to the Mediterranean diet and fresh fruit intake are associated with improved asthma control. *Allergy.* 2008 Jul;63(7):917-23.

Bartram HP, Scheppach W, Gerlach S, Ruckdeschel G, Kelber E, Kasper H. Does yogurt enriched with *Bifidobacterium longum* affect colonic microbiology and fecal metabolites in health subjects? *Am J Clin Nutr.* 1994 Feb;59(2):428-32.

Basu A, Devaraj S, Jialal I. Dietary factors that promote or retard inflammation. *Arterioscler Thromb Vasc Biol.* 2006 May;26(5):995-1001.

Basu S, Chatterjee M, Ganguly S, Chandra PK. Effect of *Lactobacillus rhamnosus* GG in persistent diarrhea in Indian children: a randomized controlled trial. *J Clin Gastroenterol.* 2007 Sep;41(8):756-60.

Basu S, Chatterjee M, Ganguly S, Chandra PK. Efficacy of *Lactobacillus rhamnosus* GG in acute watery diarrhoea of Indian children: a randomised controlled trial. *J Paediatr Child Health.* 2007 Dec;43(12):837-42.

Bateman B, Warner JO, Hutchinson E, Dean T, Rowlandson P, Gant C, Grundy J, Fitzgerald C, Stevenson J. The effects of a double blind, placebo controlled, artificial food colourings and benzoate preservative challenge on hyperactivity in a general population sample of preschool children. *Arch Dis Child.* 2004 Jun;89(6):506-11.

Bates DW, Cullen DJ, Laird N, Petersen LA, Small SD, Servi D, Laffel G, Sweitzer BJ, Shea BF, Hallisey R, et al. Incidence of adverse drug events and potential adverse drug events. Implications for prevention. ADE Prevention Study Group. *JAMA.* 1995 Jul 5;274(1):29-34.

Batista R, Martins I, Jeno P, Ricardo CP, Oliveira MM. A proteomic study to identify soya allergens—the human response to transgenic versus non-transgenic soya samples. *Int Arch Allergy Immunol.* 2007;144(1):29-38.

Batmanghelidj F. Neurotransmitter histamine: an alternative view point, *Science in Medicine Simplified.* Falls Church, VA: Foundation for the Simple in Medicine, 1990.

Batmanghelidj F. Pain: a need for paradigm change. *Anticancer Res.* 1987 Sep-Oct;7(5B):971-89.

Batmanghelidj F. *Your Body's Many Cries for Water.* 2nd Ed. Vienna, VA: Global Health, 1997.

Beasley R, Clayton T, Crane J, von Mutius E, Lai CK, Montefort S, Stewart A; ISAAC Phase Three Study Group. Association between paracetamol use in infancy and childhood, and risk of asthma, rhinoconjunctivitis, and eczema in children aged 6-7 years: analysis from Phase Three of the ISAAC programme. *Lancet.* 2008 Sep. 20;372(9643):1039-48.

Beaulieu A, Fessele K. Agent Orange: management of patients exposed in Vietnam. *Clin J Oncol Nurs.* 2003 May-Jun;7(3):320-3.

Beausoleil M, Fortier N, Guénette S, L'ecuyer A, Savoie M, Franco M, Lachaine J, Weiss K. Effect of a fermented milk combining *Lactobacillus acidophilus* Cl1285 and *Lactobacillus casei* in the prevention of antibiotic-associated diarrhea: a randomized, double-blind, placebo-controlled trial. *Can J Gastroenterol.* 2007 Nov;21(11):732-6.

Becker KG, Simon RM, Bailey-Wilson JE, Freidlin B, Biddison WE, McFarland HF, Trent JM. Clustering of non-major histocompatibility complex susceptibility candidate loci in human autoimmune diseases. *Proc Natl Acad Sci U S A.* 1998 Aug 18;95(17):9979-84.

Beddoe AF. *Biologic Ionization as Applied to Human Nutrition.* Warsaw: Wendell Whitman, 2002.

Beecher GR. Phytonutrients' role in metabolism: effects on resistance to degenerative processes. *Nutr Rev.* 1999 Sep;57(9 Pt 2):S3-6.

Belcaro G, Cesarone MR, Errichi S, Zulli C, Errichi BM, Vinciguerra G, Ledda A, Di Renzo A, Stuard S, Dugall M, Pellegrini L, Gizzi G, Ippolito E, Ricci A, Cacchio M, Cipollone G, Ruffini I, Fano F, Hosoi M, Rohdewald P. Variations in C-reactive protein, plasma free radicals and fibrinogen values in patients with osteoarthritis treated with Pycnogenol. *Redox Rep.* 2008;13(6):271-6.

Bell IR, Baldwin CM, Schwartz GE, Illness from low levels of environmental chemicals: relevance to chronic fatigue syndrome and fibromyalgia. *Am J Med.* 1998;105 (suppl 3A).:74-82. S.

245

Bell SJ, Potter PC. Milk whey-specific immune complexes in allergic and non-allergic subjects. *Allergy.* 1988 Oct;43(7):497-503.

Ben, X.M., Zhou, X.Y., Zhao, W.H., Yu, W.L., Pan, W., Zhang, W.L., Wu, S.M., Van Beusekom, C.M., Schaafsma, A. (2004) Supplementation of milk formula with galactooligosaccharides improves intestinal micro-flora and fermentation in term infants. *Chin Med J.* 117(6):927-931, 2004.

Benard A, Desreumeaux P, Huglo D, Hoorelbeke A, Tonnel AB, Wallaert B. Increased intestinal permeability in bronchial asthma. *J Allergy Clin Immunol.* 1996 Jun;97(6):1173-8.

Bengmark S. Curcumin, an atoxic antioxidant and natural NFkappaB, cyclooxygenase-2, lipooxygenase, and inducible nitric oxide synthase inhibitor: a shield against acute and chronic diseases. *JPEN J Parenter Enteral Nutr.* 2006 Jan-Feb;30(1):45-51.

Bengmark S. Immunonutrition: role of biosurfactants, fiber, and probiotic bacteria. *Nutrition.* 1998 Jul-Aug;14(7-8):585-94.

Benlounes N, Dupont C, Candalh C, Blaton MA, Darmon N, Desjeux JF, Heyman M. The threshold for immune cell reactivity to milk antigens decreases in cow's milk allergy with intestinal symptoms. *J Allergy Clin Immunol.* 1996 Oct;98(4):781-9.

Bennett WD, Zeman KL, Jarabek AM. Nasal contribution to breathing and fine particle deposition in children versus adults. *J Toxicol Environ Health A.* 2008;71(3):227-37.

Ben-Shoshan M, Harrington DW, Soller L, Fragapane J, Joseph L, St Pierre Y, Godefroy SB, Elliot SJ, Clarke AE. A population-based study on peanut, tree nut, fish, shellfish, and sesame allergy prevalence in Canada. *J Allergy Clin Immunol.* 2010 Jun;125(6):1327-35.

Ben-Shoshan M, Kagan R, Primeau MN, Alizadehfar R, Turnbull E, Harada L, Dufresne C, Allen M, Joseph L, St Pierre Y, Clarke A. Establishing the diagnosis of peanut allergy in children never exposed to peanut or with an uncertain history: a cross-Canada study. *Pediatr Allergy Immunol.* 2010 Sep;21(6):920-6.

Bensky D, Gable A, Kaptchuk T (transl.). *Chinese Herbal Medicine Materia Medica.* Seattle: Eastland Press, 1986.

Bergner P. *The Healing Power of Garlic.* Prima Publishing, Rocklin CA 1996.

Berin MC, Yang PC, Ciok L, Waserman S, Perdue MH. Role for IL-4 in macromolecular transport across human intestinal epithelium. *Am J Physiol.* 1999 May;276(5 Pt 1):C1046-52.

Berkow R., (Ed.) *The Merck Manual of Diagnosis and Therapy.* 16th Edition. Rahway, N.J.: Merck Research Labs, 1992.

Bernstein DI, Epstein T, Murphy-Berendts K, Liss GM. Surveillance of systemic reactions to subcutaneous immunotherapy injections: year 1 outcomes of the ACAAI and AAAAI collaborative study. *Ann Allergy Asthma Immunol.* 2010 Jun;104(6):530-5. .

Berseth CL, Mitmesser SH, Ziegler EE, Marunycz JD, Vanderhoof J. Tolerance of a standard intact protein formula versus a partially hydrolyzed formula in healthy, term infants. *Nutr J.* 2009 Jun 19;8:27.

Berteau O and Mulloy B. 2003. Sulfated fucans, fresh perspectives: structures, functions, and biological properties of sulfated fucans and an overview of enzymes active toward this class of polysaccharide. *Glycobiology.* Jun;13(6):29R-40R.

Beyer K, Morrow E, Li XM, Bardina L, Bannon GA, Burks AW, Sampson HA. Effects of cooking methods on peanut allergenicity. *J Allergy Clin Immunol.* 2001;107:1077-81.

Bielory BP, Perez VL, Bielory L. Treatment of seasonal allergic conjunctivitis with ophthalmic corticosteroids: in search of the perfect ocular corticosteroids in the treatment of allergic conjunctivitis. *Curr Opin Allergy Clin Immunol.* 2010 Oct;10(5):469-77.

Bielory L, Lupoli K. Herbal interventions in asthma and allergy. *J Asthma.* 1999;36:1-65.

Bielory L, Russin J, Zuckerman GB. Clinical efficacy, mechanisms of action, and adverse effects of complementary and alternative medicine therapies for asthma. *Allergy Asthma Proc.* 2004;25:283-91.

Bielory L. Complementary and alternative interventions in asthma, allergy, and immunology. *Ann Allergy Asthma Immunol.* 2004 Aug;93(2 Suppl 1):S45-54.

Billoo AG, Memon MA, Khaskheli SA, Murtaza G, Iqbal K, Saeed Shekhani M, Siddiqi AQ. Role of a probiotic (*Saccharomyces boulardii*) in management and prevention of diarrhoea. *World J Gastroenterol.* 2006 Jul 28;12(28):4557-60.

Bindslev-Jensen C, Skov PS, Roggen EL, Hvass P, Brinch DS. Investigation on possible allergenicity of 19 different commercial enzymes used in the food industry. *Food Chem Toxicol.* 2006 Nov;44(11):1909-15.

Bin-Nun A, Bromiker R, Wilschanski M, Kaplan M, Rudensky B, Caplan M, Hammerman C. Oral probiotics prevent necrotizing enterocolitis in very low birth weight neonates. *J Pediatr.* 2005 Aug;147(2):192-6.

Birch EE, Khoury JC, Berseth CL, Castañeda YS, Couch JM, Bean J, Tamer R, Harris CL, Mitmesser SH, Scalabrin DM. The impact of early nutrition on incidence of allergic manifestations and common respiratory illnesses in children. *J Pediatr.* 2010 Jun;156(6):902-6, 906.e1. 2010 Mar 15.

Bisgaard H, Loland L, Holst KK, Pipper CB. Prenatal determinants of neonatal lung function in high-risk newborns. *J Allergy Clin Immunol.* 2009 Mar;123(3):651-7, 657.e1-4. 2009 Jan 18.

Bisset N.. *Herbal Drugs and Phytopharmaceuticals.* Stuttgart: CRC, 1994.

Bjarnason I, MacPherson A, Hollander D. Intestinal permeability: an overview. *Gastroenterology.* 1995 May;108(5):1566-81.

Blackhall K, Appleton S, Cates FJ. Ionisers for chronic asthma. *Cochrane Database Syst Rev* 2003;(3):CD002986.

Blackley, CH. *Experimental Researchers on the Causes and Nature of Catarrhus Aestivus (Hay Fever or Hay-Asthma)*. London, 1873.

Bliakher MS, Fedorova IM, Lopatina TK, Arkhipov SN, Kapustin IV, Ramazanova ZK, Karpova NV, Ivanov VA, Sharapov NV. Acilact and improvement of the health status of sickly children. *Vestn Ross Akad Med Nauk*. 2005;(12):32-5.

Blood AJ, Zatorre RJ, Bermudez P, Evans AC. Emotional responses to pleasant and unpleasant music correlate with activity in paralimbic brain regions. *Nat Neurosci*. 1999;2:382-7.

Blumenthal M (ed.) *The Complete German Commission E Monographs*. Boston: Amer Botan Council, 1998.

Blumenthal M, Brinckmann J, Goldberg A (eds). *Herbal Medicine: Expanded Commission E Monographs*. Newton, MA: Integrative Med., 2000.

Boccafogli A, Vicentini L, Camerani A, Cogliati P, D'Ambrosi A, Scolozzi R. Adverse food reactions in patients with grass pollen allergic respiratory disease. *Ann Allergy*. 1994 Oct;73(4):301-8.

Bode C, Bode JC. Effect of alcohol consumption on the gut. *Best Pract Res Clin Gastroenterol*. 2003 Aug;17(4):575-92.

Bodinier M, Legoux MA, Pineau F, Triballeau S, Segain JP, Brossard C, Denery-Papini S. Intestinal translocation capabilities of wheat allergens using the Caco-2 cell line. *J Agric Food Chem*. 2007 May 30;55(11):4576-83.

Boehm, G., Lidestri, M., Casetta, P., Jelinek, J., Negretti, F., Stahl, B., Martini, A. (2002) Supplementation of a bovine milk formula with an oligosaccharide mixture increases counts of faecal bifidobacteria in preterm infants. *Arch Dis Child Fetal Neonatal Ed*. 86: F178-F181

Boivin DB, Czeisler CA. Resetting of circadian melatonin and cortisol rhythms in humans by ordinary room light. *Neuroreport*. 1998 Mar 30;9(5):779-82.

Boivin DB, Duffy JF, Kronauer RE, Czeisler CA. Dose-response relationships for resetting of human circadian clock by light. *Nature*. 1996 Feb 8;379(6565):540-2.

Bolhaar ST, Tiemessen MM, Zuidmeer L, van Leeuwen A, Hoffmann-Sommergruber K, Bruijnzeel-Koomen CA, Taams LS, Knol EF, van Hoffen E, van Ree R, Knulst AC. Efficacy of birch-pollen immunotherapy on cross-reactive food allergy confirmed by skin tests and double-blind food challenges. *Clin Exp Allergy*. 2004 May;34(5):761-9.

Bolleddula J, Goldfarb J, Wang R, Sampson H, Li XM. Synergistic Modulation Of Eotaxin And Il-4 Secretion By Constituents Of An Anti-asthma Herbal Formula (ASHMI) In Vitro. *J Allergy Clin Immunol*. 2007;119:S172.

Bonfils P, Halimi P, Malinvaud D. Adrenal suppression and osteoporosis after treatment of nasal polyposis. *Acta Otolaryngol*. 2006 Dec;126(11):1195-200.

Bongaerts GP, Severijnen RS. Preventive and curative effects of probiotics in atopic patients. *Med Hypotheses*. 2005;64(6):1089-92.

Bongartz D, Hesse A. Selective extraction of quercetin in vegetable drugs and urine by off-line coupling of boronic acid affinity chromatography and high-performance liquid chromatography. *J Chromatogr B Biomed Appl*. 1995 Nov 17;673(2):223-30.

Bonsignore MR, La Grutta S, Cibella F, Scichilone N, Cuttitta G, Interrante A, Marchese M, Veca M, Virzi' M, Bonanno A, Profita M, Morici G. Effects of exercise training and montelukast in children with mild asthma. *Med Sci Sports Exerc*. 2008 Mar;40(3):405-12.

Borchers AT, Hackman RM, Keen CL, Stern JS, Gershwin ME. Complementary medicine: a review of immunomodulatory effects of Chinese herbal medicines. *Am J Clin Nutr*. 1997 Dec;66(6):1303-12.

Borchert VE, Czyborra P, Fetscher C, Goepel M, Michel MC. Extracts from Rhois aromatica and Solidaginis virgaurea inhibit rat and human bladder contraction. *Naunyn Schmiedebergs Arch Pharmacol*. 2004 Mar;369(3):281-6.

Böttcher MF, Abrahamsson TR, Fredriksson M, Jakobsson T, Björkstén B. Low breast milk TGF-beta2 is induced by *Lactobacillus reuteri* supplementation and associates with reduced risk of sensitization during infancy. *Pediatr Allergy Immunol*. 2008 Sep;19(6):497-504.

Böttcher MF, Jenmalm MC, Voor T, Julge K, Holt PG, Björkstén B. Cytokine responses to allergens during the first 2 years of life in Estonian and Swedish children. *Clin Exp Allergy*. 2006 May;36(5):619-28.

Bottema RW, Kerkhof M, Reijmerink NE, Thijs C, Smit HA, van Schayck CP, Brunekreef B, van Oosterhout AJ, Postma DS, Koppelman GH. Gene-gene interaction in regulatory T-cell function in atopy and asthma development in childhood. *J Allergy Clin Immunol*. 2010 Aug;126(2):338-46, 346.e1-10.

Bouchez-Mahiout I, Pecquet C, Kerre S, Snégaroff J, Raison-Peyron N, Laurière M. High molecular weight entities in industrial wheat protein hydrolysates are immunoreactive with IgE from allergic patients. *J Agric Food Chem*. 2010 Apr 14;58(7):4207-15.

Bougault V, Turmel J, Boulet LP. Bronchial challenges and respiratory symptoms in elite swimmers and winter sport athletes: Airway hyperresponsiveness in asthma: its measurement and clinical significance. *Chest*. 2010 Aug;138(2 Suppl):31S-37S. 2010 Apr 2.

Boyce JA, Assa'ad A, Burks AW, Jones SM, Sampson HA, Wood RA, Plaut M, Cooper SF, Fenton MJ, Arshad SH, Bahna SL, Beck LA, Byrd-Bredbenner C, Camargo CA Jr, Eichenfield L, Furuta GT, Hanifin JM, Jones C, Kraft M, Levy BD, Lieberman P, Luccioli S, McCall KM, Schneider LC, Simon RA, Simons FE, Teach SJ, Yawn BP, Schwaninger JM. Guidelines for the diagnosis and management of food allergy in the United States: report of the NIAID-sponsored expert panel. *J Allergy Clin Immunol.* 2010 Dec;126(6 Suppl):S1-58.

Boylan R, Li Y, Simeonova L, Sherwin G, Kreismann J, Craig RG, Ship JA, McCutcheon JA. Reduction in bacterial contamination of toothbrushes using the Violight ultraviolet light activated toothbrush sanitizer. *Am J Dent.* 2008 Oct;21(5):313-7.

Bråbäck L, Breborowicz A, Julge K, Knutsson A, Riikjärv MA, Vasar M, Björkstén B. Risk factors for respiratory symptoms and atopic sensitisation in the Baltic area. *Arch Dis Child.* 1995 Jun;72(6):487-93.

Bråbäck L, Kjellman NI, Sandin A, Björkstén B. Atopy among schoolchildren in northern and southern Sweden in relation to pet ownership and early life events. *Pediatr Allergy Immunol.* 2001 Feb;12(1):4-10.

Bradette-Hébert ME, Legault J, Lavoie S, Pichette A. A new labdane diterpene from the flowers of Solidago canadensis. *Chem Pharm Bull.* 2008 Jan;56(1):82-4.

Brandtzaeg P. The mucosal immune system and its integration with the mammary glands. *J Pediatr.* 2010 Feb;156(2 Suppl):S8-15.

Brasseur JG, Nicosia MA, Pal A, Miller LS. Function of longitudinal vs circular muscle fibers in esophageal peristalsis, deduced with mathematical modeling. *World J Gastroenterol.* 2007 Mar 7;13(9):1335-46.

Braun-Fahrländer C, Gassner M, Grize L, Neu U, Sennhauser FH, Varonier HS, Vuille JC, Wüthrich B. Prevalence of hay fever and allergic sensitization in farmer's children and their peers living in the same rural community. SCARPOL team. Swiss Study on Childhood Allergy and Respiratory Symptoms with Respect to Air Pollution. *Clin Exp Allergy.* 1999 Jan;29(1):28-34.

Brehm JM, Schuemann B, Fuhlbrigge AL, Hollis BW, Strunk RC, Zeiger RS, Weiss ST, Litonjua AA; Childhood Asthma Management Program Research Group. Serum vitamin D levels and severe asthma exacerbations in the Childhood Asthma Management Program study. *J Allergy Clin Immunol.* 2010 Jul;126(1):52-8.e5. 2010 Jun 9.

Brighenti F, Valtueña S, Pellegrini N, Ardigò D, Del Rio D, Salvatore S, Piatti P, Serafini M, Zavaroni I. Total antioxidant capacity of the diet is inversely and independently related to plasma concentration of high-sensitivity C-reactive protein in adult Italian subjects. *Br J Nutr.* 2005 May;93(5):619-25.

Brinkhaus B, Witt CM, Jena S, Liecker B, Wegscheider K, Willich SN. Acupuncture in patients with allergic rhinitis: a pragmatic randomized trial. *Ann Allergy Asthma Immunol.* 2008 Nov;101(5):535-43.

Brisman J, Torén K, Lillienberg L, Karlsson G, Ahlstedt S. Nasal symptoms and indices of nasal inflammation in flour-dust-exposed bakers. *Int Arch Occup Environ Health.* 1998 Nov;71(8):525-32.

Brodtkorb TH, Zetterström O, Tinghög G. Cost-effectiveness of clean air administered to the breathing zone in allergic asthma. *Clin Respir J.* 2010 Apr;4(2):104-10.

Brody J. *Jane Brody's Nutrition Book.* New York: WW Norton, 1981.

Broekhuizen BD, Sachs AP, Hoes AW, Moons KG, van den Berg JW, Dalinghaus WH, Lammers E, Verheij TJ. Undetected chronic obstructive pulmonary disease and asthma in people over 50 years with persistent cough. *Br J Gen Pract.* 2010 Jul;60(576):489-94.

Brostoff J, Gamlin L, Brostoff J. *Food Allergies and Food Intolerance: The Complete Guide to Their Identification and Treatment.* Rochester, VT: Healing Arts, 2000.

Brownstein D. *Salt: Your Way to Health.* West Bloomfield, MI: Medical Alternatives, 2006.

Brown-Whitehorn TF, Spergel JM. The link between allergies and eosinophilic esophagitis: implications for management strategies. *Expert Rev Clin Immunol.* 2010 Jan;6(1):101-9.

Bruce S, Nyberg F, Melén E, James A, Pulkkinen V, Orsmark-Pietras C, Bergström A, Dahlén B, Wickman M, von Mutius E, Doekes G, Lauener R, Riedler J, Eder W, van Hage M, Pershagen G, Scheynius A, Kere J. The protective effect of farm animal exposure on childhood allergy is modified by NPSR1 polymorphisms. *J Med Genet.* 2009 Mar;46(3):159-67. 2008 Feb 19.

Bruneton J. *Pharmacognosy, Phytochemistry, Medicinal Plants.* Paris: Lavoisier, 1995.

Bruton A, Lewith GT. The Buteyko breathing technique for asthma: a review. *Complement Ther Med.* 2005 Mar;13(1):41-6. 2005 Apr 18.

Bruton A, Thomas M. The role of breathing training in asthma management. *Curr Opin Allergy Clin Immunol.* 2011 Feb;11(1):53-7.

Bryborn M, Halldén C, Säll T, Cardell LO. CLC- a novel susceptibility gene for allergic rhinitis? *Allergy.* 2010 Feb;65(2):220-8.

Bu LN, Chang MH, Ni YH, Chen HL, Cheng CC. *Lactobacillus casei* rhamnosus Lcr35 in children with chronic constipation. *Pediatr Int.* 2007 Aug;49(4):485-90.

Bublin M, Pfister M, Radauer C, Oberhuber C, Bulley S, Dewitt AM, Lidholm J, Reese G, Vieths S, Breiteneder H, Hoffmann-Sommergruber K, Ballmer-Weber BK. Component-resolved diagnosis of kiwifruit allergy with purified natural and recombinant kiwifruit allergens. *J Allergy Clin Immunol.* 2010 Mar;125(3):687-94, 694.e1.

REFERENCES AND BIBLIOGRAPHY

Buchanan TW, Lutz K, Mirzazade S, Specht K, Shah NJ, Zilles K, et al. Recognition of emotional prosody and verbal components of spoken language: an fMRI study. *Cogn Brain Res.* 2000;9:227-38.

Bucher X, Pichler WJ, Dahinden CA, Helbling A. Effect of tree pollen specific, subcutaneous immunotherapy on the oral allergy syndrome to apple and hazelnut. *Allergy.* 2004 Dec;59(12):1272-6.

Budzianowski J. Coumarins, caffeoyltartaric acids and their artifactual methyl esters from Taraxacum officinale leaves. *Planta Med.* 1997 Jun;63(3):288.

Bueso AK, Berntsen S, Mowinckel P, Andersen LF, Lødrup Carlsen KC, Carlsen KH. Dietary intake in adolescents with asthma - potential for improvement. *Pediatr Allergy Immunol.* 2010 Oct 20. doi: 10.1111/j.1399-3038.2010.01013.x.

Bundy R, Walker AF, Middleton RW, Booth J. Turmeric extract may improve irritable bowel syndrome symptomology in otherwise healthy adults: a pilot study. *J Altern Complement Med.* 2004 Dec;10(6):1015-8.

Burdge GC, Jones AE, Wootton SA. Eicosapentaenoic and docosapentaenoic acids are the principal products of alpha-linolenic acid metabolism in young men. *B J Nutr.* 2002 Oct;88(4):355-63.

Buret AG. How stress induces intestinal hypersensitivity. *Am J Pathol.* 2006 Jan;168(1):3-5.

Burgess CD, Bremner P, Thomson CD, Crane J, Siebers RW, Beasley R. Nebulized beta 2-adrenoceptor agonists do not affect plasma selenium or glutathione peroxidase activity in patients with asthma. *Int J Clin Pharmacol Ther.* 1994 Jun;32(6):290-2.

Burks W, Jones SM, Berseth CL, Harris C, Sampson HA, Scalabrin DM. Hypoallergenicity and effects on growth and tolerance of a new amino acid-based formula with docosahexaenoic acid and arachidonic acid. *J Pediatr.* 2008 Aug;153(2):266-71.

Burney PG, Luczynska C, Chinn S, Jarvis D. The European Community Respiratory Health Survey. *Eur Respir J.* 1994;7: 954-960.

Burr ML, Butland BK, King S, Vaughan-Williams E. Changes in asthma prevalence: two surveys 15 years apart. *Arch Dis Child.* 1989;64:1452-1456.

Busse PJ, Wen MC, Huang CK, Srivastava K, Zhang TF, Schofield B, Sampson HA, Li XM. Therapeutic effects of the Chinese herbal formula, MSSM-03d, on persistent airway hyperreactivity and airway remodeling. *J Allergy Clin Immunol.* 2004;113:S220.

Byrne AM, Malka-Rais J, Burks AW, Fleischer DM. How do we know when peanut and tree nut allergy have resolved, and how do we keep it resolved? *Clin Exp Allergy.* 2010 Sep;40(9):1303-11.

Cabanillas B, Pedrosa MM, Rodríguez J, González A, Muzquiz M, Cuadrado C, Crespo JF, Burbano C. Effects of enzymatic hydrolysis on lentil allergenicity. *Mol Nutr Food Res.* 2010 Mar 19.

Caglar E, Cildir SK, Ergeneli S, Sandalli N, Twetman S. Salivary mutans streptococci and lactobacilli levels after ingestion of the probiotic bacterium *Lactobacillus reuteri* ATCC 55730 by straws or tablets. *Acta Odontol Scand.* 2006 Oct;64(5):314-8.

Caglar E, Kavaloglu SC, Kuscu OO, Sandalli N, Holgerson PL, Twetman S. Effect of chewing gums containing xylitol or probiotic bacteria on salivary mutans streptococci and lactobacilli. *Clin Oral Investig.* 2007 Dec;11(4):425-9.

Caglar E, Kuscu OO, Cildir SK, Kuvvetli SS, Sandalli N. A probiotic lozenge administered medical device and its effect on salivary mutans streptococci and lactobacilli. *Int J Paediatr Dent.* 2008 Jan;18(1):35-9.

Caglar E, Kuscu OO, Selvi Kuvvetli S, Kavaloglu Cildir S, Sandalli N, Twetman S. Short-term effect of icecream containing *Bifidobacterium lactis* Bb-12 on the number of salivary mutans streptococci and lactobacilli. *Acta Odontol Scand.* 2008 Jun;66(3):154-8.

Cahn J, Borzeix MG. Administration of procyanidolic oligomers in rats. Observed effects on changes in the permeability of the blood-brain barrier. *Sem Hop.* 1983 Jul 7;59(27-28):2031-4.

Calder PC. Dietary modification of inflammation with lipids. *Proc Nutr Soc.* 2002 Aug;61(3):345-58.

Camargo CA Jr, Ingham T, Wickens K, Thadhani R, Silvers KM, Epton MJ, Town GI, Pattemore PK, Espinola JA, Crane J; New Zealand Asthma and Allergy Cohort Study Group. Cord-blood 25-hydroxyvitamin D levels and risk of respiratory infection, wheezing, and asthma. *Pediatrics.* 2011 Jan;127(1):e180-7.

Caminiti L, Passalacqua G, Barberi S, Vita D, Barberio G, De Luca R, Pajno GB. A new protocol for specific oral tolerance induction in children with IgE-mediated cow's milk allergy. *Allergy Asthma Proc.* 2009 Jul-Aug;30(4):443-8.

Campbell TC, Campbell TM. *The China Study.* Dallas, TX: Benbella Books, 2006.

Campieri C, Campieri M, Bertuzzi V, Swennen E, Matteuzzi D, Stefoni S, Pirovano F, Centi C, Ulisse S, Famularo G, De Simone C. Reduction of oxaluria after an oral course of lactic acid bacteria at high concentration. *Kidney Int.* 2001 Sep;60(3):1097-105.

Canakcioglu S, Tahamiler R, Saritzali G, Alimoglu Y, Isildak H, Guvenc MG, Acar GO, Inci E. Evaluation of nasal cytology in subjects with chronic rhinitis: a 7-year study. *Am J Otolaryngol.* 2009 Sep-Oct;30(5):312-7.

249

Canali R, Comitato R, Schonlau F, Virgili F. The anti-inflammatory pharmacology of Pycnogenol in humans involves COX-2 and 5-LOX mRNA expression in leukocytes. *Int Immunopharmacol.* 2009 Sep;9(10):1145-9.

Canani RB, Cirillo P, Terrin G, Cesarano L, Spagnuolo MI, De Vincenzo A, Albano F, Passariello A, De Marco G, Manguso F, Guarino A. Probiotics for treatment of acute diarrhoea in children: randomised clinical trial of five different preparations. *BMJ.* 2007 Aug 18;335(7615):340.

Canducci F, Armuzzi A, Cremonini F, Cammarota G, Bartolozzi F, Pola P, Gasbarrini G, Gasbarrini A. A lyophilized and inactivated culture of *Lactobacillus acidophilus* increases *Helicobacter pylori* eradication rates. *Aliment Pharmacol Ther.* 2000 Dec;14(12):1625-9.

Canducci F, Cremonini F, Armuzzi A, Di Caro S, Gabrielli M, Santarelli L, Nista E, Lupascu A, De Martini D, Gasbarrini A. Probiotics and Helicobacter pylori eradication. *Dig Liver Dis.* 2002 Sep;34 Suppl 2:S81-3.

Canonica GW, Passalacqua G. Noninjection routes for immunotherapy. *J Allergy Clin Immunol.* 2003 Mar;111(3):437-48; quiz 449.

Cantani A, Micera M. Natural history of cow's milk allergy. An eight-year follow-up study in 115 atopic children. *Eur Rev Med Pharmacol Sci.* 2004 Jul-Aug;8(4):153-64.

Cantani A, Micera M. The prick by prick test is safe and reliable in 58 children with atopic dermatitis and food allergy. *Eur Rev Med Pharmacol Sci.* 2006 May-Jun;10(3):115-20.

Cao G, Alessio HM, Cutler RG. Oxygen-radical absorbance capacity assay for antioxidants. *Free Radic Biol Med.* 1993 Mar;14(3):303-11.

Cao G, Shukitt-Hale B, Bickford PC, Joseph JA, McEwen J, Prior RL. Hyperoxia-induced changes in antioxidant capacity and the effect of dietary antioxidants. *J Appl Physiol.* 1999 Jun;86(6):1817-22.

Caramia G. The essential fatty acids omega-6 and omega-3: from their discovery to their use in therapy. *Minerva Pediatr.* 2008 Apr;60(2):219-33.

Carey DG, Aase KA, Pliego GJ. The acute effect of cold air exercise in determination of exercise-induced bronchospasm in apparently healthy athletes. J Strength Cond Res. 2010 Aug;24(8):2172-8.

Carpita N. C., Kanabus J., Housley T. L. Linkage structure of fructans and fructan oligomers from Triticum aestivum and Festuca arundinacea leaves. *J. Plant Physiol.* 1989;134:162-168

Carroccio A, Cavataio F, Montalto G, D'Amico D, Alabrese L, Iacono G. Intolerance to hydrolysed cow's milk proteins in infants: clinical characteristics and dietary treatment. *Clin Exp Allergy.* 2000 Nov;30(11):1597-603.

Carroll D. *The Complete Book of Natural Medicines.* New York: Summit, 1980.

Caruso M, Frasca G, Di Giuseppe PL, Pennisi A, Tringali G, Bonina FP. Effects of a new nutraceutical ingredient on allergen-induced sulphidoleukotrienes production and CD63 expression in allergic subjects. *Int Immunopharmacol.* 2008 Dec 20;8(13-14):1781-6.

Casale TB, Amin BV. Allergic rhinitis/asthma interrelationship. *Clin Rev Allergy Immunol.* 2001;21:27-49.

Cats A, Kuipers EJ, Bosschaert MA, Pot RG, Vandenbroucke-Grauls CM, Kusters JG. Effect of frequent consumption of a *Lactobacillus casei*-containing milk drink in *Helicobacter pylori*-colonized subjects. *Aliment Pharmacol Ther.* 2003 Feb;17(3):429-35.

Caughey AB, Nicholson JM, Cheng YW, Lyell DJ, Washington AE. Induction of labor and Cesarean delivery by gestational age. *Am J Obstet Gynecol.* 2006 Sep;195(3):700-5.

Celakovská J, Vaněčková J, Ettlerová K, Ettler K, Bukac J. The role of atopy patch test in diagnosis of food allergy in atopic eczema/dermatitis syndrom in patients over 14 years of age. *Acta Medica (Hradec Kralove).* 2010;53(2):101-8.

Celikel S, Karakaya G, Yurtsever N, Sorkun K, Kalyoncu AF. Bee and bee products allergy in Turkish beekeepers: determination of risk factors for systemic reactions. *Allergol Immunopathol (Madr).* 2006 Sep-Oct;34(5):180-4.

Centers for Disease Control and Prevention (CDC). Obesity prevalence among low-income, preschool-aged children - United States, 1998-2008. *MMWR Morb Mortal Wkly Rep.* 2009 Jul 24;58(28):769-73.

Centers for Disease Control and Prevention (CDC). Vital signs: nonsmokers' exposure to secondhand smoke - United States, 1999-2008. *MMWR Morb Mortal Wkly Rep.* 2010 Sep 10;59(35):1141-6.

Centre for Molecular, Environmental, Genetic and Analytic Epidemiology, School of Population Health, The UniverGumowski P, Lech B, Chaves I, Girard JP. Chronic asthma and rhinitis due to Candida albicans, epidermophyton, and trichophyton. *Ann Allergy.* 1987 Jul;59(1):48-51.

Cereijido M, Contreras RG, Flores-Benítez D, Flores-Maldonado C, Larre I, Ruiz A, Shoshani L. New diseases derived or associated with the tight junction. *Arch Med Res.* 2007 Jul;38(5):465-78.

Chafen JJ, Newberry SJ, Riedl MA, Bravata DM, Maglione M, Suttorp MJ, Sundaram V, Paige NM, Towfigh A, Hulley BJ, Shekelle PG. Diagnosing and managing common food allergies: a systematic review. *JAMA.* 2010 May 12;303(18):1848-56.

Chahine BG, Bahna SL. The role of the gut mucosal immunity in the development of tolerance versus development of allergy to food. *Curr Opin Allergy Clin Immunol.* 2010 Aug;10(4):394-9.

REFERENCES AND BIBLIOGRAPHY

Chaitow L, Trenev N. *Probiotics: The revolutionary, 'friendly bacteria way to vital health and well-being.* New York: Thorsons, 1990.

Chaitow L. *Conquer Pain the Natural Way.* San Francisco: Chronicle Books, 2002.

Chakürski I, Matev M, Koïchev A, Angelova I, Stefanov G. Treatment of chronic colitis with an herbal combination of Taraxacum officinale, Hipericum perforatum, Melissa officinaliss, Calendula officinalis and Foeniculum vulgare. *Vutr Boles.* 1981;20(6):51-4.

Chan CK, Kuo ML, Shen JJ, See LC, Chang HH, Huang JL. Ding Chuan Tang, a Chinese herb decoction, could improve airway hyper-responsiveness in stabilized asthmatic children: a randomized, double-blind clinical trial. *Pediatr Allergy Immunol.* 2006;17:316-22.

Chandra RK. Prospective studies of the effect of breast feeding on incidence of infection and allergy. *Acta Paediatr Scand.* 1979 Sep;68(5):691-4.

Chaney M, Ross M. *Nutrition.* New York: Houghton Mifflin, 1971.

Chang HT, Tseng LJ, Hung TJ, Kao BT, Lin WY, Fan TC, Chang MD, Pai TW. Inhibition of the interactions between eosinophil cationic protein and airway epithelial cells by traditional Chinese herbs. *BMC Syst Biol.* 2010 Sep 13;4 Suppl 2:S8.

Chang TT, Huang CC, Hsu CH. Clinical evaluation of the Chinese herbal medicine formula STA-1 in the treatment of allergic asthma. *Phytother Res.* 2006;20:342-7.

Chang TT, Huang CC, Hsu CH. Inhibition of mite-induced immunoglobulin E synthesis, airway inflammation, and hyperreactivity by herbal medicine STA-1. *Immunopharmacol Immunotoxicol.* 2006;28:683-95.

Chao A, Thun MJ, Connell CJ, McCullough ML, Jacobs EJ, Flanders WD, Rodriguez C, Sinha R, Calle EE. Meat consumption and risk of colorectal cancer. *JAMA.* 2005 Jan 12;293(2):172-82.

Chapat L, Chemin K, Dubois B, Bourdet-Sicard R, Kaiserlian D. Lactobacillus casei reduces CD8+ T cell-mediated skin inflammation. *Eur J Immunol.* 2004 Sep;34(9):2520-8.

Chapidze G, Kapanadze S, Dolidze N, Bachutashvili Z, Latsabidze N. Prevention of coronary atherosclerosis by the use of combination therapy with antioxidant coenzyme q10 and statins. *Georgian Med News.* 2005 Jan;(1):20-5.

Characterization and quantitation of Antioxidant Constituents of Sweet Pepper (Capsicum annuum - Cayenne). *J Agric Food Chem.* 2004 Jun 16;52(12):3861-9.

Chatzi L, Apostolaki G, Bibakis I, Skypala I, Bibaki-Liakou V, Tzanakis N, Kogevinas M, Cullinan P. Protective effect of fruits, vegetables and the Mediterranean diet on asthma and allergies among children in Crete. *Thorax.* 2007 Aug;62(8):677-83.

Chatzi L, Torrent M, Romieu I, Garcia-Esteban R, Ferrer C, Vioque J, Kogevinas M, Sunyer J. Mediterranean diet in pregnancy is protective for wheeze and atopy in childhood. *Thorax.* 2008 Jun;63(6):507-13.

Chaves TC, de Andrade e Silva TS, Monteiro SA, Watanabe PC, Oliveira AS, Grossi DB. Craniocervical posture and hyoid bone position in children with mild and moderate asthma and mouth breathing. *Int J Pediatr Otorhinolaryngol.* 2010 Sep;74(9):1021-7.

Chawes BL, Bønnelykke K, Kreiner-Møller E, Bisgaard H. Children with allergic and nonallergic rhinitis have a similar risk of asthma. *J Allergy Clin Immunol.* 2010 Sep;126(3):567-73.e1-8.

Chawes BL, Kreiner-Møller E, Bisgaard H. Objective assessments of allergic and nonallergic rhinitis in young children. *Allergy.* 2009 Oct;64(10):1547-53.

Chehade M, Aceves SS. Food allergy and eosinophilic esophagitis. *Curr Opin Allergy Clin Immunol.* 2010 Jun;10(3):231-7.

Chellini E, Talassi F, Corbo G, Berti G, De Sario M, Rusconi F, Piffer S, Caranci N, Petronio MG, Sestini P, Dell'Orco V, Bonci E, Armenio L, La Grutta S; Gruppo Collaborativo SIDRIA-2. Environmental, social and demographic characteristics of children and adolescents, resident in different Italian areas. *Epidemiol Prev.* 2005 Mar-Apr;29(2 Suppl):14-23.

Chen HJ, Shih CK, Hsu HY, Chiang W. Mast cell-dependent allergic responses are inhibited by ethanolic extract of adlay (Coix lachryma-jobi L. var. ma-yuen Stapf) testa. *J Agric Food Chem.* 2010 Feb 24;58(4):2596-601.

Chen JX, Ji B, Lu ZL, Hu LS. Effects of chai hu (radix burpleuri) containing formulation on plasma beta-endorphin, epinephrine and dopamine on patients. *Am J Chin Med.* 2005;33(5):737-45.

Chen Y, Blaser MJ. Helicobacter pylori colonization is inversely associated with childhood asthma. *J Infect Dis.* 2008 Aug 15;198(4):553-60.

Chen Y, Blaser MJ. Inverse associations of Helicobacter pylori with asthma and allergy. *Arch Intern Med.* 2007 Apr 23;167(8):821-7.

Cheney G, Waxler SH, Miller IJ. Vitamin U therapy of peptic ulcer; experience at San Quentin Prison. *Calif Med.* 1956 Jan;84(1):39-42.

Chevallier A. *Encyclopedia of Medicinal Plants.* New York, NY: DK Publishing; 1996.

Chevrier MR, Ryan AE, Lee DY, Zhongze M, Wu-Yan Z, Via CS. Boswellia carterii extract inhibits TH1 cytokines and promotes TH2 cytokines in vitro. *Clin Diagn Lab Immunol.* 2005 May;12(5):575-80.

Chiang BL, Sheih YH, Wang LH, Liao CK, Gill HS. Enhancing immunity by dietary consumption of a probiotic lactic acid bacterium (*Bifidobacterium lactis* HN019): optimization and definition of cellular immune responses. *Eur J Clin Nutr.* 2000 Nov;54(11):849-55.

Chilton F, Tucker L. *Win the War Within.* New York: Rodale, 2006.

Chilton FH, Rudel LL, Parks JS, Arm JP, Seeds MC. Mechanisms by which botanical lipids affect inflammatory disorders. *Am J Clin Nutr.* 2008 Feb;87(2):498S-503S.

Chilton FH, Tucker L. *Win the War Within.* New York: Rodale, 2006.

Chin A Paw MJ, de Jong N, Pallast EG, Kloek GC, Schouten EG, Kok FJ. Immunity in frail elderly: a randomized controlled trial of exercise and enriched foods. *Med Sci Sports Exerc.* 2000 Dec;32(12):2005-11.

Chong Neto HJ, Rosário NA; Grupo EISL Curitiba (Estudio Internacional de Sibilancias en Lactantes). Risk factors for wheezing in the first year of life. *J Pediatr.* 2008 Nov-Dec;84(6):495-502.

Chopra RN, Nayar SL, Chopra IC, eds. *Glossary of Indian Medicinal plants.* New Delhi: CSIR, 1956.

Choudhry S, Seibold MA, Borrell LN, Tang H, Serebrisky D, Chapela R, Rodriguez-Santana JR, Avila PC, Ziv E, Rodriguez-Cintron W, Risch NJ, Burchard EG. Dissecting complex diseases in complex populations: asthma in latino americans. *Proc Am Thorac Soc.* 2007 Jul;4(3):226-33.

Chouraqui JP, Grathwohl D, Labaune JM, Hascoet JM, de Montgolfier I, Leclaire M, Giarre M, Steenhout P. Assessment of the safety, tolerance, and protective effect against diarrhea of infant formulas containing mixtures of probiotics or probiotics and prebiotics in a randomized controlled trial. *Am J Clin Nutr.* 2008 May;87(5):1365-73.

Christopher JR. *School of Natural Healing.* Springville UT: Christopher Publ, 1976.

Chu YF, Liu RH. Cranberries inhibit LDL oxidation and induce LDL receptor expression in hepatocytes. *Life Sci.* 2005;77(15):1892-1901. 27.

Chu YF, Liu RH. Cranberries inhibit LDL oxidation and induce LDL receptor expression in hepatocytes. *Life Sci.* 2005;77(15):1892-1901.

Chung SY, Butts CL, Maleki SJ, Champagne ET Linking peanut allergenicity to the processes of maturation, curing, and roasting. *J Agric Food Chem.* 2003;51: 4273-4277.

Chwirot WB, Popp F. White-light-induced luminescence and mitotic activity of yeast cells. *Folia Histochemica et Cytobiologica.* 1991;29(4):155.

Cianci A, Giordano R, Delia A, Grasso E, Amodeo A, De Leo V, Caccamo F. Efficacy of *Lactobacillus rhamnosus* GR-1 and of *Lactobacillus reuteri* RC-14 in the treatment and prevention of vaginoses and bacterial vaginitis relapses. *Minerva Ginecol.* 2008 Oct;60(5):369-76.

Cibella F, Cuttitta G. Nocturnal asthma and gastroesophageal reflux. *Am J Med.* 2001 Dec 3;111 Suppl 8A:31S-36S.

Cingi C, Demirbas D, Songu M. Allergic rhinitis caused by food allergies. *Eur Arch Otorhinolaryngol.* 2010 Sep;267(9):1327-35.

Ciprandi G, De Amici M, Negrini S, Marseglia G, Tosca MA. TGF-beta and IL-17 serum levels and specific immunotherapy. *Int Immunopharmacol.* 2009 Sep;9(10):1247-9.

Cisneros C, García-Río F, Romera D, Villasante C, Girón R, Ancochea J. Bronchial reactivity indices are determinants of health-related quality of life in patients with stable asthma. *Thorax.* 2010 Sep;65(9):795-800.

Clark S, Bock SA, Gaeta TJ, Brenner BE, Cydulka RK, Camargo CA; Multicenter Airway Research Collaboration-8 Investigators. Multicenter study of emergency department visits for food allergies. *J Allergy Clin Immunol.* 2004 Feb;113(2):347-52.

Clement YN, Williams AF, Aranda D, Chase R, Watson N, Mohammed R, Stubbs O, Williamson D. Medicinal herb use among asthmatic patients attending a specialty care facility in Trinidad. *BMC Complement Altern Med.* 2005 Feb 15;5:3.

Clerici M, Balotta C, Meroni L, Ferrario E, Riva C, Trabattoni D, Ridolfo A,Villa M, Shearer GM, Moroni M, Galli M. Type 1 cytokine production and low prevalence of viral isolation correlate with long-term nonprogression in HIV infection. *AIDS Res Hum Retroviruses.* 1996 Jul 20;12(11):1053-61.

Cobo Sanz JM, Mateos JA, Muñoz Conejo A. Effect of *Lactobacillus casei* on the incidence of infectious conditions in children. *Nutr Hosp.* 2006 Jul-Aug;21(4):547-51.

Codispoti CD, Levin L, LeMasters GK, Ryan P, Reponen T, Villareal M, Burkle J, Stanforth S, Lockey JE, Khurana Hershey GK, Bernstein DI. Breast-feeding, aeroallergen sensitization, and environmental exposures during infancy are determinants of childhood allergic rhinitis. *J Allergy Clin Immunol.* 2010 May;125(5):1054-1060.e1.

Cohen RT, Raby BA, Van Steen K, Fuhlbrigge AL, Celedón JC, Rosner BA, Strunk RC, Zeiger RS, Weiss ST; Childhood Asthma Management Program Research Group. In utero smoke exposure and impaired response to inhaled corticosteroids in children with asthma. *J Allergy Clin Immunol.* 2010 Sep;126(3):491-7. 2010 Jul 31. ; .

Cohen S, Popp F. Biophoton emission of the human body. *J Photochem & Photobio.* 1997;B 40:187-189.

Colecchia A, Vestito A, La Rocca A, Pasqui F, Nikiforaki A, Festi D; Symbiotic Study Group. Effect of a symbiotic preparation on the clinical manifestations of irritable bowel syndrome, constipation-variant. Results of an open, uncontrolled multicenter study. *Minerva Gastroenterol Dietol.* 2006 Dec;52(4):349-58.

Collipp PJ, Goldzier S 3rd, Weiss N, Soleymani Y, Snyder R. Pyridoxine treatment of childhood bronchial asthma. *Ann Allergy.* 1975 Aug;35(2):93-7.

Colodner R, Edelstein H, Chazan B, Raz R. Vaginal colonization by orally administered *Lactobacillus rhamnosus* GG. *Isr Med Assoc J.* 2003 Nov;5(11):767-9.

Conquer JA, Holub BJ. Dietary docosahexaenoic acid as a source of eicosapentaenoic acid in vegetarians and omnivores. *Lipids.* 1997 Mar;32(3):341-5.

Consumer Reports. Probiotics: Are enough in your diet? *Cons Rpts Mag.* 2005:34-35.

Conway PL, Gorbach SL, Goldin BR. Survival of lactic acid bacteria in the human stomach and adhesion to intestinal cells. *J Dairy Sci.* 1987 Jan;70(1):1-12.

Cooper GS, Miller FW, Germolec DR: Occupational exposures and autoimmune diseases. *Int Immunopharm* 2002, 2:303-313.

Cooper K. *The Aerobics Program for Total Well-Being.* New York: Evans, 1980.

Corbe C, Boissin JP, Siou A. Light vision and chorioretinal circulation. Study of the effect of procyanidolic oligomers (Endotelon). *J Fr Ophtalmol.* 1988;11(5):453-60.

Corbe C, Boissin JP, Siou A. Light vision and chorioretinal circulation. Study of the effect of procyanidolic oligomers (Endotelon). *J Fr Ophtalmol.* 1988;11(5):453-60.

Corbo GM, Forastiere F, De Sario M, Brunetti L, Bonci E, Bugiani M, Chellini E, La Grutta S, Migliore E, Pistelli R, Rusconi F, Russo A, Simoni M, Talassi F, Galassi C; Sidria-2 Collaborative Group. Wheeze and asthma in children: associations with body mass index, sports, television viewing, and diet. *Epidemiology.* 2008 Sep;19(5):747-55.

Corrêa NB, Péret Filho LA, Penna FJ, Lima FM, Nicoli JR. A randomized formula controlled trial of *Bifidobacterium lactis* and *Streptococcus thermophilus* for prevention of antibiotic-associated diarrhea in infants. *J Clin Gastroenterol.* 2005 May-Jun;39(5):385-9.

Cory S, Ussery-Hall A, Griffin-Blake S, Easton A, Vigeant J, Balluz L, Garvin W, Greenlund K; Centers for Disease Control and Prevention (CDC). Prevalence of selected risk behaviors and chronic diseases and conditions-steps communities, United States, 2006-2007. *MMWR Surveill Summ.* 2010 Sep 24;59(8):1-37.

Courtney R, Cohen M. Investigating the claims of Konstantin Buteyko, M.D., Ph.D.: the relationship of breath holding time to end tidal CO_2 and other proposed measures of dysfunctional breathing. *J Altern Complement Med.* 2008 Mar;14(2):115-23.

Couto E, Boffetta P, Lagiou P, Ferrari P, Buckland G, Overvad K, Dahm CC, Tjønneland A, Olsen A, Clavel-Chapelon F, Boutron-Ruault MC, Cottet V, Trichopoulos D, Naska A, Benetou V, Kaaks R, Rohrmann S, Boeing H, von Ruesten A, Panico S, Pala V, Vineis P, Palli D, Tumino R, May A, Peeters PH, Bueno-de-Mesquita HB, Büchner FL, Lund E, Skeie G, Engeset D, Gonzalez CA, Navarro C, Rodríguez L, Sánchez MJ, Amiano P, Barricarte A, Hallmans G, Johansson I, Manjer J, Wirfärt E, Allen NE, Crowe F, Khaw KT, Wareham N, Moskal A, Slimani N, Jenab M, Romaguera D, Mouw T, Norat T, Riboli E, Trichopoulou A. Mediterranean dietary pattern and cancer risk in the EPIC cohort. *Br J Cancer.* 2011 Apr 26;104(9):1493-9.

Couzy F, Kastenmayer P, Vigo M, Clough J, Munoz-Box R, Barclay DV. Calcium bioavailability from a calcium- and sulfate-rich mineral water, compared with milk, in young adult women. *Am J Clin Nutr.* 1995 Dec;62(6):1239-44.

Covar R, Gleason M, Macomber B, Stewart L, Szefler P, Engelhardt K, Murphy J, Liu A, Wood S, DeMichele S, Gelfand EW, Szefler SJ. Impact of a novel nutritional formula on asthma control and biomarkers of allergic airway inflammation in children. *Clin Exp Allergy.* 2010 Aug;40(8):1163-74. 2010 Jun 7.

Crane J, Ellis I, Siebers R, Grimmet D, Lewis S, Fitzharris P. A pilot study of the effect of mechanical ventilation and heat exchange on house-dust mites and Der p 1 in New Zealand homes. *Allergy.* 1998 Aug;53(8):755-62.

Crescente M, Jessen G, Momi S, Höltje HD, Gresele P, Cerletti C, de Gaetano G. Interactions of gallic acid, resveratrol, quercetin and aspirin at the platelet cyclooxygenase-1 level. Functional and modelling studies. *Thromb Haemost.* 2009 Aug;102(2):336-46.

Crinnion WJ. Toxic effects of the easily avoidable phthalates and parabens. *Altern Med Rev.* 2010 Sep;15(3):190-6.

Cserhati E. Current view on the etiology of childhood bronchial asthma. *Orv Hetil.* 2000;141:759-760.

Cuesta-Herranz J, Barber D, Blanco C, Cistero-Bahíma A, Crespo JF, Fernández-Rivas M, Fernández-Sánchez J, Florido JF, Ibáñez MD, Rodríguez R, Salcedo G, Garcia BE, Lombardero M, Quiralte J, Rodriguez J, Sánchez-Monge R, Vereda A, Villalba M, Alonso Díaz de Durana MD, Basagaña M, Carrillo T, Fernández-Nieto M, Tabar AI. Differences among Pollen-Allergic Patients with and without Plant Food Allergy. *Int Arch Allergy Immunol.* 2010 Apr 23;153(2):182-192.

Cummings M. *Human Heredity: Principles and Issues.* St. Paul, MN: West, 1988.

Custovic A, Simpson BM, Simpson A, Kissen P, Woodcock A; NAC Manchester Asthma and Allergy Study Group. Effect of environmental manipulation in pregnancy and early life on respiratory symptoms and atopy during first year of life: a randomised trial. *Lancet.* 2001 Jul 21;358(9277):188-93.

D'Anneo RW, Bruno ME, Falagiani P. Sublingual allergoid immunotherapy: a new 4-day induction phase in patients allergic to house dust mites. *Int J Immunopathol Pharmacol.* 2010 Apr-Jun;23(2):553-60.

D'Auria E, Sala M, Lodi F, Radaelli G, Riva E, Giovannini M. Nutritional value of a rice-hydrolysate formula in infants with cows' milk protein allergy: a randomized pilot study. *J Int Med Res.* 2003 May-Jun;31(3):215-22.

D'Orazio N, Ficoneri C, Riccioni G, Conti P, Theoharides TC, Bollea MR. Conjugated linoleic acid: a functional food? *Int J Immunopathol Pharmacol.* 2003 Sep-Dec;16(3):215-20.

D'Urbano LE, Pellegrino K, Artesani MC, Donnanno S, Luciano R, Riccardi C, Tozzi AE, Ravà L, De Benedetti F, Cavagni G. Performance of a component-based allergen-microarray in the diagnosis of cow's milk and hen's egg allergy. *Clin Exp Allergy.* 2010 Jul 13.

Dalaly BK, Eitenmiller RR, Friend BA, Shahani KM. Human milk ribonuclease. *Biochim Biophys Acta.* 1980 Oct;615(2):381-91.

Dalaly BK, Eitenmiller RR, Vakil JR, Shahani KM. Simultaneous isolation of human milk ribonuclease and lysozyme. Anal Biochem. 1970 Sep;37(1):208-11.

Dallinga JW, Robroeks CM, van Berkel JJ, Moonen EJ, Godschalk RW, Jöbsis Q, Dompeling E, Wouters EF, van Schooten FJ. Volatile organic compounds in exhaled breath as a diagnostic tool for asthma in children. Clin Exp Allergy. 2010 Jan;40(1):68-76.

Davidson T. *Rhinology: The Collected Writings of Maurice H. Cottle, M.D.* San Diego, CA: American Rhinologic Society, 1987.

Davies G. *Timetables of Medicine.* New York: Black Dog & Leventhal, 2000.

Davin JC, Forget P, Mahieu PR. Increased intestinal permeability to (51 Cr) EDTA is correlated with IgA immune complex-plasma levels in children with IgA-associated nephropathies. *Acta Paediatr Scand.* 1988 Jan;77(1):118-24.

de Boissieu D, Dupont C, Badoual J. Allergy to nondairy proteins in mother's milk as assessed by intestinal permeability tests. *Allergy.* 1994 Dec;49(10):882-4.

De Lucca AJ, Bland JM, Vigo CB, Cushion M, Selitrennikoff CP, Peter J, Walsh TJ. CAY-I, a fungicidal saponin from Capsicum sp. fruit. *Med Mycol.* 2002 Apr;40(2):131-7.

De Preter V, Raemen H, Cloetens L, Houben E, Rutgeerts P, Verbeke K. Effect of dietary intervention with different pre- and probiotics on intestinal bacterial enzyme activities. *Eur J Clin Nutr.* 2008 Feb;62(2):225-31.

De Simone C, Ciardi A, Grassi A, Lambert Gardini S, Tzantzoglou S, Trinchieri V, Moretti S, Jirillo E. Effect of *Bifidobacterium bifidum* and *Lactobacillus acidophilus* on gut mucosa and peripheral blood B lymphocytes. *Immunopharmacol Immunotoxicol.* 1992;14(1-2):331-40.

De Smet PA. Herbal remedies. *N Engl J Med.* 2002;347:2046-2056.

de Vrese M, Rautenberg P, Laue C, Koopmans M, Herremans T, Schrezenmeir J. Probiotic bacteria stimulate virus-specific neutralizing antibodies following a booster polio vaccination. *Eur J Nutr.* 2005 Oct;44(7):406-13.

de Vrese M, Winkler P, Rautenberg P, Harder T, Noah C, Laue C, Ott S, Hampe J, Schreiber S, Heller K, Schrezenmeir J. Effect of *Lactobacillus gasseri* PA 16/8, *Bifidobacterium longum* SP 07/3, B. *bifidum* MF 20/5 on common cold episodes: a double blind, randomized, controlled trial. *Clin Nutr.* 2005 Aug;24(4):481-91.

Dean C. *Death by Modern Medicine.* Belleville, ON: Matrix Verite-Media, 2005.

Debley JS, Carter ER, Redding GJ. Prevalence and impact of gastroesophageal reflux in adolescents with asthma: a population-based study. *Pediatr Pulmonol.* 2006 May;41(5):475-81.

Dehlink E, Yen E, Leichtner AM, Hait EJ, Fiebiger E. First evidence of a possible association between gastric acid suppression during pregnancy and childhood asthma: a population-based register study. *Clin Exp Allergy.* 2009 Feb;39(2):246-53. 2008 Dec 9.

del Giudice MM, Leonardi S, Maiello N, Brunese FP. Food allergy and probiotics in childhood. *J Clin Gastroenterol.* 2010 Sep;44 Suppl 1:S22-5.

Delacourt C. Bronchial changes in untreated asthma. *Arch Pediatr.* 2004 Jun;11 Suppl 2:71s-73s.

Delia A, Morgante G, Rago G, Musacchio MC, Petraglia F, De Leo V. Effectiveness of oral administration of Lactobacillus paracasei subsp. paracasei F19 in association with vaginal suppositories of Lactobacillus acidofilus in the treatment of vaginosis and in the prevention of recurrent vaginitis. *Minerva Ginecol.* 2006 Jun;58(3):227-31.

Del-Rio-Navarro B, Berber A, Blandón-Vijil V, Ramírez-Aguilar M, Romieu I, Ramírez-Chanona N, Heras-Acevedo S, Serrano-Sierra A, Barraza-Villareal A, Baeza-Bacab M, Sienra-Monge JJ. Identification of asthma risk factors in Mexico City in an International Study of Asthma and Allergy in Childhood survey. *Allergy Asthma Proc.* 2006 Jul-Aug;27(4):325-33.

DeMan, JC, Rogosa M, Sharpe ME. A medium for the cultivation of lactobacilli. *J Bacteriol.* 1960:23;130.

Dengate S, Ruben A. Controlled trial of cumulative behavioural effects of a common bread preservative. *J Paediatr Child Health.* 2002 Aug;38(4):373-6.

Dente FL, Bacci E, Bartoli ML, Cianchetti S, Costa F, Di Franco A, Malagrinò L, Vagaggini B, Paggiaro P. Effects of oral prednisone on sputum eosinophils and cytokines in patients with severe refractory asthma. *Ann Allergy Asthma Immunol.* 2010 Jun;104(6):464-70.

Denys GA, Koch KM, Dowzicky MJ. Distribution of resistant gram-positive organisms across the census regions of the United States and in vitro activity of tigecycline, a new glycylcycline antimicrobial. *Am J Infect Control.* 2007 Oct;35(8):521-6.

Depeint F, Tzortzis G, Vulevic J, I'anson K, Gibson GR. Prebiotic evaluation of a novel galactooligosaccharide mixture produced by the enzymatic activity of *Bifidobacterium bifidum* NCIMB 41171, in healthy humans: a randomized, double-blind, crossover, placebo-controlled intervention study. *Am J Clin Nutr.* 2008 Mar;87(3):785-91.

Derebery MJ, Berliner KI. Allergy and its relation to Meniere's disease. *Otolaryngol Clin North Am.* 2010 Oct;43(5):1047-58.

Desbonnet L, Garrett L, Clarke G, Bienenstock J, Dinan TG. The probiotic Bifidobacteria infantis: An assessment of potential antidepressant properties in the rat. *J Psychiatr Res.* 2008 Dec;43(2):164-74.

Desjeux JF, Heyman M. Milk proteins, cytokines and intestinal epithelial functions in children. *Acta Paediatr Jpn.* 1994 Oct;36(5):592-6.

DesRoches A, Infante-Rivard C, Paradis L, Paradis J, Haddad E. Peanut allergy: is maternal transmission of antigens during pregnancy and breastfeeding a risk factor? *J Investig Allergol Clin Immunol.* 2010;20(4):289-94.

Deutsche Gesellschaft für Ernährung. Drink distilled water? *Med. Mo. Pharm.* 1993;16:146.

Devaraj TL. *Speaking of Ayurvedic Remedies for Common Diseases.* New Delhi: Sterling, 1985.

Devirgiliis C, Zalewski PD, Perozzi G, Murgia C. Zinc fluxes and zinc transporter genes in chronic diseases. *Mutat Res.* 2007 Sep 1;622(1-2):84-93. 2007 Feb 17.

DeWitt RC, Kudsk KA. The gut's role in metabolism, mucosal barrier function, and gut immunology. *Infect Dis Clin North Am.* 1999 Jun;13(2):465-81.

Dharmage SC, Erbas B, Jarvis D, Wjst M, Raherison C, Norbäck D, Heinrich J, Sunyer J, Svanes C. Do childhood respiratory infections continue to influence adult respiratory morbidity? *Eur Respir J.* 2009 Feb;33(2):237-44.

Di Gioacchino M, Cavallucci E, Di Stefano F, Paolini F, Ramondo S, Di Sciascio MB, Ciuffreda S, Riccioni G, Della Vecchia R, Romano A, Boscolo P. Effect of natural allergen exposure on non-specific bronchial reactivity in asthmatic farmers. *Sci Total Environ.* 2001 Apr 10;270(1-3):43-8.

Di Gioacchino M, Cavallucci E, Di Stefano F, Verna N, Ramondo S, Ciuffreda S, Riccioni G, Boscolo P. Influence of total IgE and seasonal increase of eosinophil cationic protein on bronchial hyperreactivity in asthmatic grass-sensitized farmers. *Allergy.* 2000 Nov;55(11):1030-4.

Di Marzio L, Centi C, Cinque B, Masci S, Giuliani M, Arcieri A, Zicari L, De Simone C, Cifone MG. Effect of the lactic acid bacterium *Streptococcus thermophilus* on stratum corneum ceramide levels and signs and symptoms of atopic dermatitis patients. *Exp Dermatol.* 2003 Oct;12(5):615-20.

Dierksen KP, Moore CJ, Inglis M, Wescombe PA, Tagg JR. The effect of ingestion of milk supplemented with salivaricin A-producing Streptococcus salivarius on the bacteriocin-like inhibitory activity of streptococcal populations on the tongue. *FEMS Microbiol Ecol.* 2007 Mar;59(3):584-91.

Diğrak M, Ilçim A, Hakki Alma M. Antimicrobial activities of several parts of Pinus brutia, Juniperus oxycedrus, Abies cilicia, Cedrus libani and Pinus nigra. *Phytother Res.* 1999 Nov;13(7):584-7.

DiMango E, Holbrook JT, Simpson E, Reibman J, Richter J, Narula S, Prusakowski N, Mastronarde JG, Wise RA; American Lung Association Asthma Clinical Research Centers. Effects of asymptomatic proximal and distal gastroesophageal reflux on asthma severity. *Am J Respir Crit Care Med.* 2009 Nov 1;180(9):809-16. 2009 Aug 6.

Dimitonova SP, Danova ST, Serkedjieva JP, Bakalov BV. Antimicrobial activity and protective properties of vaginal lactobacilli from healthy Bulgarian women. *Anaerobe.* 2007 Oct-Dec;13(5-6):178-84.

Din FV, Theodoratou E, Farrington SM, Tenesa A, Barnetson RA, Cetnarskyj R, Stark L, Porteous ME, Campbell H, Dunlop MG. Effect of aspirin and NSAIDs on risk and survival from colorectal cancer. *Gut.* 2010 Dec;59(12):1670-9.

Dinleyici EC, Eren M, Yargic ZA, Dogan N, Vandenplas Y. Clinical efficacy of *Saccharomyces boulardii* and metronidazole compared to metronidazole alone in children with acute bloody diarrhea caused by amebiasis: a prospective, randomized, open label study. *Am J Trop Med Hyg.* 2009 Jun;80(6):953-5.

Diop L, Guillou S, Durand H. Probiotic food supplement reduces stress-induced gastrointestinal symptoms in volunteers: a double-blind, placebo-controlled, randomized trial. *Nutr Res.* 2008 Jan;28(1):1-5.

Dixon AE, Kaminsky DA, Holbrook JT, Wise RA, Shade DM, Irvin CG. Allergic rhinitis and sinusitis in asthma: differential effects on symptoms and pulmonary function. *Chest.* 2006 Aug;130(2):429-35.

Dona A, Arvanitoyannis IS. Health risks of genetically modified foods. *Crit Rev Food Sci Nutr.* 2009 Feb;49(2):164-75.

Donato F, Monarca S, Premi S., and Gelatti, U. Drinking water hardness and chronic degenerative diseases. Part III. Tumors, urolithiasis, fetal malformations, deterioration of the cognitive function in the aged and atopic eczema. *Ann. Ig.* 2003;15:57-70.

Dooley, M.A. and Hogan S.L. Environmental epidemiology and risk factors for autoimmune disease. *Curr Opin Rheum.* 2003;15(2):99-103.

dos Santos LH, Ribeiro IO, Sánchez PG, Hetzel JL, Felicetti JC, Cardoso PF. Evaluation of pantoprazol treatment response of patients with asthma and gastroesophageal reflux: a randomized prospective double-blind placebo-controlled study. *J Bras Pneumol.* 2007 Apr;33(2):119-27.

Dotolo Institute. *The Study of Colon Hydrotherapy.* Pinellas Park, FL: Dotolo, 2003.

Dove MS, Dockery DW, Connolly GN. Smoke-free air laws and asthma prevalence, symptoms, and severity among nonsmoking youth. *Pediatrics.* 2011 Jan;127(1):102-9. 2010 Dec 13.

Dowd JB, Zajacova A, Aiello A. Early origins of health disparities: burden of infection, health, and socio-economic status in U.S. children. *Soc Sci Med.* 2009 Feb;68(4):699-707. 2009 Jan 17.

Drago L, De Vecchi E, Nicola L, Zucchetti E, Gismondo MR, Vicariotto F. Activity of a *Lactobacillus acidophilus*-based douche for the treatment of bacterial vaginosis. *J Altern Complement Med.* 2007 May;13(4):435-8.

Drouault-Holowacz S, Bieuvelet S, Burckel A, Cazaubiel M, Dray X, Marteau P. A double blind randomized controlled trial of a probiotic combination in 100 patients with irritable bowel syndrome. *Gastroenterol Clin Biol.* 2008 Feb;32(2):147-52.

Drubaix I, Maraval M, Robert L, Robert AM. Hyaluronic acid (hyaluronan) levels in pathological human saphenous veins. Effects of procyanidol oligomers, *Pathol Biol.* 1997 Jan;45(1):86-91.

Drubaix I, Robert L, Maraval M, Robert AM. Synthesis of glycoconjugates by human diseased veins: modulation by procyanidolic oligomers. *Int J Exp Pathol.* 1997 Apr;78(2):117-21.

Ducrotté P. Irritable bowel syndrome: from the gut to the brain-gut. *Gastroenterol Clin Biol.* 2009 Aug-Sep;33(8-9):703-12.

Duke J. *CRC Handbook of Medicinal Herbs.* Boca Raton: CRC; 1989.

Duke J. *The Green Pharmacy.* New York: St. Martins, 1997.

Dunstan JA, Roper J, Mitoulas L, Hartmann PE, Simmer K, Prescott SL. The effect of supplementation with fish oil during pregnancy on breast milk immunoglobulin A, soluble CD14, cytokine levels and fatty acid composition. *Clin Exp Allergy.* 2004 Aug;34(8):1237-42.

Duong M, Subbarao P, Adelroth E, Obminski G, Strinich T, Inman M, Pedersen S, O'Byrne PM. Sputum eosinophils and the response of exercise-induced bronchoconstriction to corticosteroid in asthma. *Chest.* 2008 Feb;133(2):404-11. 2007 Dec 10.

Dupont C, Barau E, Molkhou P, Raynaud F, Barbet JP, Dehennin L. Food-induced alterations of intestinal permeability in children with cow's milk-sensitive enteropathy and atopic dermatitis. *J Pediatr Gastroenterol Nutr.* 1989 May;8(4):459-65.

Dupont C, Barau E, Molkhou P. Intestinal permeability disorders in children. *Allergy Immunol.* 1991 Mar;23(3):95-103.

Dupont C, Soulaines P, Lapillonne A, Donne N, Kalach N, Benhamou P. Atopy patch test for early diagnosis of cow's milk allergy in preterm infants. *J Pediatr Gastroenterol Nutr.* 2010 Apr;50(4):463-4.

Dupuy P, Cassé M, André F, Dhivert-Donnadieu H, Pinton J, Hernandez-Pion C. Low-salt water reduces intestinal permeability in atopic patients. *Dermatology.* 1999;198(2):153-5.

Duran-Tauleria E, Vignati G, Guedan MJ, Petersson CJ. The utility of specific immunoglobulin E measurements in primary care. *Allergy.* 2004 Aug;59 Suppl 78:35-41.

Duwiejua M, Zeitlin IJ, Waterman PG, Chapman J, Mhango GJ, Provan GJ. Anti-inflammatory activity of resins from some species of the plant family Burseraceae. *Planta Med.* 1993 Feb;59(1):12-6.

Dykewicz MS, Lemmon JK, Keaney DL. Comparison of the Multi-Test II and Skintestor Omni allergy skin test devices. *Ann Allergy Asthma Immunol.* 2007 Jun;98(6):559-62.

Eastham EJ, Walker WA. Effect of cow's milk on the gastrointestinal tract: a persistent dilemma for the pediatrician. *Pediatrics.* 1977 Oct;60(4):477-81.

Eaton KK, Howard M, Howard JM. Gut permeability measured by polyethylene glycol absorption in abnormal gut fermentation as compared with food intolerance. *J R Soc Med.* 1995 Feb;88(2):63-6.

Ebers GC, Kukay K, Bulman DE, Sadovnick AD, Rice G, Anderson C, Armstrong H, Cousin K, Bell RB, Hader W, Paty DW, Hashimoto S, Oger J, Duquette P, Warren S, Gray T, O'Connor P, Nath A, Auty A, Metz L, Francis G, Paulseth JE, Murray TJ, Pryse-Phillips W, Nelson R, Freedman M, Brunet D, Bouchard JP, Hinds D, Risch N. A full genome search in multiple sclerosis. *Nat Genet.* 1996 Aug;13(4):472-6.

Eccles R. Menthol and related cooling compounds. *J Pharm Pharmacol.* 1994 Aug;46(8):618-30.

ECRHS (2002) The European Community Respiratory Health Survey II. *Eur Respir J.* 20: 1071-1079.

Edgecombe K, Latter S, Peters S, Roberts G. Health experiences of adolescents with uncontrolled severe asthma. *Arch Dis Child.* 2010 Dec;95(12):985-91. 2010 Jul 30.

Edgell PG. The psychology of asthma. *Can Med Assoc J.* 1952 Aug;67(2):121-5.

Egashira Y, Nagano H. A multicenter clinical trial of TJ-96 in patients with steroid-dependent bronchial asthma. A comparison of groups allocated by the envelope method. *Ann N Y Acad Sci.* 1993 Jun 23;685:580-3.

Ege MJ, Frei R, Bieli C, Schram-Bijkerk D, Waser M, Benz MR, Weiss G, Nyberg F, van Hage M, Pershagen G, Brunekreef B, Riedler J, Lauener R, Braun-Fahrländer C, von Mutius E; PARSIFAL Study team. Not all farming environments protect against the development of asthma and wheeze in children. *J Allergy Clin Immunol.* 2007 May;119(5):1140-7.

Ege MJ, Herzum I, Büchele G, Krauss-Etschmann S, Lauener RP, Roponen M, Hyvärinen A, Vuitton DA, Riedler J, Brunekreef B, Dalphin JC, Braun-Fahrländer C, Pekkanen J, Renz H, von Mutius E; Protection Against Allergy Study in Rural Environments (PASTURE) Study group. Prenatal exposure to a farm environment modifies atopic sensitization at birth. *J Allergy Clin Immunol.* 2008 Aug;122(2):407-12, 412.e1-4.

Eggermont E. Cow's milk protein allergy. *Tijdschr Kindergeneeskd.* 1981 Feb;49(1):16-20.

Ehling S, Hengel M, and Shibamoto T. Formation of acrylamide from lipids. *Adv Exp Med Biol* 2005, 561:223-233.

Ehnert B, Lau-Schadendorf S, Weber A, Buettner P, Schou C, Wahn U. Reducing domestic exposure to dust mite allergen reduces bronchial hyperreactivity in sensitive children with asthma. *J Allergy Clin Immunol.* 1992 Jul;90(1):135-8.

Ehren J, Morón B, Martin E, Bethune MT, Gray GM, Khosla C. A food-grade enzyme preparation with modest gluten detoxification properties. *PLoS One.* 2009 Jul 21;4(7):e6313.

Eijkemans M, Mommers M, de Vries SI, van Buuren S, Stafleu A, Bakker I, Thijs C. Asthmatic symptoms, physical activity, and overweight in young children: a cohort study. *Pediatrics.* 2008 Mar;121(3):e666-72.

Eldridge MW, Peden DB. Allergen provocation augments endotoxin-induced nasal inflammation in subjects with atopic asthma. *J Allergy Clin Immunol.* 2000 Mar;105(3):475-81.

el-Ghazaly M, Khayyal MT, Okpanyi SN, Arens-Corell M. Study of the anti-inflammatory activity of Populus tremula, Solidago virgaurea and Fraxinus excelsior. *Arzneimittelforschung.* 1992 Mar;42(3):333-6.

Ellingwood F. *American Materia Medica, Therapeutics and Pharmacognosy.* Portland: Eclectic Medical Publ., 1983.

Elliott RB, Harris DP, Hill JP, Bibby NJ, Wasmuth HE. Type I (insulin-dependent) diabetes mellitus and cow milk: casein variant consumption. *Diabetologia.* 1999 Mar;42(3):292-6.

Elmer GW, McFarland LV, Surawicz CM, Danko L, Greenberg RN. Behaviour of *Saccharomyces boulardii* in recurrent *Clostridium difficile* disease patients. *Aliment Pharmacol Ther.* 1999 Dec;13(12):1663-8.

Elwood PC. Epidemiology and trace elements. *Clin Endocrinol Metab.* 1985 Aug;14(3):617-28.

Emberlin JC, Lewis RA. Pollen challenge study of a phototherapy device for reducing the symptoms of hay fever. *Curr Med Res Opin.* 2009 Jul;25(7):1635-44.

Emmanouil E, Manios Y, Grammatikaki E, Kondaki K, Oikonomou E, Papadopoulos N, Vassilopoulou E. Association of nutrient intake and wheeze or asthma in a Greek pre-school population. *Pediatr Allergy Immunol.* 2010 Feb;21(1 Pt 1):90-5. 2009 Sep 9.

Engler RJ. Alternative and complementary medicine: a source of improved therapies for asthma? A challenge for redefining the specialty? *J Allergy Clin Immunol.* 2000;106:627-9.

Environmental Working Group. *Human Toxome Project.* 2007. http://www.ewg.org/sites/humantoxome/. Accessed: 2007 Sep.

EPA. *A Brief Guide to Mold, Moisture and Your Home.* Environmental Protection Agency, Office of Air and Radiation/Indoor Environments Division. EPA 2002;402-K-02-003.

Epstein GN, Halper JP, Barrett EA, Birdsall C, McGee M, Baron KP, Lowenstein S. A pilot study of mind-body changes in adults with asthma who practice mental imagery. *Altern Ther Health Med.* 2004 Jul-Aug;10(4):66-71.

Erkkola M, Kaila M, Nwaru BI, Kronberg-Kippilä C, Ahonen S, Nevalainen J, Veijola R, Pekkanen J, Ilonen J, Simell O, Knip M, Virtanen SM. Maternal vitamin D intake during pregnancy is inversely associated with asthma and allergic rhinitis in 5-year-old children. *Clin Exp Allergy.* 2009 Jun;39(6):875-82.

Ernst E. Frankincense: systematic review. *BMJ.* 2008 Dec 17;337:a2813.

Erwin EA, James HR, Gutekunst HM, Russo JM, Kelleher KJ, Platts-Mills TA. Serum IgE measurement and detection of food allergy in pediatric patients with eosinophilic esophagitis. *Ann Allergy Asthma Immunol.* 2010 Jun;104(6):496-502.

EuroPrevall. *WP 1.1 Birth Cohort Update.* 1st Quarter 2006. Berlin, Germany: Charité University Medical Centre.

Evans P, Forte D, Jacobs C, Fredhoi C, Aitchison E, Hucklebridge F, Clow A. Cortisol secretory activity in older people in relation to positive and negative well-being. *Psychoneuroendocrinology.* 2007 Aug 7

Everhart JE. *Digestive Diseases in the United States.* Darby, PA: Diane Pub, 1994.

FAAN. *Public Comment on 2005 Food Safety Survey: Docket No. 2004N-0516 (2005 FSS)*. Fairfax, VA: Food Allergy & Anaphylaxis Network.

Fabian E, Elmadfa I. Influence of daily consumption of probiotic and conventional yoghurt on the plasma lipid profile in young healthy women. *Ann Nutr Metab.* 2006;50(4):387-93.

Fabian E, Majchrzak D, Dieminger B, Meyer E, Elmadfa I. Influence of probiotic and conventional yoghurt on the status of vitamins B1, B2 and B6 in young healthy women. *Ann Nutr Metab.* 2008;52(1):29-36.

Fairchild SS, Shannon K, Kwan E, Mishell RI. T cell-derived glucosteroid response-modifying factor (GRMFT): a unique lymphokine made by normal T lymphocytes and a T cell hybridoma. *J Immunol.* 1984 Feb;132(2):821-7.

Fälth-Magnusson K, Kjellman NI, Magnusson KE, Sundqvist T. Intestinal permeability in healthy and allergic children before and after sodium-cromoglycate treatment assessed with different-sized poly-ethyleneglycols (PEG 400 and PEG 1000). *Clin Allergy.* 1984 May;14(3):277-86.

Fälth-Magnusson K, Kjellman NI, Odelram H, Sundqvist T, Magnusson KE. Gastrointestinal permeability in children with cow's milk allergy: effect of milk challenge and sodium cromoglycate as assessed with polyethyleneglycols (PEG 400 and PEG 1000). *Clin Allergy.* 1986 Nov;16(6):543-51.

Fan AY, Lao L, Zhang RX, Zhou AN, Wang LB, Moudgil KD, Lee DY, Ma ZZ, Zhang WY, Berman BM. Effects of an acetone extract of Boswellia carterii Birdw. (Burseraceae) gum resin on adjuvant-induced arthritis in lewis rats. *J Ethnopharmacol.* 2005 Oct 3;101(1-3):104-9.

Fanaro S, Marten B, Bagna R, Vigi V, Fabris C, Peña-Quintana, Argüelles F, Scholz-Ahrens KE, Sawatzki G, Zelenka R, Schrezenmeir J, de Vrese M and Bertino E. Galacto-oligosaccharides are bifidogenic and safe at weaning: A double-blind Randomized Multicenter study. *J Pediatr Gastroent Nutr.* 2009 48; 82-88

Fang H, Elina T, Heikki A, Seppo S. Modulation of humoral immune response through probiotic intake. *FEMS Immunol Med Microbiol.* 2000 Sep;29(1):47-52.

Fang SP, Tanaka T, Tago F, Okamoto T, Kojima S. Immunomodulatory effects of gyokuheifusan on INF-gamma/IL-4 (Th1/Th2) balance in ovalbumin (OVA)-induced asthma model mice. *Biol Pharm Bull.* 2005;28:829-33.

Fanigliulo L, Comparato G, Aragona G, Cavallaro L, Iori V, Maino M, Cavestro GM, Soliani P, Sianesi M, Franzè A, Di Mario F. Role of gut microflora and probiotic effects in the irritable bowel syndrome. *Acta Biomed.* 2006 Aug;77(2):85-9.

FAO/WHO Expert Committee. *Fats and Oils in Human Nutrition.* Food and Nutrition Paper. 1994;(57).

Farber JE, Ross J, Stephens G. Antibiotic anaphylaxis. *Calif Med.* 1954 Jul;81(1):9-11.

Farber JE, Ross J. Antibiotic anaphylaxis; a note on the treatment and prevention of severe reactions to penicillin, streptomycin and dihydrostreptomycin. *Med Times.* 1952 Jan;80(1):28-30.

Fasano A, Shea-Donohue T. Mechanisms of disease: the role of intestinal barrier function in the pathogenesis of gastrointestinal autoimmune diseases. *Nat Clin Pract Gastroenterol Hepatol.* 2005 Sep;2(9):416-22.

Fawell J, Nieuwenhuijsen MJ. Contaminants in drinking water. *Br Med Bull.* 2003;68:199-208.

Fecka I. Qualitative and quantitative determination of hydrolysable tannins and other polyphenols in herbal products from meadowsweet and dog rose. *Phytochem Anal.* 2009 May;20(3):177-90.

Felley CP, Corthésy-Theulaz I, Rivero JL, Sipponen P, Kaufmann M, Bauerfeind P, Wiesel PH, Brassart D, Pfeifer A, Blum AL, Michetti P. Favourable effect of an acidified milk (LC-1) on *Helicobacter pylori* gastritis in man. *Eur J Gastroenterol Hepatol.* 2001 Jan;13(1):25-9.

Ferencík M, Ebringer L, Mikes Z, Jahnová E, Ciznár I. Successful modification of human intestinal microflora with oral administration of lactic acid bacteria. *Bratisl Lek Listy.* 1999 May;100(5):238-45.

Ferguson BJ. Categorization of eosinophilic chronic rhinosinusitis. *Curr Opin Otolaryngol Head Neck Surg.* 2004 Jun;12(3):237-42.

Ferrari M, Benini L, Brotto E, Locatelli F, De Iorio F, Bonella F, Tacchella N, Corradini G, Lo Cascio V, Vantini I. Omeprazole reduces the response to capsaicin but not to methacholine in asthmatic patients with proximal reflux. *Scand J Gastroenterol.* 2007 Mar;42(3):299-307.

Ferrier L, Berard F, Debrauwer L, Chabo C, Langella P, Bueno L, Fioramonti J. Impairment of the intestinal barrier by ethanol involves enteric microflora and mast cell activation in rodents. *Am J Pathol.* 2006 Apr;168(4):1148-54.

Ferrier L, Berard F, Debrauwer L, Chabo C, Langella P, Bueno L, Fioramonti J. Impairment of the intestinal barrier by ethanol involves enteric microflora and mast cell activation in rodents. *Am J Pathol.* 2006 Apr;168(4):1148-54.

Field RW, Krewski D, Lubin JH, Zielinski JM, Alavanja M, Catalan VS, Klotz JB, Létourneau EG, Lynch CF, Lyon JL, Sandler DP, Schoenberg JB, Steck DJ, Stolwijk JA, Weinberg C, Wilcox HB. An overview of the North American residential radon and lung cancer case-control studies. *J Toxicol Environ Health A.* 2006 Apr;69(7):599-631.

Field T, Henteleff T, Hernandez-Reif M, Martinez E, Mavunda K, Kuhn C, Schanberg S. Children with asthma have improved pulmonary functions after massage therapy. *J Pediatr.* 1998 May;132(5):854-8.

Finkelman FD, Boyce JA, Vercelli D, Rothenberg ME. Key advances in mechanisms of asthma, allergy, and immunology in 2009. *J Allergy Clin Immunol.* 2010 Feb;125(2):312-8.

REFERENCES AND BIBLIOGRAPHY

Fiocchi, A; Restani, P; Riva, E; Qualizza, R; Bruni, P; Restelli, AR; Galli, CL. Meat allergy: I. Specific IgE to BSA and OSA in atopic, beef sensitive children. *J Am Coll Nutr*. 1995 14: 239-244.

Firmesse O, Alvaro E, Mogenet A, Bresson JL, Lemée R, Le Ruyet P, Bonhomme C, Lambert D, Andrieux C, Doré J, Corthier G, Furet JP, Rigottier-Gois L. Fate and effects of Camembert cheese microorganisms in the human colonic microbiota of healthy volunteers after regular Camembert consumption. *Int J Food Microbiol*. 2008 Jul 15;125(2):176-81.

Fjeld T, Veiersted B, Sandvik L, Riise G, Levy F. The Effect of Indoor Foliage Plants on Health and Discomfort Symptoms among Office Workers. *Ind Built Environ*. 1998 July;7(4): 204-209.

Flandrin, J, Montanari M. (eds.). *Food: A Culinary History from Antiquity to the Present*. New York: Penguin Books, 1999.

Fleischer DM, Conover-Walker MK, Christie L, Burks AW, Wood RA. Peanut allergy: recurrence and its management. *J Allergy Clin Immunol*. 2004 Nov;114(5):1195-201.

Flinterman AE, van Hoffen E, den Hartog Jager CF, Koppelman S, Pasmans SG, Hoekstra MO, Bruijnzeel-Koomen CA, Knulst AC, Knol EF. Children with peanut allergy recognize predominantly Ara h2 and Ara h6, which remains stable over time. *Clin Exp Allergy*. 2007 Aug;37(8):1221-8.

Foliaki S, Annesi-Maesano I, Tuuau-Potoi N, Waqatakirewa L, Cheng S, Douwes J, Pearce N. Risk factors for symptoms of childhood asthma, allergic rhinoconjunctivitis and eczema in the Pacific: an ISAAC Phase III study. *Int J Tuberc Lung Dis*. 2008 Jul;12(7):799-806.

Forbes EE, Groschwitz K, Abonia JP, Brandt EB, Cohen E, Blanchard C, Ahrens R, Seidu L, McKenzie A, Strait R, Finkelman FD, Foster PS, Matthaei KI, Rothenberg ME, Hogan SP. IL-9- and mast cell-mediated intestinal permeability predisposes to oral antigen hypersensitivity. *J Exp Med*. 2008 Apr 14;205(4):897-913.

Forestier C, Guelon D, Cluytens V, Gillart T, Sirot J, De Champs C. Oral probiotic and prevention of Pseudomonas aeruginosa infections: a randomized, double-blind, placebo-controlled pilot study in intensive care unit patients. *Crit Care*. 2008;12(3):R69.

Forestier C, Guelon D, Cluytens V, Gillart T, Sirot J, De Champs C. Oral probiotic and prevention of Pseudomonas aeruginosa infections: a randomized, double-blind, placebo-controlled pilot study in intensive care unit patients. *Crit Care*. 2008;12(3):R69.

Forget-Dubois N, Boivin M, Dionne G, Pierce T, Tremblay RE, Pérusse D. A longitudinal twin study of the genetic and environmental etiology of maternal hostile-reactive behavior during infancy and toddlerhood. *Infant Behav Dev*. 2007

Foster S, Hobbs C. *Medicinal Plants and Herbs*. Boston: Houghton Mifflin, 2002.

Fox RD, *Algoculture*. Doctorate Disseration, 1983 Jul.

Francavilla R, Lionetti E, Castellaneta SP, Magistà AM, Maurogiovanni G, Bucci N, De Canio A, Indrio F, Cavallo L, Ierardi E, Miniello VL. Inhibition of Helicobacter pylori infection in humans by Lactobacillus reuteri ATCC 55730 and effect on eradication therapy: a pilot study. *Helicobacter*. 2008 Apr;13(2):127-34.

Francavilla R, Lionetti E, Castellaneta SP, Magistà AM, Maurogiovanni G, Bucci N, De Canio A, Indrio F, Cavallo L, Ierardi E, Miniello VL. Inhibition of *Helicobacter pylori* infection in humans by *Lactobacillus reuteri* ATCC 55730 and effect on eradication therapy: a pilot study. *Helicobacter*. 2008 Apr;13(2):127-34.

Francis H, Fletcher G, Anthony C, Pickering C, Oldham L, Hadley E, Custovic A, Niven R. Clinical effects of air filters in homes of asthmatic adults sensitized and exposed to pet allergens. *Clin Exp Allergy*. 2003 Jan;33(1):101-5.

Frank PI, Morris JA, Hazell ML, Linehan MF, Frank TL. Long term prognosis in preschool children with wheeze: longitudinal postal questionnaire study 1993-2004. *BMJ*. 2008 Jun 21;336(7658):1423-6. 2008 Jun 16.

Frawley D, Lad V. *The Yoga of Herbs*. Sante Fe: Lotus Press, 1986.

Freedman BJ. A dietary free from additives in the management of allergic disease. *Clin Allergy*. 1977 Sep;7(5):417-21.

Fremont S, Moneret-Vautrin DA, Franck P, Morisset M, Croizier A, Codreanu F, Kanny G. Prospective study of sensitization and food allergy to flaxseed in 1317 subjects. *Eur Ann Allergy Clin Immunol*. 2010 Jun;42(3):103-11.

Frias J, Song YS, Martínez-Villaluenga C, González de Mejia E, Vidal-Valverde C. Immunoreactivity and amino acid content of fermented soybean products. *J Agric Food Chem*. 2008 Jan 9;56(1):99-105.

Friedman LS, Harvard Health Publ. Ed. *Controlling GERD and Chronic Heartburn*. Boston: Harvard Health, 2008.

Friend BA, Shahani KM, Long CA, Vaughn LA. The effect of processing and storage on key enzymes, B vitamins, and lipids of mature human milk. Evaluation of fresh samples and effects of freezing and frozen storage. *Pediatr Res*. 1983 Jan;17(1):61-4.

Friend BA, Shahani KM. Characterization and evaluation of Aspergillus oryzae lactase coupled to a regenerable support. *Biotechnol Bioeng*. 1982 Feb;24(2):329-45.

Frumkin H. Beyond toxicity: human health and the natural environment. *Am J Prev Med*. 2001;20(3):234-40.

Fu G, Zhong Y, Li C, Li Y, Lin X, Liao B, Tsang EW, Wu K, Huang S. Epigenetic regulation of peanut allergen gene Ara h 3 in developing embryos. *Planta.* 2010 Apr;231(5):1049-60.

Fu JX. Measurement of MEFV in 66 cases of asthma in the convalescent stage and after treatment with Chinese herbs. *Zhong Xi Yi Jie He Za Zhi.* 1989 Nov;9(11):658-9, 644.

Fuiano N, Fusilli S, Passalacqua G, Incorvaia C. Allergen-specific immunoglobulin E in the skin and nasal mucosa of symptomatic and asymptomatic children sensitized to aeroallergens. *J Investig Allergol Clin Immunol.* 2010;20(5):425-30.

Fujii T, Ohtsuka Y, Lee T, Kudo T, Shoji H, Sato H, Nagata S, Shimizu T, Yamashiro Y. Bifidobacterium breve enhances transforming growth factor beta1 signaling by regulating Smad7 expression in preterm in-fants. *J Pediatr Gastroenterol Nutr.* 2006 Jul;43(1):83-8.

Fujii T, Ohtsuka Y, Lee T, Kudo T, Shoji H, Sato H, Nagata S, Shimizu T, Yamashiro Y. *Bifidobacterium breve* enhances transforming growth factor beta1 signaling by regulating Smad7 expression in preterm in-fants. *J Pediatr Gastroenterol Nutr.* 2006 Jul;43(1):83-8.

Fujimori S, Gudis K, Mitsui K, Seo T, Yonezawa M, Tanaka S, Tatsuguchi A, Sakamoto C. A randomized controlled trial on the efficacy of synbiotic versus probiotic or prebiotic treatment to improve the quality of life in patients with ulcerative colitis. *Nutrition.* 2009 May;25(5):520-5.

Fulgoni VL 3rd. Current protein intake in America: analysis of the National Health and Nutrition Examination Survey, 2003-2004. *Am J Clin Nutr.* 2008 May;87(5):1554S-1557S.

Furrie E, Macfarlane S, Kennedy A, Cummings JH, Walsh SV, O'neil DA, Macfarlane GT. Synbiotic therapy (*Bifidobacterium longum*/Synergy 1) initiates resolution of inflammation in patients with active ulcerative colitis: a randomised controlled pilot trial. *Gut.* 2005 Feb;54(2):242-9.

Furrie E. Probiotics and allergy. *Proc Nutr Soc.* 2005 Nov;64(4):465-9.

Furuhjelm C, Warstedt K, Larsson J, Fredriksson M, Böttcher MF, Fälth-Magnusson K, Duchén K. Fish oil supplementation in pregnancy and lactation may decrease the risk of infant allergy. *Acta Paediatr.* 2009 Sep;98(9):1461-7.

Gabory A, Attig L, Junien C. Sexual dimorphism in environmental epigenetic programming. *Mol Cell Endocrinol.* 2009 May 25;304(1-2):8-18. 2009 Mar 9.

Gamboa PM, Cáceres O, Antepara I, Sánchez-Monge R, Ahrazem O, Salcedo G, Barber D, Lombardero M, Sanz ML. Two different profiles of peach allergy in the north of Spain. *Allergy.* 2007 Apr;62(4):408-14.

Gao X, Wang W, Wei S, Li W. Review of pharmacological effects of Glycyrrhiza radix and its bioactive compounds. *Zhongguo Zhong Yao Za Zhi.* 2009 Nov;34(21):2695-700.

Gaón D, Doweck Y, Gómez Zavaglia A, Ruiz Holgado A, Oliver G. Lactose digestion by milk fermented with *Lactobacillus acidophilus* and *Lactobacillus casei* of human origin. *Medicina (B Aires).* 1995;55(3):237-42.

Gaón D, García H, Winter L, Rodríguez N, Quintás R, González SN, Oliver G. Effect of Lactobacillus strains and *Saccharomyces boulardii* on persistent diarrhea in children. *Medicina (B Aires).* 2003;63(4):293-8.

Gaón D, Garmendia C, Murrielo NO, de Cucco Games A, Cerchio A, Quintas R, González SN, Oliver G. Effect of Lactobacillus strains (*L. casei* and *L. Acidophilus* Strains cerela) on bacterial overgrowth-related chronic diarrhea. *Medicina.* 2002;62(2):159-63.

Garaczi E, Boros-Gyevi M, Bella Z, Csoma Z, Kemény L, Koreck A. Intranasal phototherapy is more effective than fexofenadine hydrochloride in the treatment of seasonal allergic rhinitis: results of a pilot study. *Photochem Photobiol.* 2011 Mar-Apr;87(2):474-7.

Garavello W, Somigliana E, Acaia B, Gaini L, Pignataro L, Gaini RM. Nasal lavage in pregnant women with seasonal allergic rhinitis: a randomized study. *Int Arch Allergy Immunol.* 2010;151(2):137-41. 2009 Sep 15. 19752567.

Garcia Gomez LJ, Sanchez-Muniz FJ. Review: cardiovascular effect of garlic (Allium sativum). *Arch Latinoam Nutr.* 2000 Sep;50(3):219-29.

Garcia Vilela E, De Lourdes De Abreu Ferrari M, Oswaldo Da Gama Torres H, Guerra Pinto A, Carolina Carneiro Aguirre A, Paiva Martins F, Marcos Andrade Goulart E, Sales Da Cunha A. Influence of *Saccharomyces boulardii* on the intestinal permeability of patients with Crohn's disease in remission. *Scand J Gastroenterol.* 2008;43(7):842-8.

García-Compeán D, González MV, Galindo G, Mar DA, Treviño JL, Martínez R, Bosques F, Maldonado H. Prevalence of gastroesophageal reflux disease in patients with extraesophageal symptoms referred from otolaryngology, allergy, and cardiology practices: a prospective study. *Dig Dis.* 2000;18(3):178-82.

Garcia-Marcos L, Canflanca IM, Garrido JB, Varela AL, Garcia-Hernandez G, Guillen Grima F, Gonzalez-Diaz C, Carvajal-Urueña I, Arnedo-Pena A, Busquets-Monge RM, Morales Suarez-Varela M, Blanco-Quiros A. Relationship of asthma and rhinoconjunctivitis with obesity, exercise and Mediterranean diet in Spanish schoolchildren. *Thorax.* 2007 Jun;62(6):503-8.

Gardner CD, Fortmann SP, Krauss RM. Association of small low-density lipoprotein particles with the incidence of coronary artery disease in men and women. *JAMA.* 1996 Sep 18;276(11):875-81.

Gardner ML. Gastrointestinal absorption of intact proteins. *Annu Rev Nutr.* 1988;8:329-50.

Gary WK, Fanny WS, David SC. Factors associated with difference in prevalence of asthma in children from three cities in China: multicentre epidemiological survey. *BMJ.* 2004;329:1-4.

Garzi A, Messina M, Frati F, Carfagna L, Zagordo L, Belcastro M, Parmiani S, Sensi L, Marcucci F. An extensively hydrolysed cow's milk formula improves clinical symptoms of gastroesophageal reflux and reduces the gastric emptying time in infants. *Allergol Immunopathol (Madr)*. 2002 Jan-Feb;30(1):36-41.

Gawrońska A, Dziechciarz P, Horvath A, Szajewska H. A randomized double-blind placebo-controlled trial of Lactobacillus GG for abdominal pain disorders in children. *Aliment Pharmacol Ther*. 2007 Jan 15;25(2):177-84.

Gazdik F, Horvathova M, Gazdikova K, Jahnova E. The influence of selenium supplementation on the immunity of corticoid-dependent asthmatics. *Bratisl Lek Listy*. 2002;103(1):17-21.

Gazdik F, Kadrabova J, Gazdikova K. Decreased consumption of corticosteroids after selenium supplementation in corticoid-dependent asthmatics. *Bratisl Lek Listy*. 2002;103(1):22-5.

Geha RS, Beiser A, Ren C, Patterson R, Greenberger PA, Grammer LC, Ditto AM, Harris KE, Shaughnessy MA, Yarnold PR, Corren J, Saxon A. Multicenter, double-blind, placebo-controlled, multiple-challenge evaluation of reported reactions to monosodium glutamate. *J Allergy Clin Immunol*. 2000 Nov;106(5):973-80.

Gerez IF, Shek LP, Chng HH, Lee BW. Diagnostic tests for food allergy. *Singapore* Med J. 2010 Jan;51(1):4-9.

Gergen PJ, Arbes SJ Jr, Calatroni A, Mitchell HE, Zeldin DC. Total IgE levels and asthma prevalence in the US population: results from the National Health and Nutrition Examination Survey 2005-2006. *J Allergy Clin Immunol*. 2009 Sep;124(3):447-53. 2009 Aug 3.

Ghadioungui P. (transl.) The Ebers Papyrus. Academy of Scientific Research. Cairo, 1987.

Gandhi TK, Weingart SN, Borus J, Seger AC, Peterson J, Burdick E, Seger DL, Shu K, Federico F, Leape LL, Bates DW. Adverse drug events in ambulatory care. N Engl J Med. 2003 Apr 17;348(16):1556-64.

Giampietro PG, Kjellman NI, Oldaeus G, Wouters-Wesseling W, Businco L. Hypoallergenicity of an extensively hydrolyzed whey formula. *Pediatr Allergy Immunol*. 2001 Apr;12(2):83-6.

Gibbons E. *Stalking the Healthful Herbs*. New York: David McKay, 1966.

Gibson RA. Docosa-hexaenoic acid (DHA) accumulation is regulated by the polyunsaturated fat content of the diet: Is it synthesis or is it incorporation? *Asia Pac J Clin Nutr*. 2004;13(Suppl):S78.

Gilbert CR, Arum SM, Smith CM. Vitamin D deficiency and chronic lung disease. *Can Respir J*. 2009 May-Jun;16(3):75-80.

Gill HS, Rutherfurd KJ, Cross ML, Gopal PK. Enhancement of immunity in the elderly by dietary supplementation with the probiotic Bifidobacterium lactis HN019. *Am J Clin Nutr*. 2001 Dec;74(6):833-9.

Gill HS, Rutherfurd KJ, Cross ML. Dietary probiotic supplementation enhances natural killer cell activity in the elderly: an investigation of age-related immunological changes. *J Clin Immunol*. 2001 Jul;21(4):264-71.

Gillman A, Douglass JA. What do asthmatics have to fear from food and additive allergy? *Clin Exp Allergy*. 2010 Sep;40(9):1295-302.

Ginde AA, Mansbach JM, Camargo CA Jr. Association between serum 25-hydroxyvitamin D level and upper respiratory tract infection in the Third National Health and Nutrition Examination Survey. *Arch Intern Med*. 2009 Feb 23;169(4):384-90.

Gionchetti P, Rizzello F, Venturi A, Brigidi P, Matteuzzi D, Bazzocchi G, Poggioli G, Miglioli M, Campieri M. Oral bacteriotherapy as maintenance treatment in patients with chronic pouchitis: a double-blind, placebo-controlled trial. *Gastroenterology*. 2000 Aug;119(2):305-9.

Gittleman AL. *Guess What Came to Dinner*. New York: Avery, 2001.

Glück U, Gebbers J. Ingested probiotics reduce nasal colonization with pathogenic bacteria (Staphylococcus aureus, Streptococcus pneumoniae, and b-hemolytic streptococci. *Am J. Clin. Nutr*. 2003;77:517-520.

Glück U, Gebbers J. Ingested probiotics reduce nasal colonization with pathogenic bacteria (*Staphylococcus aureus, Streptococcus pneumoniae*, and b-hemolytic streptococci. *Am J. Clin. Nutr*. 2003;77:517-520.

Goedsche K, Förster M, Kroegel C, Uhlemann C. Repeated cold water stimulations (hydrotherapy according to Kneipp) in patients with COPD. *Forsch Komplementmed*. 2007 Jun;14(3):158-66.

Goel V, Dolan RJ. The functional anatomy of humor: segregating cognitive and affective components. *Nat Neurosci*. 2001;4:237-8.

Gohil K, Packer L. Bioflavonoid-Rich Botanical Extracts Show Antioxidant and Gene Regulatory Activity. *Ann N Y Acad Sci*. 2002:957:70-7.

Goldin BR, Adlercreutz H, Dwyer JT, Swenson L, Warram JH, Gorbach SL. Effect of diet on excretion of estrogens in pre- and postmenopausal women. *Cancer Res*. 1981 Sep;41(9 Pt 2):3771-3.

Goldin BR, Adlercreutz H, Gorbach SL, Warram JH, Dwyer JT, Swenson L, Woods MN. Estrogen excretion patterns and plasma levels in vegetarian and omnivorous women. *N Engl J Med*. 1982 Dec 16;307(25):1542-7.

Goldin BR, Adlercreutz H, Gorbach SL, Warram JH, Dwyer JT, Swenson L, Woods MN. Estrogen excretion patterns and plasma levels in vegetarian and omnivorous women. *N Engl J Med*. 1982 Dec 16;307(25):1542-7.

Goldin BR, Swenson L, Dwyer J, Sexton M, Gorbach SL. Effect of diet and Lactobacillus acidophilus supplements on human fecal bacterial enzymes. *J Natl Cancer Inst*. 1980 Feb;64(2):255-61.

Goldin BR, Swenson L, Dwyer J, Sexton M, Gorbach SL. Effect of diet and *Lactobacillus acidophilus* supplements on human fecal bacterial enzymes. *J Natl Cancer Inst.* 1980 Feb;64(2):255-61.

Goldstein JL, Aisenberg J, Zakko SF, Berger MF, Dodge WE. Endoscopic ulcer rates in healthy subjects associated with use of aspirin (81 mg q.d.) alone or coadministered with celecoxib or naproxen: a randomized, 1-week trial. *Dig Dis Sci.* 2008 Mar;53(3):647-56.

Golub E. *The Limits of Medicine.* New York: Times Books, 1994.

Gonzales M, Malcoe LH, Myers OB, Espinoza J. Risk factors for asthma and cough among Hispanic children in the southwestern United States of America, 2003-2004. *Rev Panam Salud Publica.* 2007 May;21(5):274-81.

González Alvarez R, Arruzazabala ML. Current views of the mechanism of action of prophylactic antiallergic drugs. *Allergol Immunopathol (Madr).* 1981 Nov-Dec;9(6):501-8.

González J, Fernández M, García Fragoso L. Exclusive breastfeeding reduces asthma in a group of children from the Caguas municipality of Puerto Rico. *Bol Asoc Med P R.* 2010 Jan-Mar;102(1):10-2.

González Morales JE, Leal de Hernández L, González Spencer D. Asthma associated with gastroesophageal reflux. *Rev Alerg Mex.* 1998 Jan-Feb;45(1):16-21.

González-Pérez A, Aponte Z, Vidaurre CF, Rodríguez LA. Anaphylaxis epidemiology in patients with and patients without asthma: a United Kingdom database review. *J Allergy Clin Immunol.* 2010 May;125(5):1098-1104.e1.

González-Sánchez R, Trujillo X, Trujillo-Hernández B, Vásquez C, Huerta M, Elizalde A. Forskolin versus sodium cromoglycate for prevention of asthma attacks: a single-blinded clinical trial. *J Int Med Res.* 2006 Mar-Apr;34(2):200-7.

Goossens D, Jonkers D, Russel M, Stobberingh E, Van Den Bogaard A, StockbrUgger R. The effect of *Lactobacillus plantarum* 299v on the bacterial composition and metabolic activity in faeces of healthy volunteers: a placebo-controlled study on the onset and duration of effects. *Aliment Pharmacol Ther.* 2003 Sep 1;18(5):495-505.

Goossens DA, Jonkers DM, Russel MG, Stobberingh EE, Stockbrügger RW. The effect of a probiotic drink with *Lactobacillus plantarum* 299v on the bacterial composition in faeces and mucosal biopsies of rectum and ascending colon. *Aliment Pharmacol Ther.* 2006 Jan 15;23(2):255-63.

Gordon BR. Patch testing for allergies. *Curr Opin Otolaryngol Head Neck Surg.* 2010 Jun;18(3):191-4.

Gore KV, Rao AK, Guruswamy MN. Physiological studies with Tylophora asthmatica in bronchial asthma. *Indian J Med Res.* 1980 Jan;71:144-8.

Goren AI, Hellmann S. Changes prevalence of asthma among schoolchildren in Israel. *Eur Respir J.* 1997;10:2279-2284.

Gotteland M, Poliak L, Cruchet S, Brunser O. Effect of regular ingestion of Saccharomyces boulardii plus inulin or Lactobacillus acidophilus LB in children colonized by Helicobacter pylori. *Acta Paediatr.* 2005 Dec;94(12):1747-51.

Gotteland M, Poliak L, Cruchet S, Brunser O. Effect of regular ingestion of *Saccharomyces boulardii* plus inulin or *Lactobacillus acidophilus* LB in children colonized by *Helicobacter pylori.* *Acta Paediatr.* 2005 Dec;94(12):1747-51.

Govindan S, Viswanathan S, Vijayasekaran V, Alagappan R. A pilot study on the clinical efficacy of Solanum xanthocarpum and Solanum trilobatum in bronchial asthma. *J Ethnopharmacol.* 1999 Aug;66(2):205-10.

Govindan S, Viswanathan S, Vijayasekaran V, Alagappan R. Further studies on the clinical efficacy of Solanum xanthocarpum and Solanum trilobatum in bronchial asthma. *Phytother Res.* 2004 Oct;18(10):805-9.

Grant WB, Holick MF. Benefits and requirements of vitamin D for optimal health: a review. *Altern Med Rev.* 2005 Jun;10(2):94-111.

Grant WB. Hypothesis—ultraviolet-B irradiance and vitamin D reduce the risk of viral infections and thus their sequelae, including autoimmune diseases and some cancers. *Photochem Photobiol.* 2008 Mar-Apr;84(2):356-65. 2008 Jan 7.

Grasso F, Grillo C, Musumeci F, Triglia A, Rodolico G, Cammisuli F, Rinzivillo C, Fragati G, Santuccio A, Rodolico M. Photon emission from normal and tumour human tissues. *Experientia.* 1992;48:10-13.

Gray H. *Anatomy, Descriptive and Surgical.* 15th Edition. New York: Random House, 1977.

Gray-Davison F. *Ayurvedic Healing.* New York: Keats, 2002.

Greskevitch M, Kullman G, Bang KM, Mazurek JM. Respiratory disease in agricultural workers: mortality and morbidity statistics. *J Agromedicine.* 2007;12(3):5-10.

Griffith HW. *Healing Herbs: The Essential Guide.* Tucson: Fisher Books, 2000.

Grimm T, Chovanová Z, Muchová J, Sumegová K, Liptáková A, Duracková Z, Högger P. Inhibition of NF-kappaB activation and MMP-9 secretion by plasma of human volunteers after ingestion of maritime pine bark extract (Pycnogenol). *J Inflamm (Lond).* 2006 Jan 27;3:1.

Grimm T, Schäfer A, Högger P. Antioxidant activity and inhibition of matrix metalloproteinases by metabolites of maritime pine bark extract (pycnogenol). *Free Radic Biol Med.* 2004 Mar 15;36(6):811-22.

Grimm T, Skrabala R, Chovanová Z, Muchová J, Sumegová K, Liptáková A, Duracková Z, Högger P. Single and multiple dose pharmacokinetics of maritime pine bark extract (pycnogenol) after oral administration to healthy volunteers. *BMC Clin Pharmacol.* 2006 Aug 3;6:4.

Grönlund MM, Gueimonde M, Laitinen K, Kociubinski G, Grönroos T, Salminen S, Isolauri E. Maternal breast-milk and intestinal bifidobacteria guide the compositional development of the *Bifidobacterium* microbiota in infants at risk of allergic disease. *Clin Exp Allergy.* 2007 Dec;37(12):1764-72.

Gropper SS, Smith JL, Groff JL. *Advanced nutrition and human metabolism.* Belmonth, CA: Wadsworth Publ, 2008.

Groppo FC, Ramacciato JC, Simões RP, Flório FM, Sartoratto A. Antimicrobial activity of garlic, tea tree oil, and chlorhexidine against oral microorganisms. *Int Dent J.* 2002 Dec;52(6):433-7.

Groschwitz KR, Ahrens R, Osterfeld H, Gurish MF, Han X, Abrink M, Finkelman FD, Pejler G, Hogan SP. Mast cells regulate homeostatic intestinal epithelial migration and barrier function by a chymase/Mcpt4-dependent mechanism. *Proc Natl Acad Sci U S A.* 2009 Dec 29;106(52):22381-6.

Grosser BI, Monti-Bloch L, Jennings-White C, Berliner DL. Behavioral and electrophysiological effects of androstadienone, a human pheromone. *Psychoneuroendocrinology.* 2000 Apr;25(3):289-99.

Grzanna R, Lindmark L, Frondoza CG. Ginger—an herbal medicinal product with broad anti-inflammatory actions. *J Med Food.* 2005 Summer;8(2):125-32.

Guandalini S. The influence of gluten: weaning recommendations for healthy children and children at risk for celiac disease. *Nestle Nutr Workshop Ser Pediatr Program.* 2007;60:139-51; discussion 151-5.

Guarino A, Canani RB, Spagnuolo MI, Albano F, Di Benedetto L. Oral bacterial therapy reduces the duration of symptoms and of viral excretion in children with mild diarrhea. *J Pediatr Gastroenterol Nutr.* 1997 Nov;25(5):516-9.

Guerin M, Huntley ME, Olaizola M. Haematococcus astaxanthin: applications for human health and nutrition. *Trends Biotechnol.* 2003 May;21(5):210-6.

Guerin-Danan C, Chabanet C, Pedone C, Popot F, Vaissade P, Bouley C, Szylit O, Andrieux C. Milk fermented with yogurt cultures and *Lactobacillus casei* compared with yogurt and gelled milk: influence on intestinal microflora in healthy infants. *Am J Clin Nutr.* 1998 Jan;67(1):111-7.

Guinot P, Brambilla C, Duchier J, Braquet P, Bonvoisin B, Cournot A. Effect of BN 52063, a specific PAF-acether antagonist, on bronchial provocation test to allergens in asthmatic patients. A preliminary study. *Prostaglandins.* 1987 Nov;34(5):723-31.

Gundermann KJ, Müller J. Phytodolor—effects and efficacy of a herbal medicine. *Wien Med Wochenschr.* 2007;157(13-14):343-7.

Gupta I, Gupta V, Parihar A, Gupta S, Lüdtke R, Safayhi H, Ammon HP. Effects of Boswellia serrata gum resin in patients with bronchial asthma: results of a double-blind, placebo-controlled, 6-week clinical study. *Eur J Med Res.* 1998 Nov 17;3(11):511-4.

Guslandi M, Giollo P, Testoni PA. A pilot trial of *Saccharomyces boulardii* in ulcerative colitis. *Eur J Gastroenterol Hepatol.* 2003 Jun;15(6):697-8.

Guslandi M, Mezzi G, Sorghi M, Testoni PA. *Saccharomyces boulardii* in maintenance treatment of Crohn's disease. *Dig Dis Sci.* 2000 Jul;45(7):1462-4.

Gutmanis J. *Hawaiian Herbal Medicine.* Waipahu, HI: Island Heritage, 2001.

Guyonnet D, Woodcock A, Stefani B, Trevisan C, Hall C. Fermented milk containing Bifidobacterium lactis DN-173 010 improved self-reported digestive comfort amongst a general population of adults. A randomized, open-label, controlled, pilot study. *J Dig Dis.* 2009 Feb;10(1):61-70.

Haarman M, Knol J. Quantitative real-time PCR assays to identify and quantify fecal *Bifidobacterium* species in infants receiving a prebiotic infant formula. *Appl Environ Microbiol.* 2005 May;71(5):2318-24.

Haggag EG, Abou-Moustafa MA, Boucher W, Theoharides TC. The effect of a herbal water-extract on histamine release from mast cells and on allergic asthma. *J Herb Pharmacother.* 2003;3(4):41-54.

Haines JL, Ter-Minassian M, Bazyk A, Gusella JF, Kim DJ, Terwedow H, Pericak-Vance MA, Rimmler JB, Haynes CS, Roses AD, Lee A, Shaner B, Menold M, Seboun E, Fitoussi RP, Gartioux C, Reyes C, Ribierre F, Gyapay G, Weissenbach J, Hauser SL, Goodkin DE, Lincoln R, Usuku K, Oksenberg JR, et al. A complete genomic screen for multiple sclerosis underscores a role for the major histocompatability complex. The Multiple Sclerosis Genetics Group. *Nat Genet.* 1996 Aug;13(4):469-71..

Halász A, Cserháti E. The prognosis of bronchial asthma in childhood in Hungary: a long-term follow-up. *J Asthma.* 2002 Dec;39(8):693-9.

Halken S, Hansen KS, Jacobsen HP, Estmann A, Faelling AE, Hansen LG, Kier SR, Lassen K, Lintrup M, Mortensen S, Ibsen KK, Osterballe O, Høst A. Comparison of a partially hydrolyzed infant formula with two extensively hydrolyzed formulas for allergy prevention: a prospective, randomized study. *Pediatr Allergy Immunol.* 2000 Aug;11(3):149-61.

Hallén A, Jarstrand C, Påhlson C. Treatment of bacterial vaginosis with lactobacilli. *Sex Transm Dis.* 1992 May-Jun;19(3):146-8.

Halpern GM, Miller AH. *Medicinal Mushrooms: Ancient Remedies for Modern Ailments.* New York: M. Evans, 2002.

Hamasaki Y, Kobayashi I, Hayasaki R, Zaitu M, Muro E, Yamamoto S, Ichimaru T, Miyazaki S. The Chinese herbal medicine, shinpi-to, inhibits IgE-mediated leukotriene synthesis in rat basophilic leukemia-2H3 cells. *J Ethnopharmacol.* 1997 Apr;56(2):123-31.

Hamelmann E, Beyer K, Gruber C, Lau S, Matricardi PM, Nickel R, Niggemann B, Wahn U. Primary prevention of allergy: avoiding risk or providing protection? *Clin Exp Allergy.* 2008 Feb;38(2):233-45.

Hamilton RG. Clinical laboratory assessment of immediate-type hypersensitivity. *J Allergy Clin Immunol.* 2010 Feb;125(2 Suppl 2):S284-96.

Hammond BG, Mayhew DA, Kier LD, Mast RW, Sander WJ. Safety assessment of DHA-rich microalgae from Schizochytrium sp. *Regul Toxicol Pharmacol.* 2002 Apr;35(2 Pt 1):255-65.

Han ER, Choi IS, Kim HK, Kang YW, Park JG, Lim JR, Seo JH, Choi JH. Inhaled corticosteroid-related tooth problems in asthmatics. *J Asthma.* 2009 Mar;46(2):160-4.

Han SN, Leka LS, Lichtenstein AH, Ausman LM, Meydani SN. Effect of a therapeutic lifestyle change diet on immune functions of moderately hypercholesterolemic humans. *J Lipid Res.* 2003 Dec;44(12):2304-10.

Hansen KS, Ballmer-Weber BK, Lüttkopf D, Skov PS, Wüthrich B, Bindslev-Jensen C, Vieths S, Poulsen LK. Roasted hazelnuts—allergenic activity evaluated by double-blind, placebo-controlled food challenge. *Allergy.* 2003 Feb;58(2):132-8.

Hansen KS, Ballmer-Weber BK, Sastre J, Lidholm J, Andersson K, Oberhofer H, Lluch-Bernal M, Ostling J, Mattsson L, Schocker F, Vieths S, Poulsen LK. Component-resolved in vitro diagnosis of hazelnut allergy in Europe. *J Allergy Clin Immunol.* 2009 May;123(5):1134-41, 1141.e1-3.

Hansen KS, Khinchi MS, Skov PS, Bindslev-Jensen C, Poulsen LK, Malling HJ. Food allergy to apple and specific immunotherapy with birch pollen. *Mol Nutr Food Res.* 2004 Nov;48(6):441-8.

Haranath PS, Shyamalakumari S. Experimental study on mode of action of Tylophora asthmatica in bronchial asthma. *Indian J Med Res.* 1975 May;63(5):661-70.

Harrington JJ, Lee-Chiong T Jr. Sleep and older patients. *Clin Chest Med.* 2007 Dec;28(4):673-84, v.

Harris LA, Chang L. Irritable bowel syndrome: new and emerging therapies. *Curr Opin Gastroenterol.* 2006 Mar;22(2):128-35.

Hartz C, Lauer I, Del Mar San Miguel Moncin M, Cistero-Bahima A, Foetisch K, Lidholm J, Vieths S, Scheurer S. Comparison of IgE-Binding Capacity, Cross-Reactivity and Biological Potency of Allergenic Non-Specific Lipid Transfer Proteins from Peach, Cherry and Hazelnut. *Int Arch Allergy Immunol.* 2010 Jun 17;153(4):335-346.

Harvald B, Hauge M: Hereditary factors elucidated by twin studies. In *Genetics and the Epidemiology of Chronic Disease.* Edited by Neel JV, Shaw MV, Schull WJ. Washington, DC: Dept Health, Education and Welfare, 1965:64-76.

Harvey HP, Solomon HJ. Acute anaphylactic shock due to para-aminosalicylic acid. *Am Rev Tuberc.* 1958 Mar;77(3):492-5.

Hassan AM. Selenium status in patients with aspirin-induced asthma. *Ann Clin Biochem.* 2008 Sep;45(Pt 5):508-12.

Hasselmark L, Malmgren R, Zetterström O, Unge G. Selenium supplementation in intrinsic asthma. *Allergy.* 1993 Jan;48(1):30-6.

Hata K, Ishikawa K, Hori K, Konishi T. Differentiation-inducing activity of lupeol, a lupane-type triterpene from Chinese dandelion root (Hokouei-kon), on a mouse melanoma cell line. *Biol Pharm Bull.* 2000 Aug;23(8):962-7.

Hata Y, Yamamoto M, Ohni M, Nakajima K, Nakamura Y, Takano T. A placebo-controlled study of the effect of sour milk on blood pressure in hypertensive subjects. *Am J Clin Nutr.* 1996 Nov;64(5):767-71.

Hatakka K, Holma R, El-Nezami H, Suomalainen T, Kuisma M, Saxelin M, Poussa T, Mykkänen H, Korpela R. The influence of *Lactobacillus rhamnosus* LC705 together with Propionibacterium freudenreichii ssp. shermanii JS on potentially carcinogenic bacterial activity in human colon. *Int J Food Microbiol.* 2008 Dec 10;128(2):406-10.

Hattori K, Sasai M, Yamamoto A, Taniuchi S, Kojima T, Kobayashi Y, Iwamoto H, Yaeshima T, Hayasawa H. Intestinal flora of infants with cow milk hypersensitivity fed on casein-hydrolyzed formula supplemented raffinose. *Arerugi.* 2000 Dec;49(12):1146-55.

Hattori K, Yamamoto A, Sasai M, Taniuchi S, Kojima T, Kobayashi Y, Iwamoto H, Namba K, Yaeshima T. Effects of administration of bifidobacteria on fecal microflora and clinical symptoms in infants with atopic dermatitis. *Arerugi.* 2003 Jan;52(1):20-30.

He M, Antoine JM, Yang Y, Yang J, Men J, Han H. Influence of live flora on lactose digestion in male adult lactose-malabsorbers after dairy products intake. *Wei Sheng Yan Jiu.* 2004 Sep;33(5):603-5.

He T, Priebe MG, Zhong Y, Huang C, Harmsen HJ, Raangs GC, Antoine JM, Welling GW, Vonk RJ. Effects of yogurt and bifidobacteria supplementation on the colonic microbiota in lactose-intolerant subjects. *J Appl Microbiol.* 2008 Feb;104(2):595-604.

REFERENCES AND BIBLIOGRAPHY

Heaney LG, Brightling CE, Menzies-Gow A, Stevenson M, Niven RM; British Thoracic Society Difficult Asthma Network. Refractory asthma in the UK: cross-sectional findings from a UK multicentre registry. *Thorax.* 2010 Sep;65(9):787-94.

Heaney RP, Dowell MS. Absorbability of the calcium in a high-calcium mineral water. *Osteoporos Int.* 1994 Nov;4(6):323-4.

Heap GA, van Heel DA. Genetics and pathogenesis of coeliac disease. *Semin Immunol.* May 13 2009.

Heine RG, Nethercote M, Rosenbaum J, Allen KJ. Emerging management concepts for eosinophilic esophagitis in children. *J Gastroenterol Hepatol.* 2011 May 4.

Hemmer W, Focke M, Marzban G, Swoboda I, Jarisch R, Laimer M. Identification of Bet v 1-related allergens in fig and other Moraceae fruits. *Clin Exp Allergy.* 2010 Apr;40(4):679-87.

Hendel B, Ferreira P. *Water & Salt: The Essence of Life.* Gaithersburg: Natural Resources, 2003.

Herbert V. Vitamin B12: Plant sources, requirements, and assay. *Am J Clin Nutr.* 1988;48:852-858.

Herman PM, Drost LM. Evaluating the clinical relevance of food sensitivity tests: a single subject experiment. *Altern Med Rev.* 2004 Jun;9(2):198-207.

Herzog AM, Black KA, Fountaine DJ, Knotts TR. Reflection and attentional recovery as two distinctive benefits of restorative environments. *J Environ Psychol.* 1997;17:165-70.

Hess-Kosa K. *Indoor Air Quality: Sampling Methodologies.* Boca Rataon: CRC Press, 2002.

Heyman M, Grasset E, Ducroc R, Desjeux JF. Antigen absorption by the jejunal epithelium of children with cow's milk allergy. *Pediatr Res.* 1988 Aug;24(2):197-202.

Hickson M, D'Souza AL, Muthu N, Rogers TR, Want S, Rajkumar C, Bulpitt CJ. Use of probiotic Lactobacillus preparation to prevent diarrhoea associated with antibiotics: randomised double blind placebo controlled trial. *BMJ.* 2007 Jul 14;335(7610):80.

Hide DW, Matthews S, Tariq S, Arshad SH. Allergen avoidance in infancy and allergy at 4 years of age. *Allergy.* 1996 Feb;51(2):89-93.

Hijazi Z, Molla AM, Al-Habashi H, Muawad WM, Molla AM, Sharma PN. Intestinal permeability is increased in bronchial asthma. *Arch Dis Child.* 2004 Mar;89(3):227-9.

Hill J, Micklewright A, Lewis S, Britton J. Investigation of the effect of short-term change in dietary magnesium intake in asthma. *Eur Respir J.* 1997 Oct;10(10):2225-9.

Hilton E, Isenberg HD, Alperstein P, France K, Borenstein MT. Ingestion of yogurt containing *Lactobacillus acidophilus* as prophylaxis for *Candida* vaginitis. *Ann Intern Med.* 1992 Mar 1;116(5):353-7.

Hirose Y, Murosaki S, Yamamoto Y, Yoshikai Y, Tsuru T. Daily intake of heat-killed *Lactobacillus plantarum* L-137 augments acquired immunity in healthy adults. *J Nutr.* 2006 Dec;136(12):3069-73.

Hlivak P, Jahnova E, Odraska J, Ferencik M, Ebringer L, Mikes Z. Long-term (56-week) oral administration of probiotic *Enterococcus faecium* M-74 decreases the expression of sICAM-1 and monocyte CD54, and increases that of lymphocyte CD49d in humans. *Bratisl Lek Listy.* 2005;106(4-5):175-81.

Hlivak P, Odraska J, Ferencik M, Ebringer L, Jahnova E, Mikes Z. One-year application of probiotic strain *Enterococcus faecium* M-74 decreases serum cholesterol levels. *Bratisl Lek Listy.* 2005;106(2):67-72.

Hobbs C. *Kombucha Manchurian Tea Mushroom: The Essential Guide.* Santa Cruz, CA: Botanica Press, 1995.

Hobbs C. *Medicinal Mushrooms.* Summertown, TN: Botanica Press, 2003.

Hobbs C. *Stress & Natural Healing.* Loveland, CO: Interweave Press, 1997.

Hoff S, Seiler H, Heinrich J, Kompauer I, Nieters A, Becker N, Nagel G, Gedrich K, Karg G, Wolfram G, Linseisen J. Allergic sensitisation and allergic rhinitis are associated with n-3 polyunsaturated fatty acids in the diet and in red blood cell membranes. *Eur J Clin Nutr.* 2005 Sep;59(9):1071-80.

Hoffmann D. *Holistic Herbal.* London: Thorsons, 2002.

Hofmann D, Hecker M, Völp A. Efficacy of dry extract of ivy leaves in children with bronchial asthma-a review of randomized controlled trials. *Phytomedicine.* 2003 Mar;10(2-3):213-20.

Höiby AS, Strand V, Robinson DS, Sager A, Rak S. Efficacy, safety, and immunological effects of a 2-year immunotherapy with Depigoid birch pollen extract: a randomized, double-blind, placebo-controlled study. *Clin Exp Allergy.* 2010 Jul;40(7):1062-70.

Holick MF. Sunlight and vitamin D for bone health and prevention of autoimmune diseases, cancers, and cardiovascular disease. *Am J Clin Nutr.* 2004 Dec;80(6 Suppl):1678S-88S.

Holick MF. The vitamin D deficiency pandemic and consequences for nonskeletal health: mechanisms of action. *Mol Aspects Med.* 2008 Dec;29(6):361-8

Holick MF. Vitamin D status: measurement, interpretation, and clinical application. *Ann Epidemiol.* 2009 Feb;19(2):73-8.

Holladay, S.D. Prenatal Immunotoxicant Exposure and Postnatal Autoimmune Disease. *Environ Health Perspect.* 1999; 107(suppl 5):687-691.

Holt GA. Food & Drug Interactions. Chicago: Precept Press, 1998, 83.

Homma M, Oka K, Niitsuma T, Itoh H. A novel 11 beta-hydroxysteroid dehydrogenase inhibitor contained in saiboku-to, a herbal remedy for steroid-dependent bronchial asthma. *J Pharm Pharmacol.* 1994 Apr;46(4):305-9.

Hönscheid A, Rink L, Haase H. T-lymphocytes: a target for stimulatory and inhibitory effects of zinc ions. *Endocr Metab Immune Disord Drug Targets.* 2009 Jun;9(2):132-44.

Hooper R, Calvert J, Thompson RL, Deetlefs ME, Burney P. Urban/rural differences in diet and atopy in South Africa. *Allergy.* 2008 Apr;63(4):425-31.

Hope BE, Massey DG, Fournier-Massey G. Hawaiian materia medica for asthma. *Hawaii Med J.* 1993 Jun;52(6):160-6.

Horak E, Morass B, Ulmer H. Association between environmental tobacco smoke exposure and wheezing disorders in Austrian preschool children. *Swiss Med Wkly.* 2007 Nov 3;137(43-44):608-13.

Horrobin DF. Effects of evening primrose oil in rheumatoid arthritis. *Ann Rheum Dis.* 1989 Nov;48(11):965-6.

Hospers IC, de Vries-Vrolijk K, Brand PL. Double-blind, placebo-controlled cow's milk challenge in children with alleged cow's milk allergies, performed in a general hospital: diagnosis rejected in two-thirds of the children. *Ned Tijdschr Geneeskd.* 2006 Jun 10;150(23):1292-7.

Hosseini S, Pishnamazi S, Sadrzadeh SM, Farid F, Farid R, Watson RR. Pycnogenol((R)) in the Management of Asthma. *J Med Food.* 2001 Winter;4(4):201-209.

Hota B, Ellenbogen C, Hayden MK, Aroutcheva A, Rice TW, Weinstein RA. Community-associated methicillin-resistant *Staphylococcus aureus* skin and soft tissue infections at a public hospital: do public housing and incarceration amplify transmission? *Arch Intern Med.* 2007 May 28;167(10):1026-33.

Hougee S, Vriesema AJ, Wijering SC, Knippels LM, Folkerts G, Nijkamp FP, Knol J, Garssen J. Oral treatment with probiotics reduces allergic symptoms in ovalbumin-sensitized mice: a bacterial strain comparative study. *Int Arch Allergy Immunol.* 2010;151(2):107-17. 2009 Sep 15.

Houle CR, Leo HL, Clark NM. A developmental, community, and psychosocial approach to food allergies in children. *Curr Allergy Asthma Rep.* 2010 Sep;10(5):381-6.

Houssen ME, Ragab A, Mesbah A, El-Samanoudy AZ, Othman G, Moustafa AF, Badria FA. Natural anti-inflammatory products and leukotriene inhibitors as complementary therapy for bronchial asthma. *Clin Biochem.* 2010 Jul;43(10-11):887-90.

Hoyme UB, Saling E. Efficient prematurity prevention is possible by pH-self measurement and immediate therapy of threatening ascending infection. *Eur J Obstet Gynecol Reprod Biol.* 2004 Aug 10;115(2):148-53.

Hoyos AB. Reduced incidence of necrotizing enterocolitis associated with enteral administration of *Lactobacillus acidophilus* and *Bifidobacterium infantis* to neonates in an intensive care unit. *Int J Infect Dis.* 1999 Summer;3(4):197-202.

Hsieh KH. Evaluation of efficacy of traditional Chinese medicines in the treatment of childhood bronchial asthma: clinical trial, immunological tests and animal study. Taiwan Asthma Study Group. *Pediatr Allergy Immunol.* 1996 Aug;7(3):130-40.

Hsu CH, Lu CM, Chang TT. Efficacy and safety of modified Mai-Men-Dong-Tang for treatment of allergic asthma. *Pediatr Allergy Immunol.* 2005;16:76-81.

Hu C, Kitts DD. Antioxidant, prooxidant, and cytotoxic activities of solvent-fractionated dandelion (Taraxacum officinale) flower extracts in vitro. *J Agric Food Chem.* 2003 Jan 1;51(1):301-10.

Hu C, Kitts DD. Dandelion (Taraxacum officinale) flower extract suppresses both reactive oxygen species and nitric oxide and prevents lipid oxidation in vitro. *Phytomedicine.* 2005 Aug;12(8):588-97.

Hu C, Kitts DD. Luteolin and luteolin-7-O-glucoside from dandelion flower suppress iNOS and COX-2 in RAW264.7 cells. *Mol Cell Biochem.* 2004 Oct;265(1-2):107-13.

Hu FB, Willett WC. Optimal diets for prevention of coronary heart disease. *JAMA.* 2002 Nov 27;288(20):2569-78.

Huang D, Ou B, Prior RL. The chemistry behind antioxidant capacity assays. *J Agric Food Chem.* 2005 Mar 23;53(6):1841-56.

Huang M, Wang W, Wei S. Investigation on medicinal plant resources of Glycyrrhiza uralensis in China and chemical assessment of its underground part. *Zhongguo Zhong Yao Za Zhi.* 2010 Apr;35(8):947-52.

Hun L. Bacillus coagulans significantly improved abdominal pain and bloating in patients with IBS. *Postgrad Med.* 2009 Mar;121(2):119-24.

Huntley A, Ernst E: Herbal medicines for asthma: a systematic review. *Thorax.* 2000, 55:925-929.

Hur YM, Rushton JP. Genetic and environmental contributions to prosocial behaviour in 2- to 9-year-old South Korean twins. *Biol Lett.* 2007 Dec 22;3(6):664-6.

Husby S. Dietary antigens: uptake and humoral immunity in man. *APMIS Suppl.* 1988;1:1-40.

Hyndman SJ, Vickers LM, Htut T, Maunder JW, Peock A, Higenbottam TW. A randomized trial of dehumidification in the control of house dust mite. *Clin Exp Allergy.* 2000 Aug;30(8):1172-80.

Ibero M, Boné J, Martín B, Martínez J. Evaluation of an extensively hydrolysed casein formula (Damira 2000) in children with allergy to cow's milk proteins. *Allergol Immunopathol (Madr).* 2010 Mar-Apr;38(2):60-8.

Ibrahim AR, Kawamoto S, Nishimura M, Pak S, Aki T, Diaz-Perales A, Salcedo G, Asturias JA, Hayashi T, Ono K. A new lipid transfer protein homolog identified as an IgE-binding antigen from Japanese cedar pollen. *Biosci Biotechnol Biochem.* 2010;74(3):504-9.

REFERENCES AND BIBLIOGRAPHY

Imase K, Tanaka A, Tokunaga K, Sugano H, Ishida H, Takahashi S. *Lactobacillus reuteri* tablets suppress *Helicobacter pylori* infection—a double-blind randomised placebo-controlled cross-over clinical study. *Kansenshogaku Zasshi.* 2007 Jul;81(4):387-93.

Inbar O, Dotan R, Dlin RA, Neuman I, Bar-Or O. Breathing dry or humid air and exercise-induced asthma during swimming. *Eur J Appl Physiol Occup Physiol.* 1980;44(1):43-50.

Indrio F, Ladisa G, Mautone A, Montagna O. Effect of a fermented formula on thymus size and stool pH in healthy term infants. *Pediatr Res.* 2007 Jul;62(1):98-100.

Indrio F, Riezzo G, Raimondi F, Bisceglia M, Cavallo L, Francavilla R. The effects of probiotics on feeding tolerance, bowel habits, and gastrointestinal motility in preterm newborns. *J Pediatr.* 2008 Jun;152(6):801-6.

Innis SM, Hansen JW. Plasma fatty acid responses, metabolic effects, and safety of microalgal and fungal oils rich in arachidonic and docosahexaenoic acids in adults. *Am J Clin Nutr.* 1996 Aug;64(2):159-67.

Innis SM, Hansen JW. Plasma fatty acid responses, metabolic effects, and safety of microalgal and fungal oils rich in arachidonic and docosahexaenoic acids in healthy adults. *Am J Clin Nutr.* 1996 Aug;64(2):159-67.

Ionescu JG. New insights in the pathogenesis of atopic disease. *J Med Life.* 2009 Apr-Jun;2(2):146-54.

Iovieno A, Lambiase A, Sacchetti M, Stampachiacchiere B, Micera A, Bonini S. Preliminary evidence of the efficacy of probiotic eye-drop treatment in patients with vernal keratoconjunctivitis. *Graefes Arch Clin Exp Ophthalmol.* 2008 Mar;246(3):435-41.

Iribarren C, Tolstykh IV, Miller MK, Eisner MD. Asthma and the prospective risk of anaphylactic shock and other allergy diagnoses in a large integrated health care delivery system. *Ann Allergy Asthma Immunol.* 2010 May;104(5):371-7.

ISAAC. The International Study of Asthma and Allergies in Childhood (ISAAC) Steering Committee. Worldwide variation in prevalence of symptoms of asthma, allergic rhinoconjunctivitis, and atopic eczema: ISAAC. *Lancet.* 1998;351:1225-1232.

Ishida Y, Nakamura F, Kanzato H, Sawada D, Hirata H, Nishimura A, Kajimoto O, Fujiwara S. Clinical effects of *Lactobacillus acidophilus* strain L-92 on perennial allergic rhinitis: a double-blind, placebo-controlled study. *J Dairy Sci.* 2005 Feb;88(2):527-33.

Ishida Y, Nakamura F, Kanzato H, Sawada D, Hirata H, Nishimura A, Kajimoto O, Fujiwara S. Clinical effects of *Lactobacillus acidophilus* strain L-92 on perennial allergic rhinitis: a double-blind, placebo-controlled study. *J Dairy Sci.* 2005 Feb;88(2):527-33.

Ishida Y, Nakamura F, Kanzato H, Sawada D, Yamamoto N, Kagata H, Oh-Ida M, Takeuchi H, Fujiwara S. Effect of milk fermented with *Lactobacillus acidophilus* strain L-92 on symptoms of Japanese cedar pollen allergy: a randomized placebo-controlled trial. *Biosci Biotechnol Biochem.* 2005 Sep;69(9):1652-60.

Ishikawa H, Akedo I, Otani T, Suzuki T, Nakamura T, Takeyama I, Ishiguro S, Miyaoka E, Sobue T, Kakizoe T. Randomized trial of dietary fiber and *Lactobacillus casei* administration for prevention of colorectal tumors. *Int J Cancer.* 2005 Sep 20;116(5):762-7.

Ishtiaq M, Hanif W, Khan MA, Ashraf M, Butt AM. An ethnomedicinal survey and documentation of important medicinal folklore food phytonims of flora of Samahni valley, (Azad Kashmir) Pakistan. *Pak J Biol Sci.* 2007 Jul 1;10(13):2241-56.

Isolauri E, Joensuu J, Suomalainen H, Luomala M, Vesikari T. Improved immunogenicity of oral D x RRV reassortant rotavirus vaccine by *Lactobacillus casei* GG. *Vaccine.* 1995 Feb;13(3):310-2.

Isolauri E, Juntunen M, Rautanen T, Sillanaukee P, Koivula T. A human Lactobacillus strain (*Lactobacillus casei* sp strain GG) promotes recovery from acute diarrhea in children. *Pediatrics.* 1991 Jul;88(1):90-7.

Isolauri E, Kaila M, Mykkänen H, Ling WH, Salminen S. Oral bacteriotherapy for viral gastroenteritis. *Dig Dis Sci.* 1994 Dec;39(12):2595-600.

Itokawa Y. Magnesium intake and cardiovascular disease. *Clin Calcium.* 2005 Feb;15(2):154-9.

Ivory K, Chambers SJ, Pin C, Prieto E, Arqués JL, Nicoletti C. Oral delivery of *Lactobacillus casei* Shirota modifies allergen-induced immune responses in allergic rhinitis. *Clin Exp Allergy.* 2008 Aug;38(8):1282-9.

Izbicki G, Chavko R, Banauch GI, Weiden MD, Berger KI, Aldrich TK, Hall C, Kelly KJ, Prezant DJ. World trade center "sarcoid-like" granulomatous pulmonary disease in New York City fire department rescue workers. *Chest.* 2007 May;131(5):1414-23.

Izquierdo JL, Martín A, de Lucas P, Rodríguez-González-Moro JM, Almonacid C, Paravisini A. Misdiagnosis of patients receiving inhaled therapies in primary care. *Int J Chron Obstruct Pulmon Dis.* 2010 Aug 9;5:241-9.

Izumi K, Aihara M, Ikezawa Z. Effects of non steroidal antiinflammatory drugs (NSAIDs) on immediate-type food allergy analysis of Japanese cases from 1998 to 2009. *Arerugi.* 2009 Dec;58(12):1629-39.

Jaber R. Respiratory and allergic diseases: from upper respiratory tract infections to asthma. *Prim Care.* 2002 Jun;29(2):231-61.

Jackson DJ, Lemanske RF Jr. The role of respiratory virus infections in childhood asthma inception. *Immunol Allergy Clin North Am.* 2010 Nov;30(4):513-22, vi.

Jacobs DE, Wilson J, Dixon SL, Smith J, Evens A. The relationship of housing and population health: a 30-year retrospective analysis. *Environ Health Perspect.* 2009 Apr;117(4):597-604. 2008 Dec 16.

Jacobsen CN, Rosenfeldt Nielsen V, Hayford AE, Møller PL, Michaelsen KF, Paerregaard A, Sandström B, Tvede M, Jakobsen M. Screening of probiotic activities of forty-seven strains of Lactobacillus spp. by in vitro techniques and evaluation of the colonization ability of five selected strains in humans. *Appl Environ Microbiol.* 1999 Nov;65(11):4949-56.

Jagetia GC, Aggarwal BB. "Spicing up" of the immune system by curcumin. *J Clin Immunol.* 2007 Jan;27(1):19-35.

Jagetia GC, Nayak V, Vidyasagar MS. Evaluation of the antineoplastic activity of guduchi (Tinospora cordifolia) in cultured HeLa cells. *Cancer Lett.* 1998 May 15;127(1-2):71-82.

Jagetia GC, Rao SK. Evaluation of Cytotoxic Effects of Dichloromethane Extract of Guduchi (Tinospora cordifolia Miers ex Hook F & THOMS) on Cultured HeLa Cells. *Evid Based Complement Alternat Med.* 2006 Jun;3(2):267-72.

Jahnova E, Horvathova M, Gazdik F, Weissova S. Effects of selenium supplementation on expression of adhesion molecules in corticoid-dependent asthmatics. *Bratisl Lek Listy.* 2002;103(1):12-6.

Jain PK, McNaught CE, Anderson AD, MacFie J, Mitchell CJ. Influence of synbiotic containing *Lactobacillus acidophilus* La5, *Bifidobacterium lactis* Bb 12, *Streptococcus thermophilus*, *Lactobacillus bulgaricus* and oligofructose on gut barrier function and sepsis in critically ill patients: a randomised controlled trial. *Clin Nutr.* 2004 Aug;23(4):467-75.

Jaiswal M, Prajapati PK, Patgiri BJ Ravishankar B. A Comparative Pharmaco - Clinical Study on Anti-Asthmatic Effect of Shirisharishta Prepared by Bark, Sapwood and Heartwood of Albizia Lebbeck. *J Res Ayurv.* 2006;27(3):67-74.

Jaiswal M, Prajapati PK, Patgiri BJ, Ravishankar B. Clinical Study on Anti-Asthmatic Effect of Shirisharishta Prepared by Bark, Sapwood and Heartwood of Albizia Lebbeck. *Pharmaco.* 2006 27(3): 67-74

Janelle KC, Barr SI. Nutrient intakes and eating behavior scores of vegetarian and nonvegetarian women. *J Am Diet Assoc.* 1995 Feb;95(2):180-6, 189, quiz 187-8.

Janson C, Anto J, Burney P, Chinn S, de Marco R, Heinrich J, Jarvis D, Kuenzli N, Leynaert B, Luczynska C, Neukirch F, Svanes C, Sunyer J, Wjst M; European Community Respiratory Health Survey II. The European Community Respiratory Health Survey: what are the main results so far? European Community Respiratory Health Survey II. *Eur Respir J.* 2001 Sep;18(3):598-611.

Jarocka-Cyrta E, Baniukiewicz A, Wasilewska J, Pawlak J, Kaczmarski M. Focal villous atrophy of the duodenum in children who have outgrown cow's milk allergy. Chromoendoscopy and magnification endoscopy evaluation. *Med Wieku Rozwoj.* 2007 Apr-Jun;11(2 Pt 1):123-7.

Jauhiainen T, Vapaatalo H, Poussa T, Kyrönpalo S, Rasmussen M, Korpela R. *Lactobacillus helveticus* fermented milk lowers blood pressure in hypertensive subjects in 24-h ambulatory blood pressure measurement. *Am J Hypertens.* 2005 Dec;18(12 Pt 1):1600-5.

Jayaprakasam B, Doddaga S, Wang R, Holmes D, Goldfarb J, Li XM. Licorice flavonoids inhibit eotaxin-1 secretion by human fetal lung fibroblasts in vitro. *J Agric Food Chem.* 2009 Feb 11;57(3):820-5.

Jennings S, Prescott SL. Early dietary exposures and feeding practices: role in pathogenesis and prevention of allergic disease? *Postgrad Med J.* 2010 Feb;86(1012):94-9.

Jensen B. *Foods that Heal.* Garden City Park, NY: Avery Publ, 1988, 1993.

Jensen B. *Nature Has a Remedy.* Los Angeles: Keats, 2001.

Jensen HK. The molecular genetic basis and diagnosis of familial hypercholesterolemia in Denmark. *Dan Med Bull.* 2002 Nov;49(4):318-45.

Jeon HJ, Kang HJ, Jung HJ, Kang YS, Lim CJ, Kim YM, Park EH. Anti-inflammatory activity of Taraxacum officinale. *J Ethnopharmacol.* 2008 Jan 4;115(1):82-8.

Jernelöv S, Höglund CO, Axelsson J, Axén J, Grönneberg R, Grunewald J, Stierna P, Lekander M. Effects of examination stress on psychological responses, sleep and allergic symptoms in atopic and non-atopic students. *Int J Behav Med.* 2009;16(4):305-10.

Jiang T, Mustapha A, Savaiano DA. Improvement of lactose digestion in humans by ingestion of unfermented milk containing *Bifidobacterium longum. J Dairy Sci.* 1996 May;79(5):750-7.

Jiménez E, Fernández L, Maldonado A, Martín R, Olivares M, Xaus J, Rodríguez JM. Oral administration of Lactobacillus strains isolated from breast milk as an alternative for the treatment of infectious mastitis during lactation. *Appl Environ Microbiol.* 2008 Aug;74(15):4650-5.

Johansson G, Holmén A, Persson L, Högstedt B, Wassén C, Ottova L, Gustafsson JA. Long-term effects of a change from a mixed diet to a lacto-vegetarian diet on human urinary and faecal mutagenic activity. *Mutagenesis.* 1998 Mar;13(2):167-71.

Johansson G, Holmén A, Persson L, Högstedt B, Wassén C, Ottova L, Gustafsson JA. Dietary influence on some proposed risk factors for colon cancer: fecal and urinary mutagenic activity and the activity of some intestinal bacterial enzymes. *Cancer Detect Prev.* 1997;21(3):258-66.

REFERENCES AND BIBLIOGRAPHY

Johansson G, Holmén A, Persson L, Högstedt R, Wassén C, Ottova L, Gustafsson JA. The effect of a shift from a mixed diet to a lacto-vegetarian diet on human urinary and fecal mutagenic activity. *Carcinogenesis.* 1992 Feb;13(2):153-7.

Johansson G, Ravald N. Comparison of some salivary variables between vegetarians and omnivores. *Eur J Oral Sci.* 1995 Apr;103(2 (Pt 1)):95-8.

Johansson GK, Ottova L, Gustafsson JA. Shift from a mixed diet to a lactovegetarian diet: influence on some cancer-associated intestinal bacterial enzyme activities. *Nutr Cancer.* 1990;14(3-4):239-46. PubMed PMID: 2128119.

Johansson ML, Nobaek S, Berggren A, Nyman M, Björck I, Ahrné S, Jeppsson B, Molin G. Survival of *Lactobacillus plantarum* DSM 9843 (299v), and effect on the short-chain fatty acid content of faeces after ingestion of a rose-hip drink with fermented oats. *Int J Food Microbiol.* 1998 Jun 30;42(1-2):29-38.

Johari H. *Ayurvedic Massage: Traditional Indian Techniques for Balancing Body and Mind.* Rochester, VT: Healing Arts, 1996.

Johnson LM. Gitksan medicinal plants—cultural choice and efficacy. *J Ethnobiol Ethnomed.* 2006 Jun 21;2:29.

Jones MA, Silman AJ, Whiting S, *et al.* Occurrence of rheumatoid arthritis is not increased in the first degree relatives of a population based inception cohort of inflammatory polyarthritis. *Ann Rheum Dis.* 1996;55(2): 89-93.

Jones SE, Versalovic J. Probiotic Lactobacillus reuteri biofilms produce antimicrobial and anti-inflammatory factors. *BMC Microbiol.* 2009 Feb 11;9:35.

José RJ, Roberts J, Bakerly ND. The effectiveness of a social marketing model on case-finding for COPD in a deprived inner city population. *Prim Care Respir J.* 2010 Jun;19(2):104-8.

Joseph SP, Borrell LN, Shapiro A. Self-reported lifetime asthma and nativity status in U.S. children and adolescents: results from the National Health and Nutrition Examination Survey 1999-2004. *J Health Care Poor Underserved.* 2010 May;21(2 Suppl):125-39.

Juergens UR, Dethlefsen U, Steinkamp G, Gillissen A, Repges R, Vetter H. Anti-inflammatory activity of 1.8-cineol (eucalyptol) in bronchial asthma: a double-blind placebo-controlled trial. *Respir Med.* 2003 Mar;97(3):250-6.

Julkunen-Tiitto R. A chemotaxonomic survey of phenolics in leaves of northern Salicaceae species. Phytochemistry. 1986;25(3):663-667.

Jung HA, Yokozawa T, Kim BW, Jung JH, Choi JS. Selective inhibition of prenylated flavonoids from Sophora flavescens against BACE1 and cholinesterases. *Am J Chin Med.* 2010;38(2):415-29.

Jurenka JS. Anti-inflammatory properties of curcumin, a major constituent of Curcuma longa: a review of preclinical and clinical research. *Altern Med Rev.* 2009 Feb;14(2):141-153.

Juvonen R, Bloigu A, Peitso A, Silvennoinen-Kassinen S, Saikku P, Leinonen M, Hassi J, Harju T. Training improves physical fitness and decreases CRP also in asthmatic conscripts. *J Asthma.* 2008 Apr;45(3):237-42.

Kähkönen MP, Hopia AI, Vuorela HJ, Rauha JP, Pihlaja K, Kujala TS, Heinonen M. Antioxidant activity of plant extracts containing phenolic compounds. *J Agric Food Chem.* 1999 Oct;47(10):3954-62.

Kaila M, Isolauri E, Saxelin M, Arvilommi H, Vesikari T. Viable versus inactivated lactobacillus strain GG in acute rotavirus diarrhoea. *Arch Dis Child.* 1995 Jan;72(1):51-3.

Kaila M, Vanto T, Valovirta E, Koivikko A, Juntunen-Backman K. Diagnosis of food allergy in Finland: survey of pediatric practices. *Pediatr Allergy Immunol.* 2000 Nov;11(4):246-9.

Kajander K, Hatakka K, Poussa T, Färkkilä M, Korpela R. A probiotic mixture alleviates symptoms in irritable bowel syndrome patients: a controlled 6-month intervention. *Aliment Pharmacol Ther.* 2005 Sep 1;22(5):387-94.

Kajander K, Korpela R. Clinical studies on alleviating the symptoms of irritable bowel syndrome. *Asia Pac J Clin Nutr.* 2006;15(4):576-80.

Kajander K, Krogius-Kurikka L, Rinttilä T, Karjalainen H, Palva A, Korpela R. Effects of multispecies probiotic supplementation on intestinal microbiota in irritable bowel syndrome. *Aliment Pharmacol Ther.* 2007 Aug 1;26(3):463-73.

Kajander K, Myllyluoma E, Rajilić-Stojanović M, Kyrönpalo S, Rasmussen M, Järvenpää S, Zoetendal EG, de Vos WM, Vapaatalo H, Korpela R. Clinical trial: multispecies probiotic supplementation alleviates the symptoms of irritable bowel syndrome and stabilizes intestinal microbiota. *Aliment Pharmacol Ther.* 2008 Jan 1;27(1):48-57.

Kalach N, Benhamou PH, Campeotto F, Dupont Ch. Anemia impairs small intestinal absorption measured by intestinal permeability in children. *Eur Ann Allergy Clin Immunol.* 2007 Jan;39(1):20-2.

Kaliner M, Shelhamer JH, Borson B, Nadel J, Patow C, Marom Z. Human respiratory mucus. *Am Rev Respir Dis.* 1986 Sep;134(3):612-21.

Kalliomäki M, Salminen S, Arvilommi H, Kero P, Koskinen P, Isolauri E. Probiotics in primary prevention of atopic disease: a randomised placebo-controlled trial. *Lancet.* 2001 Apr 7;357(9262):1076-9.

Kalliomäki M, Salminen S, Poussa T, Arvilommi H, Isolauri E. Probiotics and prevention of atopic disease: 4-year follow-up of a randomised placebo-controlled trial. *Lancet.* 2003 May 31;361(9372):1869-71.

Kalliomäki M, Salminen S, Poussa T, Isolauri E. Probiotics during the first 7 years of life: a cumulative risk reduction of eczema in a randomized, placebo-controlled trial. *J Allergy Clin Immunol.* 2007 Apr;119(4):1019-21.

Kanazawa H, Nagino M, Kamiya S, Komatsu S, Mayumi T, Takagi K, Asahara T, Nomoto K, Tanaka R, Nimura Y. Synbiotics reduce postoperative infectious complications: a randomized controlled trial in biliary cancer patients undergoing hepatectomy. *Langenbecks Arch Surg.* 2005 Apr;390(2):104-13.

Kang SK, Kim JK, Ahn SH, Oh JE, Kim JH, Lim DH, Son BK. Relationship between silent gastroesophageal reflux and food sensitization in infants and young children with recurrent wheezing. *J Korean Med Sci.* 2010 Mar;25(3):425-8.

Kankaanpää PE, Yang B, Kallio HP, Isolauri E, Salminen SJ. Influence of probiotic supplemented infant formula on composition of plasma lipids in atopic infants. *J Nutr Biochem.* 2002 Jun;13(6):364-369.

Kanny G, Grignon G, Dauca M, Guedenet JC, Moneret-Vautrin DA. Ultrastructural changes in the duodenal mucosa induced by ingested histamine in patients with chronic urticaria. *Allergy.* 1996 Dec;51(12):935-9.

Kano H, Mogami O, Uchida M. Oral administration of milk fermented with Lactobacillus delbrueckii ssp. bulgaricus OLL1073R-1 to DBA/1 mice inhibits secretion of proinflammatory cytokines. *Cytotechnology.* 2002 Nov;40(1-3):67-73.

Kapil A, Sharma S. Immunopotentiating compounds from Tinospora cordifolia. *J Ethnopharmacol.* 1997 Oct;58(2):89-95.

Kaplan C. Indoor air pollution from unprocessed solid fuels in developing countries. *Rev Environ Health.* 2010 Jul-Sep;25(3):221-42.

Kaplan M, Mutlu EA, Benson M, Fields JZ, Banan A, Keshavarzian A. Use of herbal preparations in the treatment of oxidant-mediated inflammatory disorders. *Complement Ther Med.* 2007 Sep;15(3):207-16. 2006 Aug 21.

Kaplan R. The nature of the view from home: psychological benefits. *Environ Behav.* 2001;33(4):507-42.

Kaplan R. Wilderness perception and psychological benefits: an analysis of a continuing program. *Leisure Sci.* 1984;6(3):271-90.

Karkoulias K, Patouchas D, Alahiotis S, Tsiamita M, Vrodakis K, Spiropoulos K. Specific sensitization in wheat flour and contributing factors in traditional bakers. *Eur Rev Med Pharmacol Sci.* 2007 May-Jun;11(3):141-8.

Karpińska J, Mikołuć B, Motkowski R, Piotrowska-Jastrzebska J. HPLC method for simultaneous determination of retinol, alpha-tocopherol and coenzyme Q10 in human plasma. *J Pharm Biomed Anal.* 2006 Sep 18;42(2):232-6.

Kashiwada Y, Takanaka K, Tsukada H, Miwa Y, Taga T, Tanaka S, Ikeshiro Y. Sesquiterpene glucosides from anti-leukotriene B4 release fraction of Taraxacum officinale. *J Asian Nat Prod Res.* 2001;3(3):191-7.

Katial RK, Strand M, Prasertsuntarasai T, Leung R, Zheng W, Alam R. The effect of aspirin desensitization on novel biomarkers in aspirin-exacerbated respiratory diseases. *J Allergy Clin Immunol.* 2010 Oct;126(4):738-44. 2010 Aug 21.

Kattan JD, Srivastava KD, Sampson HA, Li XM. Pharmacologic and Immunologic Effects of Individual Herbs of Food Allergy Herbal Formula 2 in a Murine Model of Peanut Allergy. *J Allergy Clin Immunol.* 2006;117(2):S34.

Kattan JD, Srivastava KD, Zou ZM, Goldfarb J, Sampson HA, Li XM. Pharmacological and immunological effects of individual herbs in the Food Allergy Herbal Formula-2 (FAHF-2) on peanut allergy. *Phytother Res.* 2008 May;22(5):651-9.

Katz DL, Cushman D, Reynolds J, Njike V, Treu JA, Walker J, Smith E, Katz C. Putting physical activity where it fits in the school day: preliminary results of the ABC (Activity Bursts in the Classroom) for fitness program. *Prev Chronic Dis.* 2010 Jul;7(4):A82. 2010 Jun 15.

Katz Y, Rajuan N, Goldberg MR, Eisenberg E, Heyman E, Cohen A, Leshno M. Early exposure to cow's milk protein is protective against IgE-mediated cow's milk protein allergy. *J Allergy Clin Immunol.* 2010 Jul;126(1):77-82.e1.

Kawase M, Hashimoto H, Hosoda M, Morita H, Hosono A. Effect of administration of fermented milk containing whey protein concentrate to rats and healthy men on serum lipids and blood pressure. *J Dairy Sci.* 2000 Feb;83(2):255-63.

Kazaks AG, Uriu-Adams JY, Albertson TE, Shenoy SF, Stern JS. Effect of oral magnesium supplementation on measures of airway resistance and subjective assessment of asthma control and quality of life in men and women with mild to moderate asthma: a randomized placebo controlled trial. *J Asthma.* 2010 Feb;47(1):83-92.

Kazansky DB. MHC restriction and allogeneic immune responses. *J Immunotoxicol.* 2008 Oct;5(4):369-84.

Kazłowska K, Hsu T, Hou CC, Yang WC, Tsai GJ. Anti-inflammatory properties of phenolic compounds and crude extract from Porphyra dentata. *J Ethnopharmacol.* 2010 Mar 2;128(1):123-30.

REFERENCES AND BIBLIOGRAPHY

Ke X, Qian D, Zhu L, Hong S. [Analysis on quality of life and personality characteristics of allergic rhinitis]. *Lin Chung Er Bi Yan Hou Tou Jing Wai Ke Za Zhi*. 2010 Mar;24(5):200-2.

Kecskés G, Belágyi T, Oláh A. Early jejunal nutrition with combined pre- and probiotics in acute pancreatitis—prospective, randomized, double-blind investigations. *Magy Seb*. 2003 Feb;56(1):3-8.

Keita AV, Söderholm JD. The intestinal barrier and its regulation by neuroimmune factors. *Neurogastroenterol Motil*. 2010 Jul;22(7):718-33.

Kekkonen RA, Lummela N, Karjalainen H, Latvala S, Tynkkynen S, Jarvenpaa S, Kautiainen H, Julkunen I, Vapaatalo H, Korpela R. Probiotic intervention has strain-specific anti-inflammatory effects in healthy adults. *World J Gastroenterol*. 2008 Apr 7;14(13):2029-36.

Kekkonen RA, Sysi-Aho M, Seppanen-Laakso T, Julkunen I, Vapaatalo H, Oresic M, Korpela R. Effect of probiotic *Lactobacillus rhamnosus* GG intervention on global serum lipidomic profiles in healthy adults. *World J Gastroenterol*. 2008 May 28;14(20):3188-94.

Kekkonen RA, Vasankari TJ, Vuorimaa T, Haahtela T, Julkunen I, Korpela R. The effect of probiotics on respiratory infections and gastrointestinal symptoms during training in marathon runners. *Int J Sport Nutr Exerc Metab*. 2007 Aug;17(4):352-63.

Kekkonen RA, Vasankari TJ, Vuorimaa T, Haahtela T, Julkunen I, Korpela R. The effect of probiotics on respiratory infections and gastrointestinal symptoms during training in marathon runners. *Int J Sport Nutr Exerc Metab*. 2007 Aug;17(4):352-63.

Kelder P. *Ancient Secret of the Fountain of Youth*. New York: Doubleday, 1998.

Kelly HW, Van Natta ML, Covar RA, Tonascia J, Green RP, Strunk RC; CAMP Research Group. Effect of long-term corticosteroid use on bone mineral density in children: a prospective longitudinal assessment in the childhood Asthma Management Program (CAMP) study. *Pediatrics*. 2008 Jul;122(1):e53-61.

Kelly-Pieper K, Patil SP, Busse P, Yang N, Sampson H, Li XM, Wisnivesky JP, Kattan M. Safety and tolerability of an antiasthma herbal Formula (ASHMI) in adult subjects with asthma: a randomized, double-blinded, placebo-controlled, dose-escalation phase I study. *J Altern Complement Med*. 2009 Jul;15(7):735-43.

Kenia P, Houghton T, Beardsmore C. Does inhaling menthol affect nasal patency or cough? *Pediatr Pulmonol*. 2008 Jun;43(6):532-7.

Keogh JB, Grieger JA, Noakes M, Clifton PM. Flow-Mediated Dilatation Is Impaired by a High-Saturated Fat Diet but Not by a High-Carbohydrate Diet. *Arterioscler Thromb Vasc Biol*. 2005 Mar 17

Keogh JB, Grieger JA, Noakes M, Clifton PM. Flow-Mediated Dilatation Is Impaired by a High-Saturated Fat Diet but Not by a High-Carbohydrate Diet. *Arterioscler Thromb Vasc Biol*. 2005 Mar:17

Kerckhoffs DA, Brouns F, Hornstra G, Mensink RP. Effects on the human serum lipoprotein profile of beta-glucan, soy protein and isoflavones, plant sterols and stanols, garlic and tocotrienols. *J Nutr*. 2002 Sep;132(9):2494-505.

Kerckhoffs DA, Brouns F, Hornstra G, Mensink RP. Effects on the human serum lipoprotein profile of beta-glucan, soy protein and isoflavones, plant sterols and stanols, garlic and tocotrienols. *J Nutr*. 2002 Sep;132(9):2494-505.

Kerkhof M, Postma DS, Brunekreef B, Reijmerink NE, Wijga AH, de Jongste JC, Gehring U, Koppelman GH. Toll-like receptor 2 and 4 genes influence susceptibility to adverse effects of traffic-related air pollution on childhood asthma. *Thorax*. 2010 Aug;65(8):690-7.

Key T, Appleby P, Davey G, Allen N, Spencer E, Travis R. Mortality in British vegetarians: review and preliminary results from EPIC-Oxford. *Amer. Jour. Clin. Nutr. Suppl*. 2003;78(3): 533S-538S.

Kiecolt-Glaser JK, Heffner KL, Glaser R, Malarkey WB, Porter K, Atkinson C, Laskowski B, Lemeshow S, Marshall GD. How stress and anxiety can alter immediate and late phase skin test responses in allergic rhinitis. *Psychoneuroendocrinology*. 2009 Jun;34(5):670-80.

Kiefte-de Jong JC, Escher JC, Arends LR, Jaddoe VW, Hofman A, Raat H, Moll HA. Infant nutritional factors and functional constipation in childhood: the Generation R study. *Am J Gastroenterol*. 2010 Apr;105(4):940-5.

Kiessling G, Schneider J, Jahreis G. Long-term consumption of fermented dairy products over 6 months increases HDL cholesterol. *Eur J Clin Nutr*. 2002 Sep;56(9):843-9.

Kilara A, Shahani KM. The use of immobilized enzymes in the food industry: a review. *CRC Crit Rev Food Sci Nutr*. 1979 Dec;12(2):161-98.

Kim HM, Shin HY, Lim KH, Ryu ST, Shin TY, Chae HJ, Kim HR, Lyu YS, An NH, Lim KS. Taraxacum officinale inhibits tumor necrosis factor-alpha production from rat astrocytes. *Immunopharmacol Immunotoxicol*. 2000 Aug;22(3):519-30.

Kim JH, An S, Kim JE, Choi GS, Ye YM, Park HS. Beef-induced anaphylaxis confirmed by the basophil activation test. *Allergy Asthma Immunol Res*. 2010 Jul;2(3):206-8.

Kim JH, Ellwood PE, Asher MI. Diet and asthma: looking back, moving forward. *Respir Res*. 2009 Jun 12;10:49.

Kim JH, Kim JE, Choi GS, Hwang EK, An S, Ye YM, Park HS. A case of occupational rhinitis caused by rice powder in the grain industry. *Allergy Asthma Immunol Res*. 2010 Apr;2(2):141-3.

Kim JH, Lee SY, Kim HB, Jin HS, Yu JH, Kim BJ, Kim BS, Kang MJ, Jang SO, Hong SJ. TBXA2R gene polymorphism and responsiveness to leukotriene receptor antagonist in children with asthma. *Clin Exp Allergy.* 2008 Jan;38(1):51-9.

Kim JI, Lee MS, Jung SY, Choi JY, Lee S, Ko JM, Zhao H, Zhao J, Kim AR, Shin MS, Kang KW, Jung HJ, Kim TH, Liu B, Choi SM. Acupuncture for persistent allergic rhinitis: a multi-centre, randomised, controlled trial protocol. *Trials.* 2009 Jul 14;10:54.

Kim JY, Kim DY, Lee YS, Lee BK, Lee KH, Ro JY. DA-9601, Artemisia asiatica herbal extract, ameliorates airway inflammation of allergic asthma in mice. *Mol Cells.* 2006;22:104-12.

Kim LS, Waters RF, Burkholder PM. Immunological activity of larch arabinogalactan and Echinacea: a preliminary, randomized, double-blind, placebo-controlled trial. *Altern Med Rev.* 2002 Apr;7(2):138-49.

Kim MN, Kim N, Lee SH, Park YS, Hwang JH, Kim JW, Jeong SH, Lee DH, Kim JS, Jung HC, Song IS. The effects of probiotics on PPI-triple therapy for *Helicobacter pylori* eradication. *Helicobacter.* 2008 Aug;13(4):261-8.

Kim NI, Jo Y, Ahn SB, Son BK, Kim SH, Park YS, Kim SH, Ju JE. A case of eosinophilic esophagitis with food hypersensitivity. *J Neurogastroenterol Motil.* 2010 Jul;16(3):315-8.

Kim SJ, Jung JY, Kim HW, Park T. Anti-obesity effects of Juniperus chinensis extract are associated with increased AMP-activated protein kinase expression and phosphorylation in the visceral adipose tissue of rats. *Biol Pharm Bull.* 2008 Jul;31(7):1415-21.

Kim TE, Park SW, Noh G, Lee S. Comparison of skin prick test results between crude allergen extracts from foods and commercial allergen extracts in atopic dermatitis by double-blind placebo-controlled food challenge for milk, egg, and soybean. *Yonsei Med J.* 2002 Oct;43(5):613-20.

Kim YG, Moon JT, Lee KM, Chon NR, Park H. The effects of probiotics on symptoms of irritable bowel syndrome. *Korean J Gastroenterol.* 2006 Jun;47(6):413-9.

Kim YH, Kim KS, Han CS, Yang HC, Park SH, Ko KI, Lee SH, Kim KH, Lee NH, Kim JM, Son K. Inhibitory effects of natural plants of Jeju Island on elastase and MMP-1 expression. *Int J Cosmet Sci.* 2007 Dec;29(6):487-8.

Kimata H. Differential effects of laughter on allergen-specific immunoglobulin and neurotrophin levels in tears. *Percept Mot Skills.* 2004 Jun;98(3 Pt 1):901-8.

Kimata H. Effect of viewing a humorous vs. nonhumorous film on bronchial responsiveness in patients with bronchial asthma. *Physiol Behav.* 2004 Jun;81(4):681-4.

Kimata H. Emotion with tears decreases allergic responses to latex in atopic eczema patients with latex allergy. *J Psychosom Res.* 2006 Jul;61(1):67-9.

Kimata H. Increase in dermcidin-derived peptides in sweat of patients with atopic eczema caused by a humorous video. *J Psychosom Res.* 2007 Jan;62(1):57-9.

Kimata H. Laughter counteracts enhancement of plasma neurotrophin levels and allergic skin wheal responses by mobile phone-mediated stress. *Behav Med.* 2004 Winter;29(4):149-52.

Kimata H. Modulation of fecal polyamines by viewing humorous films in patients with atopic dermatitis. *Eur J Gastroenterol Hepatol.* 2010 Jun;22(6):724-8.

Kimata H. Reduction of allergic responses in atopic infants by mother's laughter. *Eur J Clin Invest.* 2004 Sep;34(9):645-6.

Kimata H. Viewing a humorous film decreases IgE production by seminal B cells from patients with atopic eczema. *J Psychosom Res.* 2009 Feb;66(2):173-5.

Kimata H. Viewing humorous film improves nighttime wakening in children with atopic dermatitis. *Indian Pediatr.* 2007 Apr;44(4):281-5.

Kimata M, Inagaki N, Nagai H. Effects of luteolin and other flavonoids on IgE-mediated allergic reactions. *Planta Med.* 2000 Feb;66(1):25-9.

Kimata M, Shichijo M, Miura T, Serizawa I, Inagaki N, Nagai H. Effects of luteolin, quercetin and baicalein on immunoglobulin E-mediated mediator release from human cultured mast cells. *Clin Exp Allergy.* 2000 Apr;30(4):501-8.

Kimmatkar N, Thawani V, Hingorani L, Khiyani R. Efficacy and tolerability of Boswellia serrata extract in treatment of osteoarthritis of knee—a randomized double blind placebo controlled trial. *Phytomedicine.* 2003 Jan;10(1):3-7.

Kinaciyan T, Jahn-Schmid B, Radakovics A, Zwölfer B, Schreiber C, Francis JN, Ebner C, Bohle B. Successful sublingual immunotherapy with birch pollen has limited effects on concomitant food allergy to apple and the immune response to the Bet v 1 homolog Mal d 1. *J Allergy Clin Immunol.* 2007 Apr;119(4):937-43.

Kinross JM, von Roon AC, Holmes E, Darzi A, Nicholson JK. The human gut microbiome: implications for future health care. *Curr Gastroenterol Rep.* 2008 Aug;10(4):396-403.

Kippelen P, Larsson J, Anderson SD, Brannan JD, Dahlén B, Dahlén SE. Effect of sodium cromoglycate on mast cell mediators during hyperpnea in athletes. *Med Sci Sports Exerc.* 2010 Oct;42(10):1853-60.

Kirjavainen PV, Arvola T, Salminen SJ, Isolauri E. Aberrant composition of gut microbiota of allergic infants: a target of bifidobacterial therapy at weaning? *Gut.* 2002 Jul;51(1):51-5.

REFERENCES AND BIBLIOGRAPHY

Kirjavainen PV, Salminen SJ, Isolauri E. Probiotic bacteria in the management of atopic disease: underscoring the importance of viability. *J Pediatr Gastroenterol Nutr.* 2003 Feb;36(2):223-7.

Kirpich IA, Solovieva NV, Leikhter SN, Shidakova NA, Lebedeva OV, Sidorov PI, Bazhukova TA, Soloviev AG, Barve SS, McClain CJ, Cave M. Probiotics restore bowel flora and improve liver enzymes in human alcohol-induced liver injury: a pilot study. *Alcohol.* 2008 Dec;42(8):675-82.

Kisiel W, Barszcz B. Further sesquiterpenoids and phenolics from Taraxacum officinale. *Fitoterapia.* 2000 Jun;71(3):269-73.

Kisiel W, Michalska K. Sesquiterpenoids and phenolics from Taraxacum hondoense. *Fitoterapia.* 2005 Sep;76(6):520-4.

Kitajima H, Sumida Y, Tanaka R, Yuki N, Takayama H, Fujimura M. Early administration of *Bifidobacterium breve* to preterm infants: randomised controlled trial. *Arch Dis Child Fetal Neonatal Ed.* 1997 Mar;76(2):F101-7.

Klarin B, Johansson ML, Molin G, Larsson A, Jeppsson B. Adhesion of the probiotic bacterium *Lactobacillus plantarum* 299v onto the gut mucosa in critically ill patients: a randomised open trial. *Crit Care.* 2005 Jun;9(3):R285-93.

Klarin B, Molin G, Jeppsson B, Larsson A. Use of the probiotic *Lactobacillus plantarum* 299 to reduce pathogenic bacteria in the oropharynx of intubated patients: a randomised controlled open pilot study. *Crit Care.* 2008;12(6):R136.

Klein A, Friedrich U, Vogelsang H, Jahreis G. *Lactobacillus acidophilus* 74-2 and *Bifidobacterium animalis* subsp *lactis* DGCC 420 modulate unspecific cellular immune response in healthy adults. *Eur J Clin Nutr.* 2008 May;62(5):584-93.

Klein E, Smith D, Laxminarayan R. Trends in Hospitalizations and Deaths in the United States Associated with Infections Caused by Staphylococcus aureus and MRSA, 1999-2004. *Emerging Infectious Diseases.* University of Florida Rel. 2007 Dec 3.

Klein R, Landau MG. *Healing: The Body Betrayed.* Minneapolis: DCI:Chronimed, 1992.

Klein U, Kanellis MJ, Drake D. Effects of four anticaries agents on lesion depth progression in an in vitro caries model. *Pediatr Dent.* 1999 May-Jun;21(3):176-80.

Klein-Galczinsky C. Pharmacological and clinical effectiveness of a fixed phytogenic combination trembling poplar (Populus tremula), true goldenrod (Solidago virgaurea) and ash (Fraxinus excelsior) in mild to moderate rheumatic complaints. *Wien Med Wochenschr.* 1999;149(8-10):248-53.

Klemola T, Vanto T, Juntunen-Backman K, Kalimo K, Korpela R, Varjonen E. Allergy to soy formula and to extensively hydrolyzed whey formula in infants with cow's milk allergy: a prospective, randomized study with a follow-up to the age of 2 years. *J Pediatr.* 2002 Feb;140(2):219-24.

Klima H, Haas O, Roschger P. Photon emission from blood cells and its possible role in immune system regulation. In: Jezowska-Trzebiatowska B. (ed.): *Photon Emission from Biological Systems. Singapore: World Sci.* 1987:153-169.

Klingberg TD, Budde BB. The survival and persistence in the human gastrointestinal tract of five potential probiotic lactobacilli consumed as freeze-dried cultures or as probiotic sausage. *Int J Food Microbiol.* 2006 May 25;109(1-2):157-9.

Kloss J. *Back to Eden.* Twin Oaks, WI: Lotus Press, 1939-1999.

Knutson TW, Bengtsson U, Dannaeus A, Ahlstedt S, Knutson L. Effects of luminal antigen on intestinal albumin and hyaluronan permeability and ion transport in atopic patients. *J Allergy Clin Immunol.* 1996 Jun;97(6):1225-32.

Ko J, Busse PJ, Shek L, Noone SA, Sampson HA, Li XM. Effect of Chinese Herbal Formulas on T Cell Responses in Patients with Peanut Allergy or Asthma. *J Allergy Clin Immunol* .2005;115:S34.

Ko J, Lee JI, Munoz-Furlong A, Li XM, Sicherer SH. Use of complementary and alternative medicine by food-allergic patients. *Ann Allergy Asthma Immunol.* 2006;97:365-9.

Kobayashi I, Hamasaki Y, Sato R, Zaitu M, Muro E, Yamamoto S, Ichimaru T, Miyazaki S. Saiboku-To, a herbal extract mixture, selectively inhibits 5-lipoxygenase activity in leukotriene synthesis in rat basophilic leukemia-1 cells. *J Ethnopharmacol.* 1995 Aug 11;48(1):33-41.

Kohlhammer Y, Döring A, Schäfer T, Wichmann HE, Heinrich J; KORA Study Group. Swimming pool attendance and hay fever rates later in life. *Allergy.* 2006 Nov;61(11):1305-9. PubMed PMID: 17002706.

Kohlhammer Y, Zutavern A, Rzehak P, Woelke G, Heinrich J. Influence of physical inactivity on the prevalence of hay fever. *Allergy.* 2006 Nov;61(11):1310-5.

Kokwaro JO. *Medicinal Plants of East Africa.* Nairobi: Univ of Neirobi Press, 2009.

Kollaritsch H, Holst H, Grobara P, Wiedermann G. Prevention of traveler's diarrhea with *Saccharomyces boulardii.* Results of a placebo controlled double-blind study. *Fortschr Med.* 1993 Mar 30;111(9):152-6.

Kong LF, Guo LH, Zheng XY. Effect of yiqi bushen huoxue herbs in treating children asthma and on levels of nitric oxide, endothelin-1 and serum endothelial cells. *Zhongguo Zhong Xi Yi Jie He Za Zhi.* 2001 Sep;21(9):667-9.

THE LIVING CLEANSE

Koo HN, Hong SH, Song BK, Kim CH, Yoo YH, Kim HM. Taraxacum officinale induces cytotoxicity through TNF-alpha and IL-1alpha secretion in Hep G2 cells. *Life Sci.* 2004 Jan 16;74(9):1149-57.

Koop H, Bachem MG. Serum iron, ferritin, and vitamin B12 during prolonged omeprazole therapy. *J Clin Gastroenterol.* 1992;14:288-92.

Kootstra HS, Vlieg-Boerstra BJ, Dubois AE. Assessment of the reduced allergenic properties of the Santana apple. *Ann Allergy Asthma Immunol.* 2007 Dec;99(6):522-5.

Korschunov VM, Smeianov VV, Efimov BA, Tarabrina NP, Ivanov AA, Baranov AE. Therapeutic use of an antibiotic-resistant *Bifidobacterium* preparation in men exposed to high-dose gamma-irradiation. *J Med Microbiol.* 1996 Jan;44(1):70-4.

Kositz C, Schroecksnadel K, Grander G, Schennach H, Kofler H, Fuchs D. High serum tryptophan concentration in pollinosis patients is associated with unresponsiveness to pollen extract therapy. *Int Arch Allergy Immunol.* 2008;147(1):35-40.

Kotowska M, Albrecht P, Szajewska H. *Saccharomyces boulardii* in the prevention of antibiotic-associated diarrhoea in children: a randomized double-blind placebo-controlled trial. *Aliment Pharmacol Ther.* 2005 Mar 1;21(5):583-90.

Kotzampassi K, Giamarellos-Bourboulis EJ, Voudouris A, Kazamias P, Eleftheriadis E. Benefits of a synbiotic formula (Synbiotic 2000Forte) in critically Ill trauma patients: early results of a randomized controlled trial. *World J Surg.* 2006 Oct;30(10):1848-55.

Kotzampassi K, Giamarellos-Bourboulis EJ, Voudouris A, Kazamias P, Eleftheriadis E. Benefits of a synbiotic formula (Synbiotic 2000Forte) in critically Ill trauma patients: early results of a randomized controlled trial. *World J Surg.* 2006 Oct;30(10):1848-55.

Kovács T, Mette H, Per B, Kun L, Schmelczer M, Barta J, Jean-Claude D, Nagy J. Relationship between intestinal permeability and antibodies against food antigens in IgA nephropathy. *Orv Hetil.* 1996 Jan 14;137(2):65-9.

Kowalchik C, Hylton W (eds). *Rodale's Illustrated Encyclopedia of Herbs.* Emmaus, PA: 1987.

Kowalczyk E, Krzesiński P, Kura M, Niedworok J, Kowalski J, Błaszczyk J. Pharmacological effects of flavonoids from Scutellaria baicalensis. *Przegl Lek.* 2006;63(2):95-6.

Kozlowski LT, Mehta NY, Sweeney CT, Schwartz SS, Vogler GP, Jarvis MJ, West RJ. Filter ventilation and nicotine content of tobacco in cigarettes from Canada, the United Kingdom, and the United States. *Tob Control.* 1998 Winter;7(4):369-75.

Krasse P, Carlsson B, Dahl C, Paulsson A, Nilsson A, Sinkiewicz G. Decreased gum bleeding and reduced gingivitis by the probiotic *Lactobacillus reuteri. Swed Dent J.* 2006;30(2):55-60.

Kreig M. *Black Market Medicine.* New York: Bantam, 1968.

Kremmyda LS, Vlachava M, Noakes PS, Diaper ND, Miles EA, Calder PC. Atopy Risk in Infants and Children in Relation to Early Exposure to Fish, Oily Fish, or Long-Chain Omega-3 Fatty Acids: A Systematic Review. *Clin Rev Allergy Immunol.* 2009 Dec 9.

Krogulska A, Dynowski J, Wasowska-Królikowska K. Bronchial reactivity in schoolchildren allergic to food. *Ann Allergy Asthma Immunol.* 2010 Jul;105(1):31-8.

Krogulska A, Wasowska-Królikowska K, Dynowski J. Evaluation of bronchial hyperreactivity in children with asthma undergoing food challenges. *Pol Merkur Lekarski.* 2007 Jul;23(133):30-5.

Krogulska A, Wasowska-Królikowska K, Polakowska E, Chrul S. Cytokine profile in children with asthma undergoing food challenges. *J Investig Allergol Clin Immunol.* 2009;19(1):43-8.

Krogulska A, Wasowska-Królikowska K, Polakowska E, Chrul S. Evaluation of receptor expression on immune system cells in the peripheral blood of asthmatic children undergoing food challenges. Int Arch Allergy Immunol. 2009;150(4):377-88. 2009 Jul 1.

Krogulska A, Wasowska-Królikowska K, Trzeźwińska B. Food challenges in children with asthma. *Pol Merkur Lekarski.* 2007 Jul;23(133):22-9.

Kroidl RF, Schwichtenberg U, Frank E. Bronchial asthma due to storage mite allergy. Pneumologie. 2007 Aug;61(8):525-30.

Krueger AP, Reed EJ. Biological impact of small air ions. Science. 1976 Sep 24;193(4259):1209-13.

Kruger K, Kamilli I, Schattenkirchner M. Blastocystis hominis as a rare arthritogenic pathogen. *Z Rheumatol.* 1994 Mar-Apr;53(2):83-5.

Krüger P, Kanzer J, Hummel J, Fricker G, Schubert-Zsilavecz M, Abdel-Tawab M. Permeation of Boswellia extract in the Caco-2 model and possible interactions of its constituents KBA and AKBA with OATP1B3 and MRP2. *Eur J Pharm Sci.* 2009 Feb 15;36(2-3):275-84.

Kubota A, He F, Kawase M, Harata G, Hiramatsu M, Iino H. Diversity of intestinal bifidobacteria in patients with Japanese cedar pollinosis and possible influence of probiotic intervention. *Curr Microbiol.* 2011 Jan;62(1):71-7.

Kubota A, He F, Kawase M, Harata G, Hiramatsu M, Salminen S, Iino H. Lactobacillus strains stabilize intestinal microbiota in Japanese cedar pollinosis patients. *Microbiol Immunol.* 2009 Apr;53(4):198-205.

REFERENCES AND BIBLIOGRAPHY

Kuitunen M, Kukkonen K, Juntunen-Backman K, Korpela R, Poussa T, Tuure T, Haahtela T, Savilahti E. Probiotics prevent IgE-associated allergy until age 5 years in Cesarean-delivered children but not in the total cohort. *J Allergy Clin Immunol.* 2009 Feb;123(2):335-41.

Kuitunen M, Savilahti E, Sarnesto A. Human alpha-lactalbumin and bovine beta-lactoglobulin absorption in infants. *Allergy.* 1994 May;49(5):354-60.

Kuitunen M, Savilahti E. Mucosal IgA, mucosal cow's milk antibodies, serum cow's milk antibodies and gastrointestinal permeability in infants. *Pediatr Allergy Immunol.* 1995 Feb;6(1):30-5.

Kukkonen K, Kuitunen M, Haahtela T, Korpela R, Poussa T, Savilahti E. High intestinal IgA associates with reduced risk of IgE-associated allergic diseases. *Pediatr Allergy Immunol.* 2010 Feb;21(1 Pt 1):67-73.

Kukkonen K, Nieminen T, Poussa T, Savilahti E, Kuitunen M. Effect of probiotics on vaccine antibody responses in infancy—a randomized placebo-controlled double-blind trial. *Pediatr Allergy Immunol.* 2006 Sep;17(6):416-21.

Kukkonen K, Savilahti E, Haahtela T, Juntunen-Backman K, Korpela R, Poussa T, Tuure T, Kuitunen M. Probiotics and prebiotic galacto-oligosaccharides in the prevention of allergic diseases: a randomized, double-blind, placebo-controlled trial. *J Allergy Clin Immunol.* 2007 Jan;119(1):192-8.

Kukkonen K, Savilahti E, Haahtela T, Juntunen-Backman K, Korpela R, Poussa T, Tuure T, Kuitunen M. Long-term safety and impact on infection rates of postnatal probiotic and prebiotic (synbiotic) treatment: randomized, double-blind, placebo-controlled trial. *Pediatrics.* 2008 Jul;122(1):8-12.

Kukkonen K, Savilahti E, Haahtela T, Juntunen-Backman K, Korpela R, Poussa T, Tuure T, Kuitunen M. Probiotics and prebiotic galacto-oligosaccharides in the prevention of allergic diseases: a randomized, double-blind, placebo-controlled trial. *J Allergy Clin Immunol.* 2007 Jan;119(1):192-8.

Kulka M. The potential of natural products as effective treatments for allergic inflammation: implications for allergic rhinitis. *Curr Top Med Chem.* 2009;9(17):1611-24.

Kull I, Bergström A, Lilja G, Pershagen G, Wickman M. Fish consumption during the first year of life and development of allergic diseases during childhood. *Allergy.* 2006 Aug;61(8):1009-15.

Kull I, Melen E, Alm J, Hallberg J, Svartengren M, van Hage M, Pershagen G, Wickman M, Bergström A. Breast-feeding in relation to asthma, lung function, and sensitization in young schoolchildren. *J Allergy Clin Immunol.* 2010 May;125(5):1013-9.

Kullo IJ, Ballantyne CM. Conditional risk factors for atherosclerosis. *Mayo Clin Proc.* 2005 Feb;80(2):219-30.

Kumar A, Panghal S, Mallapur SS, Kumar M, Ram V, Singh BK. Antiinflammatory Activity of Piper longum Fruit Oil. *Indian J Pharm Sci.* 2009 Jul;71(4):454-6.

Kumar A, Saluja AK, Shah UD, Mayavanshi AV. Pharmacological potential of Albizzia lebbeck: A Review. *Pharmacog.* 2007 Jan-May; 1(1) 171-174.

Kumar R, Singh BP, Srivastava P, Sridhara S, Arora N, Gaur SN. Relevance of serum IgE estimation in allergic bronchial asthma with special reference to food allergy. *Asian Pac J Allergy Immunol.* 2006 Dec;24(4):191-9.

Kummeling I, Mills EN, Clausen M, Dubakiene R, Pérez CF, Fernández-Rivas M, Knulst AC, Kowalski ML, Lidholm J, Le TM, Metzler C, Mustakov T, Popov T, Potts J, van Ree R, Sakellariou A, Töndury B, Tzannis K, Burney P. The EuroPrevall surveys on the prevalence of food allergies in children and adults: background and study methodology. *Allergy.* 2009 Oct;64(10):1493-7.

Kung HC, Hoyert DL, Xu J, Murphy SL. Deaths: Final Data for 2005. *National Vital Statistics Reports.* 2008;56(10). http://www.cdc.gov/nchs/data/ nvsr/nvsr56/nvsr56_10.pdf. Accessed: 2008 Jun.

Kunisawa J, Kiyono H. Aberrant interaction of the gut immune system with environmental factors in the development of food allergies. *Curr Allergy Asthma Rep.* 2010 May;10(3):215-21.

Kurth T, Barr RG, Gaziano JM, Buring JE. Randomised aspirin assignment and risk of adult-onset asthma in the Women's Health Study. *Thorax.* 2008 Jun;63(6):514-8. 2008 Mar 13.

Kurugöl Z, Koturoğlu G. Effects of *Saccharomyces boulardii* in children with acute diarrhoea. *Acta Paediatr.* 2005 Jan;94(1):44-7.

Kusunoki T, Morimoto T, Nishikomori R, Yasumi T, Heike T, Mukaida K, Fujii T, Nakahata T. Breastfeeding and the prevalence of allergic diseases in schoolchildren: Does reverse causation matter? *Pediatr Allergy Immunol.* 2010 Feb;21(1 Pt 1):60-6.

Kuvaeva IB. Permeability of the gastrointestinal tract for macromolecules in health and disease. *Hum Physiol.* 1979 Mar-Apr;4(2):272-83.

Kuz'mina IaS, Vavilova NN. Kinesitherapy of patients with bronchial asthma and excessive body weight at the early stage of rehabilitation treatment. *Vopr Kurortol Fizioter Lech Fiz Kult.* 2009 Sep-Oct;(5):17-20.

Kuznetsov VF, Iushchuk ND, Iurko LP, Nabokova NIu. Intestinal dysbacteriosis in yersiniosis patients and the possibility of its correction with biopreparations. *Ter Arkh.* 1994;66(11):17-8.

Kuznetsova TA, Shevchenko NM, Zviagintseva TN, Besednova NN. Biological activity of fucoidans from brown algae and the prospects of their use in medicine]. *Antibiot Khimioter.* 2004;49(5):24-30.

Kvamme JM, Wilsgaard T, Florholmen J, Jacobsen BK. Body mass index and disease burden in elderly men and women: the Tromsø Study. *Eur J Epidemiol.* 2010 Mar;25(3):183-93. 2010 Jan 20.

Lad V. *Ayurveda: The Science of Self-Healing.* Twin Lakes, WI: Lotus Press.

Laitinen K, Isolauri E. Management of food allergy: vitamins, fatty acids or probiotics? *Eur J Gastroenterol Hepatol.* 2005 Dec;17(12):1305-11.

Laitinen K, Poussa T, Isolauri E; Nutrition, Allergy, Mucosal Immunology and Intestinal Microbiota Group. Probiotics and dietary counselling contribute to glucose regulation during and after pregnancy: a randomised controlled trial. *Br J Nutr.* 2009 Jun;101(11):1679-87.

Lamaison JL, Carnat A, Petitjean-Freytet C. Tannin content and inhibiting activity of elastase in Rosaceae. *Ann Pharm Fr.* 1990;48(6):335-40.

Landmark K, Reikvam A. Do vitamins C and E protect against the development of carotid stenosis and cardiovascular disease? *Tidsskr Nor Laegeforen.* 2005 Jan 20;125(2):159-62.

Laney AS, Cragin LA, Blevins LZ, Sumner AD, Cox-Ganser JM, Kreiss K, Moffatt SG, Lohff CJ. Sarcoidosis, asthma, and asthma-like symptoms among occupants of a historically water-damaged office building. *Indoor Air.* 2009 Feb;19(1):83-90.

Lang CJ, Hansen M, Roscioli E, Jones J, Murgia C, Leigh Ackland M, Zalewski P, Anderson G, Ruffin R. Dietary zinc mediates inflammation and protects against wasting and metabolic derangement caused by sustained cigarette smoke exposure in mice. *Biometals.* 2011 Feb;24(1):23-39. 2010 Aug 29.

Lange NE, Rifas-Shiman SL, Camargo CA Jr, Gold DR, Gillman MW, Litonjua AA. Maternal dietary pattern during pregnancy is not associated with recurrent wheeze in children. *J Allergy Clin Immunol.* 2010 Aug;126(2):250-5, 255.e1-4.

Langhendries JP, Detry J, Van Hees J, Lamboray JM, Darimont J, Mozin MJ, Secretin MC, Senterre J. Effect of a fermented infant formula containing viable bifidobacteria on the fecal flora composition and pH of healthy full-term infants. *J Pediatr Gastroenterol Nutr.* 1995 Aug;21(2):177-81.

Lappe FM. *Diet for a Small Planet.* New York: Ballantine, 1971.

Lara-Villoslada F, Sierra S, Boza J, Xaus J, Olivares M. Beneficial effects of consumption of a dairy product containing two probiotic strains, Lactobacillus coryniformis CECT5711 and *Lactobacillus gasseri* CECT5714 in healthy children. *Nutr Hosp.* 2007 Jul-Aug;22(4):496-502.

Larenas-Linnemann D, Matta JJ, Shah-Hosseini K, Michels A, Mösges R. Skin prick test evaluation of Dermatophagoides pteronyssinus diagnostic extracts from Europe, Mexico, and the United States. *Ann Allergy Asthma Immunol.* 2010 May;104(5):420-5.

Lau BH, Riesen SK, Truong KP, Lau EW, Rohdewald P, Barreta RA. Pycnogenol as an adjunct in the management of childhood asthma. *J Asthma.* 2004;41(8):825-32.

Laubereau B, Filipiak-Pittroff B, von Berg A, Grübl A, Reinhardt D, Wichmann HE, Koletzko S; GINI Study Group. Caesarean section and gastrointestinal symptoms, atopic dermatitis, and sensitisation during the first year of life. *Arch Dis Child.* 2004 Nov;89(11):993-7.

Laurière M, Pecquet C, Bouchez-Mahiout I, Snégaroff J, Bayrou O, Raison-Peyron N, Vigan M. Hydrolysed wheat proteins present in cosmetics can induce immediate hypersensitivities. *Contact Dermatitis.* 2006 May;54(5):283-9.

LaValle JB. *The Cox-2 Connection.* Rochester, VT: Healing Arts, 2001.

Lazarou J, Pomeranz BH, Corey PN. Incidence of adverse drug reactions in hospitalized patients: a meta-analysis of prospective studies. *JAMA.* 1998 Apr.

Leal AL, Eslava-Schmalbach J, Alvarez C, Buitrago G, Méndez M; Grupo para el Control de la Resistencia Bacteriana en Bogotá. Endemic tendencies and bacterial resistance markers in third-level hospitals in Bogotá, Colombia. Rev Salud Publica (Bogota). 2006 May;8 Suppl 1:59-70.

Lean G. US study links more than 200 diseases to pollution. *London Independent.* 2004 Nov 14.

Leander M, Cronqvist A, Janson C, Uddenfeldt M, Rask-Andersen A. Health-related quality of life predicts onset of asthma in a longitudinal population study. *Respir Med.* 2009 Feb;103(2):194-200.

Lecheler J, Pfannebecker B, Nguyen DT, Petzold U, Munzel U, Kremer HJ, Maus J. Prevention of exercise-induced asthma by a fixed combination of disodium cromoglycate plus reproterol compared with montelukast in young patients. *Arzneimittelforschung.* 2008;58(6):303-9.

Lee E, Haa K, Yook JM, Jin MH, Seo CS, Son KH, Kim HP, Bae KH, Kang SS, Son JK, Chang HW. Anti-asthmatic activity of an ethanol extract from Saururus chinensis. *Biol Pharm Bull.* 2006 Feb;29(2):211-5.

Lee JH, Noh J, Noh G, Kim HS, Mun SH, Choi WS, Cho S, Lee S. Allergen-specific B cell subset responses in cow's milk allergy of late eczematous reactions in atopic dermatitis. *Cell Immunol.* 2010;262(1):44-51.

Lee JY, Kim CJ. Determination of allergenic egg proteins in food by protein-, mass spectrometry-, and DNA-based methods. *J AOAC Int.* 2010 Mar-Apr;93(2):462-77.

Lee KH, Yeh MH, Kao ST, Hung CM, Chen BC, Liu CJ, Yeh CC. Xia-bai-san inhibits lipopolysaccharide-induced activation of intercellular adhesion molecule-1 and nuclear factor-kappa B in human lung cells. *J Ethnopharmacol.* 2009 Jul 30;124(3):530-8.

Lee MC, Lin LH, Hung KL, Wu HY. Oral bacterial therapy promotes recovery from acute diarrhea in children. *Acta Paediatr Taiwan.* 2001 Sep-Oct;42(5):301-5.

Lee SJ, Cho SJ, Park EA. Effects of probiotics on enteric flora and feeding tolerance in preterm infants. *Neonatology.* 2007;91(3):174-9.

Lee SJ, Shim YH, Cho SJ, Lee JW. Probiotics prophylaxis in children with persistent primary vesicoureteral reflux. *Pediatr Nephrol.* 2007 Sep;22(9):1315-20.

Lee TH, Hsueh PR, Yeh WC, Wang HP, Wang TH, Lin JT. Low frequency of bacteremia after endoscopic mucosal resection. *Gastrointest Endosc.* 2000 Aug;52(2):223-5.

Lee YS, Kim SH, Jung SH, Kim JK, Pan CH, Lim SS. Aldose reductase inhibitory compounds from Glycyrrhiza uralensis. *Biol Pharm Bull.* 2010;33(5):917-21.

Léger D, Annesi-Maesano I, Carat F, Rugina M, Chanal I, Pribil C, El Hasnaoui A, Bousquet J. Allergic rhinitis and its consequences on quality of sleep: An unexplored area. *Arch Intern Med.* 2006 Sep 18;166(16):1744-8.

Lehmann B. The vitamin D3 pathway in human skin and its role for regulation of biological processes. *Photochem Photobiol.* 2005 Nov-Dec;81(6):1246-51.

Lehto M, Airaksinen L, Puustinen A, Tillander S, Hannula S, Nyman T, Toskala E, Alenius H, Lauerma A. Thaumatin-like protein and baker's respiratory allergy. *Ann Allergy Asthma Immunol.* 2010 Feb;104(2):139-46.

Leitzmann C. Vegetarian diets: what are the advantages? *Forum Nutr.* 2005;(57):147-56.

Léonard R, Wopfner N, Pabst M, Stadlmann J, Petersen BO, Duus JØ, Himly M, Radauer C, Gadermaier G, Razzazi-Fazeli E, Ferreira F, Altmann F. A new allergen from ragweed (Ambrosia artemisiifolia) with homology to art v 1 from mugwort. *J Biol Chem.* 2010 Aug 27;285(35):27192-200.

Lerman RH, Minich DM, Darland G, Lamb JJ, Chang JL, Hsi A, Bland JS, Tripp ML. Subjects with elevated LDL cholesterol and metabolic syndrome benefit from supplementation with soy protein, phytosterols, hops rho iso-alpha acids, and Acacia nilotica proanthocyanidins. J Clin Lipidol. 2010 Jan-Feb;4(1):59-68.

Leu YL, Shi LS, Damu AG. Chemical constituents of Taraxacum formosanum. Chem *Pharm Bull.* 2003 May;51(5):599-601.

Leu YL, Wang YL, Huang SC, Shi LS. Chemical constituents from roots of Taraxacum formosanum. *Chem Pharm Bull.* 2005 Jul;53(7):853-5.

Leung DY, Sampson HA, Yunginger JW, Burks AW Jr, Schneider LC, Wortel CH, Davis FM, Hyun JD, Shanahan WR Jr; Avon Longitudinal Study of Parents and Children Study Team. Effect of anti-IgE therapy in patients with peanut allergy. *N Engl J Med.* 2003 Mar 13;348(11):986-93.

Leung DY, Shanahan WR Jr, Li XM, Sampson HA. New approaches for the treatment of anaphylaxis. *Novartis Found Symp.* 2004;257:248-60; discussion 260-4, 276-85.

Lewerin C, Jacobsson S, Lindstedt G, Nilsson-Ehle H. Serum biomarkers for atrophic gastritis and antibodies against Helicobacter pylori in the elderly: Implications for vitamin B12, folic acid and iron status and response to oral vitamin therapy. *Scand J Gastroenterol.* 2008;43(9):1050-6.

Lewis SA, Grimshaw KE, Warner JO, Hourihane JO. The promiscuity of immunoglobulin E binding to peanut allergens, as determined by Western blotting, correlates with the severity of clinical symptoms. *Clin Exp Allergy.* 2005 Jun;35(6):767-73.

Lewis WH, Elvin-Lewis MPF. *Medical Botany: Plants Affecting Man's Health.* New York: Wiley, 1977.

Lewontin R. *The Genetic Basis of Evolutionary Change.* New York: Columbia Univ Press, 1974.

Leyel CF. *Culpeper's English Physician & Complete Herbal.* Hollywood, CA: Wilshire, 1971.

Leynadier F. Mast cells and basophils in asthma. Ann Biol Clin (Paris). 1989;47(6):351-6.

Li J, Sun B, Huang Y, Lin X, Zhao D, Tan G, Wu J, Zhao H, Cao L, Zhong N. A multicentre study assessing the prevalence of sensitizations in patients with asthma and/or rhinitis in China. *Allergy.* 2009;64:1083-1092.

Li MH, Zhang HL, Yang BY. Effects of ginkgo leaf concentrated oral liquor in treating asthma. *Zhongguo Zhong Xi Yi Jie He Za Zhi.* 1997 Apr;17(4):216-8. 5.

Li Q, Li XL, Yang X, Bao JM, Shen XH. Effects of antiallergic herbal agents on cystic fibrosis transmembrane conductance regulator in nasal mucosal epithelia of allergic rhinitis rabbits. *Chin Med J (Engl).* 2009 Dec 20;122(24):3020-4.

Li S, Li W, Wang Y, Asada Y, Koike K. Prenylflavonoids from Glycyrrhiza uralensis and their protein tyrosine phosphatase-1B inhibitory activities. *Bioorg Med Chem Lett.* 2010 Sep 15;20(18):5398-401.

Li XM, Huang CK, Zhang TF, Teper AA, Srivastava K, Schofield BH, Sampson HA. The chinese herbal medicine formula MSSM-002 suppresses allergic airway hyperreactivity and modulates TH1/TH2 responses in a murine model of allergic asthma. *J Allergy Clin Immunol.* 2000;106:660-8.

Li XM, Srivastava K. Traditional Chinese medicine for the therapy of allergic disorders. *Curr Opin Otolaryngol Head Neck Surg.* 2006 Jun;14(3):191-6.

Li XM, Zhang TF, Huang CK, Srivastava K, Teper AA, Zhang L, Schofield BH, Sampson HA. Food Allergy Herbal Formula-1 (FAHF-1) blocks peanut-induced anaphylaxis in a murine model. *J Allergy Clin Immunol.* 2001;108:639-46.

Li XM, Zhang TF, Sampson H, Zou ZM, Beyer K, Wen MC, Schofield B. The potential use of Chinese herbal medicines in treating allergic asthma. *Ann Allergy Asthma Immunol.* 2004;93:S35-S44.

Li XM. Beyond allergen avoidance: update on developing therapies for peanut allergy. *Curr Opin Allergy Clin Immunol.* 2005;5:287-92.

Li YQ, Yuan W, Zhang SL. Clinical and experimental study of xiao er ke cuan ling oral liquid in the treatment of infantile bronchopneumonia. *Zhongguo Zhong Xi Yi Jie He Za Zhi.* 1992 Dec;12(12):719-21, 737, 708.

Lied GA, Lillestøl K, Valeur J, Berstad A. Intestinal B cell-activating factor: an indicator of non-IgE-mediated hypersensitivity reactions to food? *Aliment Pharmacol Ther.* 2010 Jul;32(1):66-73.

Lieske JC, Goldfarb DS, De Simone C, Regnier C. Use of a probiotic to decrease enteric hyperoxaluria. *Kidney Int.* 2005 Sep;68(3):1244-9.

Lillestøl K, Berstad A, Lind R, Florvaag E, Arslan Lied G, Tangen T. Anxiety and depression in patients with self-reported food hypersensitivity. *Gen Hosp Psychiatry.* 2010 Jan-Feb;32(1):42-8.

Lima JA, Fischer GB, Sarria EE, Mattiello R, Solé D. Prevalence of and risk factors for wheezing in the first year of life. *J Bras Pneumol.* 2010 Oct;36(5):525-31. English, Portuguese.

Limb SL, Brown KC, Wood RA, Wise RA, Eggleston PA, Tonascia J, Hamilton RG, Adkinson NF Jr. Adult asthma severity in individuals with a history of childhood asthma. *J Allergy Clin Immunol.* 2005 Jan;115(1):61-6.

Lin HC, Hsu CH, Chen HL, Chung MY, Hsu JF, Lien RI, Tsao LY, Chen CH, Su BH. Oral probiotics prevent necrotizing enterocolitis in very low birth weight preterm infants: a multicenter, randomized, controlled trial. *Pediatrics.* 2008 Oct;122(4):693-700.

Lin HC, Su BH, Chen AC, Lin TW, Tsai CH, Yeh TF, Oh W. Oral probiotics reduce the incidence and severity of necrotizing enterocolitis in very low birth weight infants. *Pediatrics.* 2005 Jan;115(1):1-4.

Lin JS, Chiu YH, Lin NT, Chu CH, Huang KC, Liao KW, Peng KC. Different effects of probiotic species/strains on infections in preschool children: A double-blind, randomized, controlled study. *Vaccine.* 2009 Feb 11;27(7):1073-9.

Lin SY, Ayres JW, Winkler W Jr, Sandine WE. Lactobacillus effects on cholesterol: in vitro and in vivo results. *J Dairy Sci.* 1989 Nov;72(11):2885-99.

Lindahl O, Lindwall L, Spångberg A, Stenram A, Ockerman PA. Vegan regimen with reduced medication in the treatment of bronchial asthma. *J Asthma.* 1985;22(1):45-55.

Ling WH, Hänninen O. Shifting from a conventional diet to an uncooked vegan diet reversibly alters fecal hydrolytic activities in humans. *J Nutr.* 1992 Apr;122(4):924-30.

Ling WH, Hänninen O. Shifting from a conventional diet to an uncooked vegan diet reversibly alters fecal hydrolytic activities in humans. *J Nutr.* 1992 Apr;122(4):924-30.

Lininger S, Gaby A, Austin S, Brown D, Wright J, Duncan A. *The Natural Pharmacy.* New York: Three Rivers, 1999.

Lininger S, Gaby A, Austin S, Brown D, Wright J, Duncan A. *The Natural Pharmacy.* New York: Three Rivers, 1999.

Linsalata M, Russo F, Berloco P, Caruso ML, Matteo GD, Cifone MG, Simone CD, Ierardi E, Di Leo A. The influence of Lactobacillus brevis on ornithine decarboxylase activity and polyamine profiles in Helicobacter pylori-infected gastric mucosa. Helicobacter. 2004 Apr;9(2):165-72.

Linsalata M, Russo F, Berloco P, Caruso ML, Matteo GD, Cifone MG, Simone CD, Ierardi E, Di Leo A. The influence of *Lactobacillus brevis* on ornithine decarboxylase activity and polyamine profiles in *Helicobacter pylori*-infected gastric mucosa. *Helicobacter.* 2004 Apr;9(2):165-72.

Lipkind M. Registration of spontaneous photon emission from virus-infected cell cultures: development of experimental system. *Indian J Exp Biol.* 2003 May;41(5):457-72.

Lipski E. *Digestive Wellness.* Los Angeles, CA: Keats, 2000.

Lipski E. *Digestive Wellness.* Los Angeles, CA: Keats, 2000.

Liu AH, Jaramillo R, Sicherer SH, Wood RA, Bock SA, Burks AW, Massing M, Cohn RD, Zeldin DC. National prevalence and risk factors for food allergy and relationship to asthma: results from the National Health and Nutrition Examination Survey 2005-2006. *J Allergy Clin Immunol.* 2010 Oct;126(4):798-806.e13.

Liu F, Zhang J, Liu Y, Zhang N, Holtappels G, Lin P, Liu S, Bachert C. Inflammatory profiles in nasal mucosa of patients with persistent vs intermittent allergic rhinitis. *Allergy.* 2010 Sep;65(9):1149-57.

Liu GM, Cao MJ, Huang YY, Cai QF, Weng WY, Su WJ. Comparative study of in vitro digestibility of major allergen tropomyosin and other food proteins of Chinese mitten crab (Eriocheir sinensis). *J Sci Food Agric.* 2010 Aug 15;90(10):1614-20.

Liu HY, Giday Z, Moore BF. Possible pathogenetic mechanisms producing bovine milk protein inducible malabsorption: a hypothesis. *Ann Allergy.* 1977 Jul;39(1):1-7.

Liu J, Zhang J, Shi Y, Grimsgaard S, Alraek T, Fønnebø V. Chinese red yeast rice (Monascus purpureus) for primary hyperlipidemia: a meta-analysis of randomized controlled trials. *Chin Med.* 2006 Nov 23;1:4.

Liu JY, Hu JH, Zhu QG, Li FQ, Wang J, Sun HJ. Effect of matrine on the expression of substance P receptor and inflammatory cytokines production in human skin keratinocytes and fibroblasts. *Int Immunopharmacol.* 2007 Jun;7(6):816-23.

REFERENCES AND BIBLIOGRAPHY

Liu T, Valdez R, Yoon PW, Crocker D, Moonesinghe R, Khoury MJ. The association between family history of asthma and the prevalence of asthma among US adults: National Health and Nutrition Examination Survey, 1999-2004. *Genet Med.* 2009 May;11(5):323-8.

Liu X, Beaty TH, Deindl P, Huang SK, Lau S, Sommerfeld C, Fallin MD, Kao WH, Wahn U, Nickel R. Associations between specific serum IgE response and 6 variants within the genes IL4, IL13, and IL4RA in German children: the German Multicenter Atopy Study. *J Allergy Clin Immunol.* 2004 Mar;113(3):489-95.

Liu XJ, Cao MA, Li WH, Shen CS, Yan SQ, Yuan CS. Alkaloids from Sophora flavescens Aition. *Fitoterapia.* 2010 Sep;81(6):524-7.

Liu Z, Bhattacharyya S, Ning B, Midoro-Horiuti T, Czerwinski EW, Goldblum RM, Mort A, Kearney CM. Plant-expressed recombinant mountain cedar allergen Jun a 1 is allergenic and has limited pectate lyase activity. *Int Arch Allergy Immunol.* 2010;153(4):347-58.

Lloyd JU. *American Materia Medica, Therapeutics and Pharmacognosy.* Portland, OR: Eclectic Medical Publications, 1989-1983.

Lloyd Spencer J. Immunization via the anal mucosa and adjacent skin to protect against respiratory virus infections and allergic rhinitis: a hypothesis. *Med Hypotheses.* 2010 Mar;74(3):542-6.

Lloyd-Still JD, Powers CA, Hoffman DR, Boyd-Trull K, Lester LA, Benisek DC, Arterburn LM. Bioavailability and safety of a high dose of docosahexaenoic acid triacylglycerol of algal origin in cystic fibrosis patients: a randomized, controlled study. *Nutrition.* 2006 Jan;22(1):36-46.

Locke GR 3rd, Talley NJ, Fett SL, Zinsmeister AR, Melton LJ 3rd. Prevalence and clinical spectrum of gastroesophageal reflux: a population-based study in Olmsted County, Minnesota. *Gastroenterology.* 1997 May;112(5):1448-56.

Loguercio C, Abbiati R, Rinaldi M, Romano A, Del Vecchio Blanco C, Coltorti M. Long-term effects of *Enterococcus faecium* SF68 versus lactulose in the treatment of patients with cirrhosis and grade 1-2 hepatic encephalopathy. *J Hepatol.* 1995 Jul;23(1):39-46.

Loguercio C, Del Vecchio Blanco C, Coltorti M. Enterococcus lactic acid bacteria strain SF68 and lactulose in hepatic encephalopathy: a controlled study. *J Int Med Res.* 1987 Nov-Dec;15(6):335-43.

Loizzo MR, Saab AM, Tundis R, Statti GA, Menichini F, Lampronti I, Gambari R, Cinatl J, Doerr HW. Phytochemical analysis and in vitro antiviral activities of the essential oils of seven Lebanon species. *Chem Biodivers.* 2008 Mar;5(3):461-70.

Lomax AR, Calder PC. Probiotics, immune function, infection and inflammation: a review of the evidence from studies conducted in humans. *Curr Pharm Des.* 2009;15(13):1428-518.

Longo G, Barbi E, Berti I, Meneghetti R, Pittalis A, Ronfani L, Ventura A. Specific oral tolerance induction in children with very severe cow's milk-induced reactions. *J Allergy Clin Immunol.* 2008 Feb;121(2):343-7.

Lopes EA, Fanelli-Galvani A, Prisco CC, Gonçalves RC, Jacob CM, Cabral AL, Martins MA, Carvalho CR. Assessment of muscle shortening and static posture in children with persistent asthma. *Eur J Pediatr.* 2007 Jul;166(7):715-21.

López N, de Barros-Mazón S, Vilela MM, Silva CM, Ribeiro JD. Genetic and environmental influences on atopic immune response in early life. *J Investig Allergol Clin Immunol.* 1999 Nov-Dec;9(6):392-8.

Lopez-Garcia E, Schulze MB, Meigs JB, Manson JE, Rifai N, Stampfer MJ, Willett WC, Hu FB. Consumption of trans fatty acids is related to plasma biomarkers of inflammation and endothelial dysfunction. *J Nutr.* 2005 Mar;135(3):562-6.

Lopez-Garcia E, Schulze MB, Meigs JB, Manson JE, Rifai N, Stampfer MJ, Willett WC, Hu FB. Consumption of trans fatty acids is related to plasma biomarkers of inflammation and endothelial dysfunction. *J Nutr.* 2005 Mar;135(3):562-6.

Lorea Baroja M, Kirjavainen PV, Hekmat S, Reid G. Anti-inflammatory effects of probiotic yogurt in inflammatory bowel disease patients. *Clin Exp Immunol.* 2007 Sep;149(3):470-9.

Lu MK, Shih YW, Chang Chien TT, Fang LH, Huang HC, Chen PS. α-Solanine inhibits human melanoma cell migration and invasion by reducing matrix metalloproteinase-2/9 activities. *Biol Pharm Bull.* 2010;33(10):1685-91.

Lucas A, Brooke OG, Cole TJ, Morley R, Bamford MF. Food and drug reactions, wheezing, and eczema in preterm infants. *Arch Dis Child.* 1990 Apr;65(4):411-5. 8; .

Lucendo AJ, Lucendo B. An update on the immunopathogenesis of eosinophilic esophagitis. *Expert Rev Gastroenterol Hepatol.* 2010 Apr;4(2):141-8.

Lunardi AC, Marques da Silva CC, Rodrigues Mendes FA, Marques AP, Stelmach R, Fernandes Carvalho CR. Musculoskeletal dysfunction and pain in adults with asthma. *J Asthma.* 2011 Feb;48(1):105-10.

Lv X, Xi L, Han D, Zhang L. Evaluation of the psychological status in seasonal allergic rhinitis patients. *ORL J Otorhinolaryngol Relat Spec.* 2010;72(2):84-90.

Lykken DT, Tellegen A, DeRubeis R: Volunteer bias in twin research: the rule of two-thirds. *Soc Biol* 1978, 25(1): 1-9. Phillips DI: Twin studies in medical research: can they tell us whether diseases are genetically determined? *Lancet* 1993;341(8851): 1008-1009.

Lythcott GI. Anaphylaxis to viomycin. *Am Rev Tuberc.* 1957 Jan;75(1):135-8.

Ma J, Xiao L, Knowles SB. Obesity, insulin resistance and the prevalence of atopy and asthma in US adults. *Allergy.* 2010 Nov;65(11):1455-63.

Ma XP, Muzhapaer D. Efficacy of sublingual immunotherapy in children with dust mite allergic asthma. *Zhongguo Dang Dai Er Ke Za Zhi.* 2010 May;12(5):344-7.

Mabey R, ed. *The New Age Herbalist.* New York: Simon & Schuster, 1941.

Macdonald TT, Monteleone G. Immunity, inflammation, and allergy in the gut. *Science.* 2005 Mar 25;307(5717):1920-5.

Maciorkowska E, Kaczmarski M, Andrzej K. Endoscopic evaluation of upper gastrointestinal tract mucosa in children with food hypersensitivity. *Med Wieku Rozwoj.* 2000 Jan-Mar;4(1):37-48.

Mackerras D, Cunningham J, Hunt A, Brent P. Re: "effect of supplemental folic acid in pregnancy on childhood asthma: a prospective birth cohort study". *Am J Epidemiol.* 2010 Mar 15;171(6):746-7; author reply 747. 2010 Feb 9.

MacRedmond R, Singhera G, Attridge S, Bahzad M, Fava C, Lai Y, Hallstrand TS, Dorscheid DR. Conjugated linoleic acid improves airway hyper-reactivity in overweight mild asthmatics. *Clin Exp Allergy.* 2010 Jul;40(7):1071-8.

Macsali F, Real FG, Omenaas ER, Bjorge L, Janson C, Franklin K, Svanes C. Oral contraception, body mass index, and asthma: a cross-sectional Nordic-Baltic population survey. *J Allergy Clin Immunol.* 2009 Feb;123(2):391-7.

Madden JA, Plummer SF, Tang J, Garaiova I, Plummer NT, Herbison M, Hunter JO, Shimada T, Cheng L, Shirakawa T. Effect of probiotics on preventing disruption of the intestinal microflora following antibiotic therapy: a double-blind, placebo-controlled pilot study. *Int Immunopharmacol.* 2005 Jun;5(6):1091-7.

Maeda N, Inomata N, Morita A, Kirino M, Ikezawa Z. Correlation of oral allergy syndrome due to plant-derived foods with pollen sensitization in Japan. *Ann Allergy Asthma Immunol.* 2010 Mar;104(3):205-10.

Maes HH, Silberg JL, Neale MC, Eaves LJ. Genetic and cultural transmission of antisocial behavior: an extended twin parent model. *Twin Res Hum Genet.* 2007 Feb;10(1):136-50.

Mah KW, Chin VI, Wong WS, Lay C, Tannock GW, Shek LP, Aw MM, Chua KY, Wong HB, Panchalingham A, Lee BW. Effect of a milk formula containing probiotics on the fecal microbiota of asian infants at risk of atopic diseases. *Pediatr Res.* 2007 Dec;62(6):674-9.

Mai XM, Kull I, Wickman M, Bergström A. Antibiotic use in early life and development of allergic diseases: respiratory infection as the explanation. *Clin Exp Allergy.* 2010 Aug;40(8):1230-7.

Mainardi T, Kapoor S, Bielory L. Complementary and alternative medicine: herbs, phytochemicals and vitamins and their immunologic effects. *J Allergy Clin Immunol.* 2009 Feb;123(2):283-94; quiz 295-6.

Majamaa H, Isolauri E, Saxelin M, Vesikari T. Lactic acid bacteria in the treatment of acute rotavirus gastroenteritis. *J Pediatr Gastroenterol Nutr.* 1995 Apr;20(3):333-8.

Majamaa H, Isolauri E. Probiotics: a novel approach in the management of food allergy. *J Allergy Clin Immunol.* 1997 Feb;99(2):179-85.

Makrides M, Neumann M, Gibson R. Effect of maternal docosahexaenoic acid (DHA) supplementation on breast milk composition. *Europ Jrnl of Clin Nutr.* 1996;50:352-357.

Maliakal PP, Wanwimolruk S. Effect of herbal teas on hepatic drug metabolizing enzymes in rats. *J Pharm Pharmacol.* 2001 Oct;53(10):1323-9.

Mälkönen T, Alanko K, Jolanki R, Luukkonen R, Aalto-Korte K, Lauerma A, Susitaival P. Long-term follow-up study of occupational hand eczema. Br J Dermatol. 2010 Aug 13.

Mallol J, Solé D, Baeza-Bacab M, Aguirre-Camposano V, Soto-Quiros M, Baena-Cagnani C; Latin American ISAAC Group. Regional variation in asthma symptom prevalence in Latin American children. *J Asthma.* 2010 Aug;47(6):644-50.

Maneechotesuwan K, Supawita S, Kasetsinsombat K, Wongkajornsilp A, Barnes PJ. Sputum indoleamine-2, 3-dioxygenase activity is increased in asthmatic airways by using inhaled corticosteroids. *J Allergy Clin Immunol.* 2008 Jan;121(1):43-50.

Manley KJ, Fraenkel MB, Mayall BC, Power DA. Probiotic treatment of vancomycin-resistant enterococci: a randomised controlled trial. *Med J Aust.* 2007 May 7;186(9):454-7.

Mansfield LE, Posey CR. Daytime sleepiness and cognitive performance improve in seasonal allergic rhinitis treated with intranasal fluticasone propionate. *Allergy Asthma Proc.* 2007 Mar-Apr;28(2):226-9.

Mansson HL. Fatty acids in bovine milk fat. *Food Nutr Res.* 2008;52. doi: 10.3402/fnr.v52i0.1821.

Manz F. Hydration and disease. *J Am Coll Nutr.* 2007 Oct;26(5 Suppl):535S-541S.

Manzoni P, Mostert M, Leonessa ML, Priolo C, Farina D, Monetti C, Latino MA, Gomirato G. Oral supplementation with *Lactobacillus casei* subspecies *rhamnosus* prevents enteric colonization by *Candida* species in preterm neonates: a randomized study. *Clin Infect Dis.* 2006 Jun 15;42(12):1735-42.

Marcos A, Wärnberg J, Nova E, Gómez S, Alvarez A, Alvarez R, Mateos JA, Cobo JM. The effect of milk fermented by yogurt cultures plus *Lactobacillus casei* DN-114001 on the immune response of subjects under academic examination stress. *Eur J Nutr.* 2004 Dec;43(6):381-9.

REFERENCES AND BIBLIOGRAPHY

Marcucci F, Duse M, Frati F, Incorvaia C, Marseglia GL, La Rosa M. The future of sublingual immunotherapy. *Int J Immunopathol Pharmacol.* 2009 Oct-Dec;22(4 Suppl):31-3.

Margioris AN. Fatty acids and postprandial inflammation. *Curr Opin Clin Nutr Metab Care.* 2009 Mar;12(2):129-37.

Maria KW, Behrens T, Brasky TM. Are asthma and allergies in children and adolescents increasing? Results from ISAAC Phase I and Phase II surveys in Munster, Germany. *Allergy.* 2003;58:572-579.

Marin C, Ramirez R, Delgado-Lista J, Yubero-Serrano EM, Perez-Martinez P, Carracedo J, Garcia-Rios A, Rodriguez F, Gutierrez-Mariscal FM, Gomez P, Perez-Jimenez F, Lopez-Miranda J. Mediterranean diet reduces endothelial damage and improves the regenerative capacity of endothelium. *Am J Clin Nutr.* 2011 Feb;93(2):267-74.

Marteau P, Pochart P, Bouhnik Y, Zidi S, Goderel I, Rambaud JC. Survival of *Lactobacillus acidophilus* and *Bifidobacterium* sp. in the small intestine following ingestion in fermented milk. A rational basis for the use of probiotics in man. *Gastroenterol Clin Biol.* 1992;16(1):25-8.

Marth K, Novatchkova M, Focke-Tejkl M, Jenisch S, Jäger S, Kabelitz D, Valenta R. Tracing antigen signatures in the human IgE repertoire. *Mol Immunol.* 2010 Aug;47(14):2323-9.

Martin IR, Wickens K, Patchett K, Kent R, Fitzharris P, Siebers R, Lewis S, Crane J, Holbrook N, Town GI, Smith S. Cat allergen levels in public places in New Zealand. *N Z Med J.* 1998 Sep 25;111(1074):356-8.

Martinez M. Docosahexaenoic acid therapy in docosahexaenoic acid-deficient patients with disorders of peroxisomal biogenesis. *Versicherungsmedizin.* 1996;31 Suppl:145-152

Martínez-Augustin O, Boza JJ, Del Pino JI, Lucena J, Martínez-Valverde A, Gil A. Dietary nucleotides might influence the humoral immune response against cow's milk proteins in preterm neonates. *Biol Neonate.* 1997;71(4):215-23.

Martin-Venegas R, Roig-Perez S, Ferrer R, Moreno JJ. Arachidonic acid cascade and epithelial barrier function during Caco-2 cell differentiation. J Lipid Res. 2006 Apr;3.

Martin-Venegas R, Roig-Perez S, Ferrer R, Moreno JJ. Arachidonic acid cascade and epithelial barrier function during Caco-2 cell differentiation. *J Lipid Res.* 2006 Apr;3.

Marushko IuV. The development of a treatment method for streptococcal tonsillitis in children. *Lik Sprava.* 2000 Jan-Feb;(1):79-82.

Maslowski KM, Mackay CR. Diet, gut microbiota and immune responses. *Nat Immunol.* 2011 Jan;12(1):5-9.

Masoli M, Fabian D, Holt S, Beasley R. The global burden of asthma: executive summary of the GINA Dissemination Committee Report. *Allergy.* 2004;59:469-478.

Massey DG, Chien YK, Fournier-Massey G. Mamane: scientific therapy for asthma? *Hawaii Med J.* 1994;53:350-1. 363.

Massicot JG, Cohen SG. Epidemiologic and socioeconomic aspects of allergic diseases. *J Allergy Clin Immunol.* 1986 Nov;78(5 Pt 2):954-8.

Masuno T, Kishimoto S, Ogura T, Honma T, Niitani H, Fukuoka M, Ogawa N. A comparative trial of LC9018 plus doxorubicin and doxorubicin alone for the treatment of malignant pleural effusion secondary to lung cancer. *Cancer.* 1991 Oct 1;68(7):1495-500.

Matasar MJ, Neugut AI. Epidemiology of anaphylaxis in the United States. *Curr Allergy Asthma Rep.* 2003;3:30-35.

Mater DD, Bretigny L, Firmesse O, Flores MJ, Mogenet A, Bresson JL, Corthier G. *Streptococcus thermophilus* and *Lactobacillus delbrueckii* subsp. bulgaricus survive gastrointestinal transit of healthy volunteers consuming yogurt. *FEMS Microbiol Lett.* 2005 Sep 15;250(2):185-7.

Matheson MC, Haydn Walters E, Burgess JA, Jenkins MA, Giles GG, Hopper JL, Abramson MJ, Dharmage SC. Childhood immunization and atopic disease into middle-age—a prospective cohort study. *Pediatr Allergy Immunol.* 2010 Mar;21(2 Pt 1):301-6.

Mathur NB, Shahani KM. Use of total whey constituents for human food. *J Dairy Sci.* 1979 Jan;62(1):99-105.

Matricardi PM, Bockelbrink A, Beyer K, Keil T, Niggemann B, Grüber C, Wahn U, Lau S. Primary versus secondary immunoglobulin E sensitization to soy and wheat in the Multi-Centre Allergy Study cohort. *Clin Exp Allergy.* 2008 Mar;38(3):493-500.

Matsui EC, Matsui W. Higher serum folate levels are associated with a lower risk of atopy and wheeze. *J Allergy Clin Immunol.* 2009 Jun;123(6):1253-9.e2. 2009 May 5.

Matsumoto M, Benno Y. Anti-inflammatory metabolite production in the gut from the consumption of probiotic yogurt containing *Bifidobacterium animalis* subsp. *lactis* LKM512. *Biosci Biotechnol Biochem.* 2006 Jun;70(6):1287-92.

Matsumoto M, Benno Y. Consumption of *Bifidobacterium lactis* LKM512 yogurt reduces gut mutagenicity by increasing gut polyamine contents in healthy adult subjects. *Mutat Res.* 2004 Dec 21;568(2):147-53.

Matsumoto Y, Noguchi E, Imoto Y, Nanatsue K, Takeshita K, Shibasaki M, Arinami T, Fujieda S. Upregulation of IL17RB during natural allergen exposure in patients with seasonal allergic rhinitis. *Allergol Int.* 2011 Mar;60(1):87-92.

Matsuzaki T, Saito M, Usuku K, Nose H, Izumo S, Arimura K, Osame M. A prospective uncontrolled trial of fermented milk drink containing viable *Lactobacillus casei* strain Shirota in the treatment of HTLV-1 associated myelopathy/tropical spastic paraparesis. *J Neurol Sci.* 2005 Oct 15;237(1-2):75-81.

Mattila P, Renkonen J, Toppila-Salmi S, Parviainen V, Joenväärä S, Alff-Tuomala S, Nicorici D, Renkonen R. Time-series nasal epithelial transcriptomics during natural pollen exposure in healthy subjects and allergic patients. *Allergy.* 2010 Feb;65(2):175-83.

Maurer HR. Bromelain: biochemistry, pharmacology and medical use. *Cell Mol Life Sci.* 2001 Aug;58(9):1234-45.

Mayes MD. Epidemiologic studies of environmental agents and systemic autoimmune diseases. *Environ Health Perspect.* 1999 Oct;107 Suppl 5:743-8.

McAlindon TE. Nutraceuticals: do they work and when should we use them? *Best Pract Res Clin Rheumatol.* 2006 Feb;20(1):99-115.

McCarney RW, Lasserson TJ, Linde K, Brinkhaus B. An overview of two Cochrane systematic reviews of complementary treatments for chronic asthma: acupuncture and homeopathy. *Respir Med.* 2004 Aug;98(8):687-96.

McCarney RW, Linde K, Lasserson TJ. Homeopathy for chronic asthma. *Cochrane Database Syst Rev.* 2004;(1):CD000353.

McConnaughey E. *Sea Vegetables.* Happy Camp, CA: Naturegraph, 1985.

McDougall J, McDougall M. *The McDougal Plan.* Clinton, NJ: New Win, 1983.

McGuire BW, Sia LL, Haynes JD, Kisicki JC, Gutierrez ML, Stokstad EL. Absorption kinetics of orally administered leucovorin calcium. *NCI Monogr.* 1987;(5):47-56.

McGuire BW, Sia LL, Leese PT, Gutierrez ML, Stokstad EL. Pharmacokinetics of leucovorin calcium after intravenous, intramuscular, and oral administration. *Clin Pharm.* 1988 Jan;7(1):52-8.

McHugh MK, Symanski E, Pompeii LA, Delclos GL. Prevalence of asthma by industry and occupation in the U.S. working population. *Am J Ind Med.* 2010 May;53(5):463-75.

McHugh MK, Symanski E, Pompeii LA, Delclos GL. Prevalence of asthma among adult females and males in the United States: results from the National Health and Nutrition Examination Survey (NHANES), 2001-2004. *J Asthma.* 2009 Oct;46(8):759-66.

McKeever TM, Lewis SA, Cassano PA, Ocké M, Burney P, Britton J, Smit HA. Patterns of dietary intake and relation to respiratory disease, forced expiratory volume in 1 s, and decline in 5-y forced expiratory volume. *Am J Clin Nutr.* 2010 Aug;92(2):408-15. 2010 Jun 16.

McKenzie H, Main J, Pennington CR, Parratt D. Antibody to selected strains of Saccharomyces cerevisiae (baker's and brewer's yeast) and Candida albicans in Crohn's disease. *Gut.* 1990 May;31(5):536-8.

McLachlan CN. beta-casein A1, ischaemic heart disease mortality, and other illnesses. *Med Hypotheses.* 2001 Feb;56(2):262-72.

McNally ME, Atkinson SA, Cole DE. Contribution of sulfate and sulfoesters to total sulfur intake in infants fed human milk. *J Nutr.* 1991 Aug;121(8):1250-4.

McNaught CE, Woodcock NP, Anderson AD, MacFie J. A prospective randomised trial of probiotics in critically ill patients. *Clin Nutr.* 2005 Apr;24(2):211-9.

McNaught CE, Woodcock NP, Anderson AD, MacFie J. A prospective randomised trial of probiotics in critically ill patients. *Clin Nutr.* 2005 Apr;24(2):211-9.

McNaught CE, Woodcock NP, MacFie J, Mitchell CJ. A prospective randomised study of the probiotic *Lactobacillus plantarum* 299V on indices of gut barrier function in elective surgical patients. *Gut.* 2002 Dec;51(6):827-31.

Meglio P, Bartone E, Plantamura M, Arabito E, Giampietro PG. A protocol for oral desensitization in children with IgE-mediated cow's milk allergy. *Allergy.* 2004 Sep;59(9):980-7.

Mehra PN, Puri HS. Studies on Gaduchi satwa. *Indian J Pharm.* 1969;31:180-2.

Meier B, Shao Y, Julkunen-Tiitto R, Bettschart A, Sticher O. A chemotaxonomic survey of phenolic compounds in Swiss willow species. Planta Med. 1992;58:A698.

Meier B, Sticher O, Julkunen-Tiitto R. Pharmaceutical aspects of the use of willows in herbal remedies. Planta Med. 1988;54(6):559-560.

Melcion C, Verroust P, Baud L, Ardaillou N, Morel-Maroger L, Ardaillou R. Protective effect of procyanidolic oligomers on the heterologous phase of glomerulonephritis induced by anti-glomerular basement membrane antibodies. *C R Seances Acad Sci III.* 1982 Dec 6;295(12):721-6.

Melcion C, Verroust P, Baud L, Ardaillou N, Morel-Maroger L, Ardaillou R. Protective effect of procyanidolic oligomers on the heterologous phase of glomerulonephritis induced by anti-glomerular basement membrane antibodies. *C R Seances Acad Sci III.* 1982 Dec 6;295(12):721-6.

Men, Research, And The History Of Hay Fever. *OldAndSold.com*, 1943; Accessed May 16, 2011

Merchant RE and Andre CA. 2001. A review of recent clinical trials of the nutritional supplement Chlorella pyrenoidosa in the treatment of fibromyalgia, hypertension, and ulcerative colitis. *Altern Ther Health Med.* May-Jun;7(3):79-91.

Messina M. Insights gained from 20 years of soy research. *J Nutr.* 2010 Dec;140(12):2289S-2295S. 2010 Oct 27.

Metsälä J, Lundqvist A, Kaila M, Gissler M, Klaukka T, Virtanen SM. Maternal and perinatal characteristics and the risk of cow's milk allergy in infants up to 2 years of age: a case-control study nested in the Finnish population. *Am J Epidemiol.* 2010 Jun 15;171(12):1310-6.

Meyer A, Kirsch H, Domergue F, Abbadi A, Sperling P, Bauer J, Cirpus P, Zank TK, Moreau H, Roscoe TJ, Zahringer U, Heinz E. Novel fatty acid elongases and their use for the reconstitution of docosahexaenoic acid biosynthesis. *J Lipid Res.* 2004 Oct;45(10):1899-909.

Meyer AL, Elmadfa I, Herbacek I, Micksche M. Probiotic, as well as conventional yogurt, can enhance the stimulated production of proinflammatory cytokines. J Hum Nutr Diet. 2007;20(6):590-8.

Meyer AL, Elmadfa I, Herbacek I, Micksche M. Probiotic, as well as conventional yogurt, can enhance the stimulated production of proinflammatory cytokines. *J Hum Nutr Diet.* 2007 Dec;20(6):590-8.

Michaelsen KF. Probiotics, breastfeeding and atopic eczema. *Acta Derm Venereol Suppl (Stockh).* 2005 Nov;(215):21-4.

Michail S. The role of probiotics in allergic diseases. Allergy Asthma Clin Immunol. 2009 Oct 22;5(1):5.

Michalska K, Kisiel W. Sesquiterpene lactones from Taraxacum obovatum. *Planta Med.* 2003 Feb;69(2):181-3.

Michelson PH, Williams LW, Benjamin DK, Barnato AE. Obesity, inflammation, and asthma severity in childhood: data from the National Health and Nutrition Examination Survey 2001-2004. *Ann Allergy Asthma Immunol.* 2009 Nov;103(5):381-5.

Michetti P, Dorta G, Wiesel PH, Brassart D, Verdu E, Herranz M, Felley C, Porta N, Rouvet M, Blum AL, Corthésy-Theulaz I. Effect of whey-based culture supernatant of *Lactobacillus acidophilus* (johnsonii) La1 on *Helicobacter pylori* infection in humans. *Digestion.* 1999;60(3):203-9.

Michielutti F, Bertini M, Presciuttini B, Andreotti G. Clinical assessment of a new oral bacterial treatment for children with acute diarrhea. *Minerva Med.* 1996 Nov;87(11):545-50.

Mickleborough TD, Lindley MR, Ray S. Dietary salt, airway inflammation, and diffusion capacity in exercise-induced asthma. *Med Sci Sports Exerc.* 2005 Jun;37(6):904-14.

Mikoluc B, Motkowski R, Karpinska J, Piotrowska-Jastrzebska J. Plasma levels of vitamins A and E, coenzyme Q10, and anti-ox-LDL antibody titer in children treated with an elimination diet due to food hypersensitivity. *Int J Vitam Nutr Res.* 2009 Sep;79(5-6):328-36.

Milgrom P, Ly KA, Roberts MC, Rothen M, Mueller G, Yamaguchi DK. Mutans streptococci dose response to xylitol chewing gum. *J Dent Res.* 2006 Feb;85(2):177-81.

Miller AL. The etiologies, pathophysiology, and alternative/complementary treatment of asthma. *Altern Med Rev.* 2001 Feb;6(1):20-47.

Miller GT. *Living in the Environment.* Belmont, CA: Wadsworth, 1996.

Miller JD, Morin LP, Schwartz WJ, Moore RY. New insights into the mammalian circadian clock. *Sleep.* 1996 Oct;19(8):641-67.

Miller K. Cholesterol and In-Hospital Mortality in Elderly Patients. *Am Family Phys.* 2004 May.

Mindell E, Hopkins V. *Prescription Alternatives.* New Canaan, CT: Keats, 1998.

Miranda H, Outeiro TF. The sour side of neurodegenerative disorders: the effects of protein glycation. *J Pathol.* 2010 May;221(1):13-25.

Mitchell AE, Hong YJ, Koh E, Barrett DM, Bryant DE, Denison RF, Kaffka S. Ten-year comparison of the influence of organic and conventional crop management practices on the content of flavonoids in tomatoes. *J Agric Food Chem.* 2007 Jul 25;55(15):6154-9.

Mittag D, Akkerdaas J, Ballmer-Weber BK, Vogel L, Wensing M, Becker WM, Koppelman SJ, Knulst AC, Helbling A, Hefle SL, Van Ree R, Vieths S. Ara h 8, a Bet v 1-homologous allergen from peanut, is a major allergen in patients with combined birch pollen and peanut allergy. *J Allergy Clin Immunol.* 2004 Dec;114(6):1410-7.

Mittag D, Vieths S, Vogel L, Becker WM, Rihs HP, Helbling A, Wüthrich B, Ballmer-Weber BK. Soybean allergy in patients allergic to birch pollen: clinical investigation and molecular characterization of allergens. *J Allergy Clin Immunol.* 2004 Jan;113(1):148-54.

Miyake Y, Sasaki S, Tanaka K, Hirota Y. Dairy food, calcium and vitamin D intake in pregnancy, and wheeze and eczema in infants. *Eur Respir J.* 2010 Jun;35(6):1228-34. 2009 Oct 19.

Miyazawa T, Itahashi K, Imai T. Management of neonatal cow's milk allergy in high-risk neonates. *Pediatr Int.* 2009 Aug;51(4):544-7.

Moattari A, Aleyasin S, Arabpour M, Sadeghi S. Prevalence of Human Metapneumovirus (hMPV) in Children with Wheezing in Shiraz-Iran. *Iran J Allergy Asthma Immunol.* 2010 Dec;9(4):250-4.

Modern Biology. Austin: Harcourt Brace, 1993.

Mohammad MA, Molloy A, Scott J, Hussein L. Plasma cobalamin and folate and their metabolic markers methylmalonic acid and total homocysteine among Egyptian children before and after nutritional supplementation with the probiotic bacteria *Lactobacillus acidophilus* in yoghurt matrix. *Int J Food Sci Nutr.* 2006 Nov-Dec;57(7-8):470-80.

Mohan R, Koebnick C, Schildt J, Mueller M, Radke M, Blaut M. Effects of *Bifidobacterium lactis* Bb12 supplementation on body weight, fecal pH, acetate, lactate, calprotectin, and IgA in preterm infants. *Pediatr Res.* 2008 Oct;64(4):418-22.

Mohan R, Koebnick C, Schildt J, Schmidt S, Mueller M, Possner M, Radke M, Blaut M. Effects of *Bifidobacterium lactis* Bb12 supplementation on intestinal microbiota of preterm infants: a double-blind, placebo-controlled, randomized study. *J Clin Microbiol.* 2006 Nov;44(11):4025-31.

Mokhtar N, Chan SC. Use of complementary medicine amongst asthmatic patients in primary care. *Med J Malaysia.* 2006 Mar;61(1):125-7.

Monarca S. Zerbini I, Simonati C, Gelatti U. Drinking water hardness and chronic degenerative diseases. Part II. Cardiovascular diseases. *Ann. Ig.* 2003;15:41-56.

Moneret-Vautrin DA, Kanny G, Thévenin F. Asthma caused by food allergy. *Rev Med Interne.* 1996;17(7):551-7.

Moneret-Vautrin DA, Morisset M. Adult food allergy. *Curr Allergy Asthma Rep.* 2005 Jan;5(1):80-5.

Monks H, Gowland MH, Mackenzie H, Erlewyn-Lajeunesse M, King R, Lucas JS, Roberts G. How do teenagers manage their food allergies? *Clin Exp Allergy.* 2010 Aug 2.

Moorhead KJ, Morgan HC. *Spirulina: Nature's Superfood.* Kailua-Kona, HI: Nutrex, 1995.

Moreira A, Delgado L, Haahtela T, Fonseca J, Moreira P, Lopes C, Mota J, Santos P, Rytilä P, Castel-Branco MG. Physical training does not increase allergic inflammation in asthmatic children. Eur Respir J. 2008 Dec;32(6):1570-5.

Moreira P, Moreira A, Padrão P, Delgado L. The role of economic and educational factors in asthma: evidence from the Portuguese health survey. *Public Health.* 2008 Apr;122(4):434-9. 2007 Oct 17.

Morel AF, Dias GO, Porto C, Simionatto E, Stuker CZ, Dalcol II. Antimicrobial activity of extractives of Solidago microglossa. *Fitoterapia.* 2006 Sep;77(6):453-5.

Morimoto K, Takeshita T, Nanno M, Tokudome S, Nakayama K. Modulation of natural killer cell activity by supplementation of fermented milk containing *Lactobacillus casei* in habitual smokers. *Prev Med.* 2005 May;40(5):589-94.

Morisset M, Moneret-Vautrin DA, Kanny G, Guénard L, Beaudouin E, Flabbée J, Hatahet R. Thresholds of clinical reactivity to milk, egg, peanut and sesame in immunoglobulin E-dependent allergies: evaluation by double-blind or single-blind placebo-controlled oral challenges. *Clin Exp Allergy.* 2003 Aug;33(8):1046-51.

Moss M. E. Coli Path Shows Flaws in Ground Beef Inspection. *NY Times* 2009 Oct 3.

Moussaieff A, Shein NA, Tsenter J, Grigoriadis S, Simeonidou C, Alexandrovich AG, Trembovler V, Ben-Neriah Y, Schmitz ML, Fiebich BL, Munoz E, Mechoulam R, Shohami E. Incensole acetate: a novel neuroprotective agent isolated from Boswellia carterii. *J Cereb Blood Flow Metab.* 2008 Jul;28(7):1341-52.

Moyle A. *Nature Cure for Asthma and Hay Fever.* Wellingborough, U.K.: Thorsons, 1978.

Mozafar A. Is there vitamin B12 in plants or not? A plant nutritionist's view. *Veg Nutr.* 1997;1/2:50-52.

Mozaffarian D, Aro A, Willett WC. Health effects of trans-fatty acids: experimental and observational evidence. *Eur J Clin Nutr.* 2009 May;63 Suppl 2:S5-21.

Muller H, Lindman AS, Blomfeldt A, Seljeflot I, Pedersen JI. A diet rich in coconut oil reduces diurnal postprandial variations in circulating tissue plasminogen activator antigen and fasting lipoprotein (a) compared with a diet rich in unsaturated fat in women. *J Nutr.* 2003 Nov;133(11):3422-7.

Müller S, Pühl S, Vieth M, Stolte M. Analysis of symptoms and endoscopic findings in 117 patients with histological diagnoses of eosinophilic esophagitis. *Endoscopy.* 2007 Apr;39(4):339-44.

Mullié C, Yazourh A, Thibault H, Odou MF, Singer E, Kalach N, Kremp O, Romond MB. Increased poliovirus-specific intestinal antibody response coincides with promotion of *Bifidobacterium longum*-infantis and *Bifidobacterium breve* in infants: a randomized, double-blind, placebo-controlled trial. *Pediatr Res.* 2004 Nov;56(5):791-5.

Murray M and Pizzorno J. *Encyclopedia of Natural Medicine.* 2nd Edition. Roseville, CA: Prima Publishing, 1998.

Murray M, Pizzorno J. *Encyclopedia of Natural Medicine.* 2nd Edition. Roseville, CA: Prima Publishing, 1998.

Mustapha A, Jiang T, Savaiano DA. Improvement of lactose digestion by humans following ingestion of unfermented acidophilus milk: influence of bile sensitivity, lactose transport, and acid tolerance of *Lactobacillus acidophilus.* J Dairy Sci. 1997 Aug;80(8):1537-45.

Myllyluoma E, Ahonen AM, Korpela R, Vapaatalo H, Kankuri E. Effects of multispecies probiotic combination on helicobacter pylori infection in vitro. *Clin Vaccine Immunol.* 2008 Sep;15(9):1472-82.

Nadkarni AK, Nadkarni KM. *Indian Materia Medica.* (Vols 1 and 2). Bombay, India: Popular Pradashan, 1908, 1976.

Nagai T, Arai Y, Emori M, Nunome SY, Yabe T, Takeda T, Yamada H. Anti-allergic activity of a Kampo (Japanese herbal) medicine "Sho-seiryu-to (Xiao-Qing-Long-Tang)" on airway inflammation in a mouse model. *Int Immunopharmacol.* 2004 Oct;4(10-11):1353-65.

Nagel G, Linseisen J. Dietary intake of fatty acids, antioxidants and selected food groups and asthma in adults. *Eur J Clin Nutr.* 2005 Jan;59(1):8-15.

REFERENCES AND BIBLIOGRAPHY

Nagel G, Weinmayr G, Kleiner A, Garcia-Marcos L, Strachan DP; ISAAC Phase Two Study Group. Effect of diet on asthma and allergic sensitisation in the International Study on Allergies and Asthma in Childhood (ISAAC) Phase Two. Thorax. 2010 Jun;65(6):516-22.

Naghii MR, Samman S. The role of boron in nutrition and metabolism. *Prog Food Nutr Sci.* 1993 Oct-Dec;17(4):331-49.

Nair PK, Rodriguez S, Ramachandran R, Alamo A, Melnick SJ, Escalon E, Garcia PI Jr, Wnuk SF, Ramachandran C. Immune stimulating properties of a novel polysaccharide from the medicinal plant Tinospora cordifolia. *Int Immunopharmacol.* 2004 Dec 15;4(13):1645-59.

Naito S, Koga H, Yamaguchi A, Fujimoto N, Hasui Y, Kuramoto H, Iguchi A, Kinukawa N; Kyushu University Urological Oncology Group. Prevention of recurrence with epirubicin and *Lactobacillus casei* after transurethral resection of bladder cancer. *J Urol.* 2008 Feb;179(2):485-90.

Nakano T, Shimojo N, Morita Y, Arima T, Tomiita M, Kohno Y. Sensitization to casein and beta-lactoglobulin (BLG) in children with cow's milk allergy (CMA). *Arerugi.* 2010 Feb;59(2):117-22.

Napoli, J.E., Brand-Miller, J.C., Conway, P. (2003) Bifidogenic effects of feeding infant formula containing galactooligosaccharides in healthy formula-fed infants. *Asia Pac J Clin Nutr.* 12(Suppl): S60

Nariya M, Shukla V, Jain S, Ravishankar B. Comparison of enteroprotective efficacy of triphala formulations (Indian Herbal Drug) on methotrexate-induced small intestinal damage in rats. *Phytother Res.* 2009 Aug;23(8):1092-8.

Naruszewicz M, Daniewski M, Nowicka G, Kozlowska-Wojciechowska M. Trans-unsaturated fatty acids and acrylamide in food as potential atherosclerosis progression factors. Based on own studies. *Acta Microbiol Pol.* 2003;52 Suppl:75-81.

Naruszewicz M, Johansson ML, Zapolska-Downar D, Bukowska H. Effect of Lactobacillus plantarum 299v on cardiovascular disease risk factors in smokers. *Am J Clin Nutr.* 2002 Dec;76(6):1249-55.

Naruszewicz M, Johansson ML, Zapolska-Downar D, Bukowska H. Effect of *Lactobacillus plantarum* 299v on cardiovascular disease risk factors in smokers. *Am J Clin Nutr.* 2002 Dec;76(6):1249-55.

Narva M, Nevala R, Poussa T, Korpela R. The effect of *Lactobacillus helveticus* fermented milk on acute changes in calcium metabolism in postmenopausal women. *Eur J Nutr.* 2004 Apr;43(2):61-8.

Näse L, Hatakka K, Savilahti E, Saxelin M, Pönkä A, Poussa T, Korpela R, Meurman JH. Effect of long-term consumption of a probiotic bacterium, *Lactobacillus rhamnosus* GG, in milk on dental caries and caries risk in children. *Caries Res.* 2001 Nov-Dec;35(6):412-20.

National Cooperation Group on Childhood Asthma. A nationwide survey in China on prevalence of asthma in urban children. Chin J Pediatr. pp. 123-127.

National Toxicology Program. Final Report on Carcinogens Background Document for Formaldehyde. *Rep Carcinog Backgr Doc.* 2010 Jan;(10-5981):i-512.

NDL, BHNRC, ARS, USDA. *Oxygen Radical Absorbance Capacity (ORAC) of Selected Foods - 2007.* Beltsville, MD: USDA-ARS. 2007.

Nentwich I, Michková E, Nevoral J, Urbanek R, Szépfalusi Z. Cow's milk-specific cellular and humoral immune responses and atopy skin symptoms in infants from atopic families fed a partially (pHF) or extensively (eHF) hydrolyzed infant formula. *Allergy.* 2001 Dec;56(12):1144-56.

Nestel PJ. Adulthood - prevention: Cardiovascular disease. Med J Aust. 2002 Jun 3;176(11 Suppl):S118-9.

Newall CA, Anderson LA, Phillipson JD (eds). *Herbal Medicines: A Guide for Health-Care Professionals.* London: Pharmaceut Press; 1996.

Newmark T, Schulick P. *Beyond Aspirin.* Prescott, AZ: Holm, 2000.

Neyestani TR, Shariatzadeh N, Gharavi A, Kalayi A, Khalaji N. Physiological dose of lycopene suppressed oxidative stress and enhanced serum levels of immunoglobulin M in patients with Type 2 diabetes mellitus: a possible role in the prevention of long-term complications. *J Endocrinol Invest.* 2007 Nov;30(10):833-8.

Ngai SP, Jones AY, Hui-Chan CW, Ko FW, Hui DS. Effect of Acu-TENS on post-exercise expiratory lung volume in subjects with asthma-A randomized controlled trial. *Respir Physiol Neurobiol.* 2009 Jul 31;167(3):348-53. 2009 Jun 18.

Nicholls SJ, Lundman P, Harmer JA, Cutri B, Griffiths KA, Rye KA, Barter PJ, Celermajer DS. Consumption of saturated fat impairs the anti-inflammatory properties of high-density lipoproteins and endothelial function. *J Am Coll Cardiol.* 2006 Aug 15;48(4):715-20.

Nicolaou N, Poorafshar M, Murray C, Simpson A, Winell H, Kerry G, Härlin A, Woodcock A, Ahlstedt S, Custovic A. Allergy or tolerance in children sensitized to peanut: prevalence and differentiation using component-resolved diagnostics. *J Allergy Clin Immunol.* 2010 Jan;125(1):191-7.e1-13.

Niederau C, Göpfert E. The effect of chelidonium- and turmeric root extract on upper abdominal pain due to functional disorders of the biliary system. Results from a placebo-controlled double-blind study. *Med Klin.* 1999 Aug 15;94(8):425-30.

Niedzielin K, Kordecki H, Birkenfeld B. A controlled, double-blind, randomized study on the efficacy of *Lactobacillus plantarum* 299V in patients with irritable bowel syndrome. *Eur J Gastroenterol Hepatol.* 2001 Oct;13(10):1143-7.

Nielsen OH, Jørgensen S, Pedersen K, Justesen T. Microbiological evaluation of jejunal aspirates and faecal samples after oral administration of bifidobacteria and lactic acid bacteria. *J Appl Bacteriol.* 1994 May;76(5):469-74.

Nielsen RG, Bindslev-Jensen C, Kruse-Andersen S, Husby S. Severe gastroesophageal reflux disease and cow milk hypersensitivity in infants and children: disease association and evaluation of a new challenge procedure. J *Pediatr Gastroenterol Nutr.* 2004 Oct;39(4):383-91.

Niggemann B, von Berg A, Bollrath C, Berdel D, Schauer U, Rieger C, Haschke-Becher E, Wahn U. Safety and efficacy of a new extensively hydrolyzed formula for infants with cow's milk protein allergy. *Pediatr Allergy Immunol.* 2008 Jun;19(4):348-54.

Nightingale JA, Rogers DF, Hart LA, Kharitonov SA, Chung KF, Barnes PJ. Effect of inhaled endotoxin on induced sputum in normal, atopic, and atopic asthmatic subjects. *Thorax.* 1998 Jul;53(7):563-71.

Niimi A, Nguyen LT, Usmani O, Mann B, Chung KF. Reduced pH and chloride levels in exhaled breath condensate of patients with chronic cough. *Thorax.* 2004 Jul;59(7):608-12.

Nilson KM, Vakil JR, Shahani KM. B-complex vitamin content of cheddar cheese. *J Nutr.* 1965 Aug;86:362-8.

Ninan TK, Russell G. Respiratory symptoms and atopy in Aberdeen schoolchildren: evidence from two surveys 25 years apart. BMJ. 1992;304:873-875.

Njoroge GN, Bussmann RW. Traditional management of ear, nose and throat (ENT) diseases in Central Kenya. *J Ethnobiol Ethnomed.* 2006 Dec 27;2:54.

Nobaek S, Johansson ML, Molin G, Ahrné S, Jeppsson B. Alteration of intestinal microflora is associated with reduction in abdominal bloating and pain in patients with irritable bowel syndrome. *Am J Gastroenterol.* 2000 May;95(5):1231-8.

Nodake Y, Fukumoto S, Fukasawa M, Sakakibara R, Yamasaki N. Reduction of the immunogenicity of beta-lactoglobulin from cow's milk by conjugation with a dextran derivative. *Biosci Biotechnol Biochem.* 2010;74(4):721-6.

Noh J, Lee JH, Noh G, Bang SY, Kim HS, Choi WS, Cho S, Lee SS. Characterisation of allergen-specific responses of IL-10-producing regulatory B cells (Br1) in Cow Milk Allergy. *Cell Immunol.* 2010;264(2):143-9.

Noone EJ, Roche HM, Nugent AP, Gibney MJ. The effect of dietary supplementation using isomeric blends of conjugated linoleic acid on lipid metabolism in healthy human subjects. *Br J Nutr.* 2002 Sep;88(3):243-51.

Noorbakhsh R, Mortazavi SA, Sankian M, Shahidi F, Assarehzadegan MA, Varasteh A. Cloning, expression, characterization, and computational approach for cross-reactivity prediction of manganese superoxide dismutase allergen from pistachio nut. *Allergol Int.* 2010 Sep;59(3):295-304.

Nopchinda S, Varavithya W, Phuapradit P, Sangchai R, Suthutvoravut U, Chantraruksa V, Haschke F. Effect of bifidobacterium Bb12 with or without *Streptococcus thermophilus* supplemented formula on nutritional status. *J Med Assoc Thai.* 2002 Nov;85 Suppl 4:S1225-31.

Norris R. "Flush-free niacin": Dietary supplement may be "benefit-free." *Prev Cardio.* 2006 Winter: 64.

Nova E, Toro O, Varela P, López-Vidriero I, Morandé G, Marcos A. Effects of a nutritional intervention with yogurt on lymphocyte subsets and cytokine production capacity in anorexia nervosa patients. *Eur J Nutr.* 2006 Jun;45(4):225-33.

Novembre E, Dini L, Bernardini R, Resti M, Vierucci A. Unusual reactions to food additives. *Pediatr Med Chir.* 1992 Jan-Feb;14(1):39-42.

Nowak-Wegrzyn A, Fiocchi A. Is oral immunotherapy the cure for food allergies? *Curr Opin Allergy Clin Immunol.* 2010 Jun;10(3):214-9.

Nsouli TM. Long-term use of nasal saline irrigation: harmful or helpful? *Amer Acad of Allergy, Asthma and Immunol.* 2009; Abstract O32.

Nurmatov U, Devereux G, Sheikh A. Nutrients and foods for the primary prevention of asthma and allergy: Systematic review and meta-analysis. *J Allergy Clin Immunol.* 2010 Dec 23.

Nusem D, Panasoff J. Beer anaphylaxis. *Isr Med Assoc J.* 2009 Jun;11(6):380-1.

Nwaru BI, Erkkola M, Ahonen S, Kaila M, Haapala AM, Kronberg-Kippilä C, Salmelin R, Veijola R, Ilonen J, Simell O, Knip M, Virtanen SM. Age at the introduction of solid foods during the first year and allergic sensitization at age 5 years. *Pediatrics.* 2010 Jan;125(1):50-9. 2009 Dec 7.

O'Connor J., Bensky D. (ed). *Shanghai College of Traditional Chinese Medicine: Acupuncture: A Comprehensive Text.* Seattle: Eastland Press, 1981.

O'Neil C, Helbling AA, Lehrer SB. Allergic reactions to fish. *Clin Rev Allergy.* 1993 Summer;11(2):183-200.

O'Neil C, Helbling AA, Lehrer SB. Allergic reactions to fish. *Clin Rev Allergy.* 1993;11(2):183-200.

O'Brien SJ, Shannon JE, Gail MH. A molecular approach to the identification and individualization of human and animal cells in culture: isozyme and allozyme genetic signatures. *In Vitro.* 1980 Feb;16(2):119-35.

Odamaki T, Xiao JZ, Iwabuchi N, Sakamoto M, Takahashi N, Kondo S, Miyaji K, Iwatsuki K, Togashi H, Enomoto T, Benno Y. Influence of Bifidobacterium longum BB536 intake on faecal microbiota in individuals with Japanese cedar pollinosis during the pollen season. *J Med Microbiol.* 2007 Oct;56(Pt 10):1301-8.

Odamaki T, Xiao JZ, Iwabuchi N, Sakamoto M, Takahashi N, Kondo S, Iwatsuki K, Kokubo S, Togashi H, Enomoto T, Benno Y. Fluctuation of fecal microbiota in individuals with Japanese cedar pollinosis during the pollen season and influence of probiotic intake. *J Investig Allergol Clin Immunol.* 2007;17(2):92-100.

Oehme FW (ed.). *Toxicity of heavy metals in the environment. Part 1.* New York: M.Dekker, 1979.

Ogawa T, Hashikawa S, Asai Y, Sakamoto H, Yasuda K, Makimura Y. A new synbiotic, Lactobacillus casei subsp. casei together with dextran, reduces murine and human allergic reaction. *FEMS Immunol Med Microbiol.* 2006 Apr;46(3):400-9.

Ogawa T, Hashikawa S, Asai Y, Sakamoto H, Yasuda K, Makimura Y. A new synbiotic, *Lactobacillus casei* subsp. casei together with dextran, reduces murine and human allergic reaction. *FEMS Immunol Med Microbiol.* 2006 Apr;46(3):400-9.

Oh CK, Lücker PW, Wetzelsberger N, Kuhlmann F. The determination of magnesium, calcium, sodium and potassium in assorted foods with special attention to the loss of electrolytes after various forms of food preparations. *Mag.-Bull.* 1986;8:297-302.

Oh SY, Chung J, Kim MK, Kwon SO, Cho BH. Antioxidant nutrient intakes and corresponding biomarkers associated with the risk of atopic dermatitis in young children. *Eur J Clin Nutr.* 2010 Mar;64(3):245-52. 2010 Jan 27.

Ohashi Y, Nakai S, Tsukamoto T, Masumori N, Akaza H, Miyanaga N, Kitamura T, Kawabe K, Kotake T, Kuroda M, Naito S, Koga H, Saito Y, Nomata K, Kitagawa M, Aso Y. Habitual intake of lactic acid bacteria and risk reduction of bladder cancer. *Urol Int.* 2002;68(4):273-80.

Ok IS, Kim SH, Kim BK, Lee JC, Lee YC. Pinellia ternata, Citrus reticulata, and their combinational prescription inhibit eosinophil infiltration and airway hyperresponsiveness by suppressing CCR3+ and Th2 cytokines production in the ovalbumin-induced asthma model. *Mediators Inflamm.* 2009;2009:413270.

Okamura T, Maehara Y, Sugimachi K. Phase II clinical study of LC9018 on carcinomatous peritonitis of gastric cancer. Subgroup for Carcinomatous Peritonitis, Cooperative, Study Group of LC9018. *Gan To Kagaku Ryoho.* 1989 Jun;16(6):2257-62.

Okawa T, Niibe H, Arai T, Sekiba K, Noda K, Takeuchi S, Hashimoto S, Ogawa N. Effect of LC9018 combined with radiation therapy on carcinoma of the uterine cervix. A phase III, multicenter, randomized, controlled study. *Cancer.* 1993 Sep 15;72(6):1949-54.

Oláh A, Belágyi T, Issekutz A, Gamal ME, Bengmark S. Randomized clinical trial of specific lactobacillus and fibre supplement to early enteral nutrition in patients with acute pancreatitis. *Br J Surg.* 2002 Sep;89(9):1103-7.

Ołdak E, Kurzatkowska B, Stasiak-Barmuta A. Natural course of sensitization in children: follow-up study from birth to 6 years of age, I. Evaluation of total serum IgE and specific IgE antibodies with regard to atopic family history. *Rocz Akad Med Bialymst.* 2000;45:87-95.

Oleïnichenko EV, Mitrokhin SD, Nonikov VE, Minaev VI. Effectiveness of acipole in prevention of enteric dysbacteriosis due to antibacterial therapy. *Antibiot Khimioter.* 1999;44(1):23-5.

Olivares M, Díaz-Ropero MA, Gómez N, Lara-Villoslada F, Sierra S, Maldonado JA, Martín R, López-Huertas E, Rodríguez JM, Xaus J. Oral administration of two probiotic strains, *Lactobacillus gasseri* CECT5714 and Lactobacillus coryniformis CECT5711, enhances the intestinal function of healthy adults. *Int J Food Microbiol.* 2006 Mar 15;107(2):104-11.

Olivares M, Paz Díaz-Ropero M, Gómez N, Sierra S, Lara-Villoslada F, Martín R, Miguel Rodríguez J, Xaus J. Dietary deprivation of fermented foods causes a fall in innate immune response. Lactic acid bacteria can counteract the immunological effect of this deprivation. *J Dairy Res.* 2006 Nov;73(4):492-8.

O'Mahony L, McCarthy J, Kelly P, Hurley G, Luo F, Chen K, O'Sullivan GC, Kiely B, Collins JK, Shanahan F, Quigley EM. Lactobacillus and bifidobacterium in irritable bowel syndrome: symptom responses and relationship to cytokine profiles. *Gastroenterology.* 2005 Mar;128(3):541-51.

Onbasi K, Sin AZ, Doganavsargil B, Onder GF, Bor S, Sebik F. Eosinophil infiltration of the oesophageal mucosa in patients with pollen allergy during the season. *Clin Exp Allergy.* 2005 Nov;35(11):1423-31.

Onder G, et al. Serum cholesterol levels and in-hospital mortality in the elderly. *Am J Med.* 2003 Sept;115:265-71.

Onwulata CI, Rao DR, Vankineni P. Relative efficiency of yogurt, sweet acidophilus milk, hydrolyzed-lactose milk, and a commercial lactase tablet in alleviating lactose maldigestion. *Am J Clin Nutr.* 1989 Jun;49(6):1233-7.

Oozeer R, Leplingard A, Mater DD, Mogenet A, Michelin R, Seksek I, Marteau P, Doré J, Bresson JL, Corthier G. Survival of *Lactobacillus casei* in the human digestive tract after consumption of fermented milk. *Appl Environ Microbiol.* 2006 Aug;72(8):5615-7.

Oreskovic NM, Sawicki GS, Kinane TB, Winickoff JP, Perrin JM. Travel patterns to school among children with asthma. *Clin Pediatr.* 2009 Jul;48(6):632-40. 2009 May 6.

Ortiz-Andrellucchi A, Sánchez-Villegas A, Rodríguez-Gallego C, Lemes A, Molero T, Soria A, Peña-Quintana L, Santana M, Ramírez O, García J, Cabrera F, Cobo J, Serra-Majem L. Immunomodulatory effects of the intake of fermented milk with Lactobacillus casei DN114001 in lactating mothers and their children. *Br J Nutr.* 2008 Oct;100(4):834-45.

Osguthorpe JD. Immunotherapy. *Curr Opin Otolaryngol Head Neck Surg.* 2010 Jun;18(3):206-12.

Otto SJ, van Houwelingen AC, Hornstra G. The effect of supplementation with docosahexaenoic and arachidonic acid derived from single cell oils on plasma and erythrocyte fatty acids of pregnant women in the second trimester. *Prostaglandins Leukot Essent Fatty Acids.* 2000 Nov;63(5):323-8.

Ou CC, Tsao SM, Lin MC, Yin MC. Protective action on human LDL against oxidation and glycation by four organosulfur compounds derived from garlic. *Lipids.* 2003 Mar;38(3):219-24.

Ouwehand AC, Bergsma N, Parhiala R, Lahtinen S, Gueimonde M, Finne-Soveri H, Strandberg T, Pitkälä K, Salminen S. *Bifidobacterium* microbiota and parameters of immune function in elderly subjects. *FEMS Immunol Med Microbiol.* 2008 Jun;53(1):18-25.

Ouwehand AC, Nermes M, Collado MC, Rautonen N, Salminen S, Isolauri E. Specific probiotics alleviate allergic rhinitis during the birch pollen season. *World J Gastroenterol.* 2009 Jul 14;15(26):3261-8.

Ouwehand AC, Tiihonen K, Saarinen M, Putaala H, Rautonen N. Influence of a combination of *Lactobacillus acidophilus* NCFM and lactitol on healthy elderly: intestinal and immune parameters. *Br J Nutr.* 2009 Feb;101(3):367-75.

Ouwehand AC. Antiallergic effects of probiotics. *J Nutr.* 2007 Mar;137(3 Suppl 2):794S-7S.

Ozdemir O. Any benefits of probiotics in allergic disorders? *Allergy Asthma Proc.* 2010 Mar;31(2):103-11.

Ozkan TB, Sahin E, Erdemir G, Budak F. Effect of *Saccharomyces boulardii* in children with acute gastroenteritis and its relationship to the immune response. *J Int Med Res.* 2007 Mar-Apr;35(2):201-12.

Paganelli R, Pallone F, Montano S, Le Moli S, Matricardi PM, Fais S, Paoluzi P, D'Amelio R, Aiuti F. Isotypic analysis of antibody response to a food antigen in inflammatory bowel disease. *Int Arch Allergy Appl Immunol.* 1985;78(1):81-5.

Pahud JJ, Schwarz K. Research and development of infant formulae with reduced allergenic properties. *Ann Allergy.* 1984 Dec;53(6 Pt 2):609-14.

Paineau D, Carcano D, Leyer G, Darquy S, Alyanakian MA, Simoneau G, Bergmann JF, Brassart D, Bornet F, Ouwehand AC. Effects of seven potential probiotic strains on specific immune responses in healthy adults: a double-blind, randomized, controlled trial. *FEMS Immunol Med Microbiol.* 2008 Jun;53(1):107-13.

Pakhale S, Doucette S, Vandemheen K, Boulet LP, McIvor RA, Fitzgerald JM, Hernandez P, Lemiere C, Sharma S, Field SK, Alvarez GG, Dales RE, Aaron SD. A comparison of obese and nonobese people with asthma: exploring an asthma-obesity interaction. *Chest.* 2010 Jun;137(6):1316-23. 2010 Feb 12.

Palacin A, Bartra J, Muñoz R, Diaz-Perales A, Valero A, Salcedo G. Anaphylaxis to wheat flour-derived foodstuffs and the lipid transfer protein syndrome: a potential role of wheat lipid transfer protein Tri a 14. *Int Arch Allergy Immunol.* 2010;152(2):178-83.

Palacios R, Sugawara I. Hydrocortisone abrogates proliferation of T cells in autologous mixed lymphocyte reaction by rendering the interleukin-2 Producer T cells unresponsive to interleukin-1 and unable to synthesize the T-cell growth factor. *Scand J Immunol.* 1982 Jan;15(1):25-31. 7.

Palacios R. HLA-DR antigens render interleukin-2-producer T lymphocytes sensitive to interleukin-1. *Scand J Immunol.* 1981 Sep;14(3):321-6.

Palmer DJ, Gold MS, Makrides M. Effect of cooked and raw egg consumption on ovalbumin content of human milk: a randomized, double-blind, cross-over trial. *Clin Exp Allergy.* 2005 Feb;35(2):173-8.

Panghal S, Mallapur SS, Kumar M, Ram V, Singh BK. Antiinflammatory Activity of Piper longum Fruit Oil. *Indian J Pharm Sci.* 2009 Jul;71(4):454-6.

Panigrahi P, Parida S, Pradhan L, Mohapatra SS, Misra PR, Johnson JA, Chaudhry R, Taylor S, Hansen NI, Gewolb IH. Long-term colonization of a *Lactobacillus plantarum* synbiotic preparation in the neonatal gut. *J Pediatr Gastroenterol Nutr.* 2008 Jul;47(1):45-53.

Pant H, Ferguson BJ, Macardle PJ. The role of allergy in rhinosinusitis. *Curr Opin Otolaryngol Head Neck Surg.* 2009 Jun;17(3):232-8.

Pant H, Kette FE, Smith WB, Wormald PJ, Macardle PJ. Fungal-specific humoral response in eosinophilic mucus chronic rhinosinusitis. *Laryngoscope.* 2005 Apr;115(4):601-6.

Panzani R, Ariano R, Mistrello G. Cypress pollen does not cross-react to plant-derived foods. *Eur Ann Allergy Clin Immunol.* 2010 Jun;42(3):125-6.

Parcell S. Sulfur in human nutrition and applications in medicine. *Altern Med Rev.* 2002 Feb;7(1):22-44.

Park BJ, Tsunetsugu Y, Kasetani T, Kagawa T, Miyazaki Y. The physiological effects of Shinrin-yoku (taking in the forest atmosphere or forest bathing): evidence from field experiments in 24 forests across Japan. *Environ Health Prev Med.* 2010 Jan;15(1):18-26.

Parra D, De Morentin BM, Cobo JM, Mateos A, Martinez JA. Monocyte function in healthy middle-aged people receiving fermented milk containing *Lactobacillus casei. J Nutr Health Aging.* 2004;8(4):208-11.

Parra MD, Martínez de Morentin BE, Cobo JM, Mateos A, Martínez JA. Daily ingestion of fermented milk containing Lactobacillus casei DN114001 improves innate-defense capacity in healthy middle-aged people. *J Physiol Biochem.* 2004 Jun;60(2):85-91.

Parra MD, Martínez de Morentin BE, Cobo JM, Mateos A, Martínez JA. Daily ingestion of fermented milk containing *Lactobacillus casei* DN114001 improves innate-defense capacity in healthy middle-aged people. *J Physiol Biochem.* 2004 Jun;60(2):85-91.

Partridge MR, Dockrell M, Smith NM: The use of complementary medicines by those with asthma. Respir Med 2003, 97:436-438.

Passeron T, Lacour JP, Fontas E, Ortonne JP. Prebiotics and synbiotics: two promising approaches for the treatment of atopic dermatitis in children above 2 years. *Allergy.* 2006 Apr;61(4):431-7.

Pastorello EA, Farioli L, Conti A, Pravettoni V, Bonomi S, Iametti S, Fortunato D, Scibilia J, Bindslev-Jensen C, Ballmer-Weber B, Robino AM, Ortolani C. Wheat IgE-mediated food allergy in European patients: alpha-amylase inhibitors, lipid transfer proteins and low-molecular-weight glutenins. Allergenic molecules recognized by double-blind, placebo-controlled food challenge. *Int Arch Allergy Immunol.* 2007;144(1):10-22.

Pastorello EA, Pompei C, Pravettoni V, Farioli L, Calamari AM, Scibilia J, Robino AM, Conti A, Iametti S, Fortunato D, Bonomi S, Ortolani C. Lipid-transfer protein is the major maize allergen maintaining IgE-binding activity after cooking at 100 degrees C, as demonstrated in anaphylactic patients and patients with positive double-blind, placebo-controlled food challenge results. *J Allergy Clin Immunol.* 2003 Oct;112(4):775-83.

Patchett K, Lewis S, Crane J, Fitzharris P. Cat allergen (Fel d 1) levels on school children's clothing and in primary school classrooms in Wellington, New Zealand. *J Allergy Clin Immunol.* 1997 Dec;100(6 Pt 1):755-9.

Patel DS, Rafferty GF, Lee S, Hannam S, Greenough A. Work of breathing and volume targeted ventilation in respiratory distress. *Arch Dis Child Fetal Neonatal Ed.* 2010 Nov;95(6):F443-6.

Patriarca G, Nucera E, Pollastrini E, Roncallo C, De Pasquale T, Lombardo C, Pedone C, Gasbarrini G, Buonomo A, Schiavino D. Oral specific desensitization in food-allergic children. *Dig Dis Sci.* 2007 Jul;52(7):1662-72.

Patriarca G, Nucera E, Roncallo C, Pollastrini E, Bartolozzi F, De Pasquale T, Buonomo A, Gasbarrini G, Di Campli C, Schiavino D. Oral desensitizing treatment in food allergy: clinical and immunological results. *Aliment Pharmacol Ther.* 2003 Feb;17(3):459-65.

Patterson DB. Anaphylactic shock from chloromycetin. Northwest Med. 1950 May;49(5):352-3.Agarwal KN, Bhasin SK. Feasibility studies to control acute diarrhoea in children by feeding fermented milk preparations Actimel and Indian Dahi. *Eur J Clin Nutr.* 2002 Dec;56 Suppl 4:S56-9.

Patwardhan B, Gautam M. Botanical immunodrugs: scope and opportunities. *Drug Discov Today.* 2005 Apr 1;10(7):495-502.

Paul M, Somkuti GA. Hydrolytic breakdown of lactoferricin by lactic acid bacteria. J Ind Microbiol Biotechnol. 2010 Feb;37(2):173-8. Epub 2009 Nov 19.

Payment P, Franco E, Richardson L, Siemiatyck, J. Gastrointestinal health effects associated with the consumption of drinking water produced by point-of-use domestic reverse-osmosis filtration units. *Appl. Environ. Microbiol.* 1991;57:945-948.

Peat JK, van den Berg RH, Green WF, Mellis CM, Leeder SR, Woolcock AJ. Changing prevalence of asthma in Australian children. *BMJ.* 1994;308:1591-1596.

Peat JK. The rising trend in allergic illness: which environmental factors are important? Clin Exp Allergy. 1994 Sep;24(9):797-800.

Pedone CA, Arnaud CC, Postaire ER, Bouley CF, Reinert P. Multicentric study of the effect of milk fermented by *Lactobacillus casei* on the incidence of diarrhoea. *Int J Clin Pract.* 2000 Nov;54(9):568-71.

Pedone CA, Bernabeu AO, Postaire ER, Bouley CF, Reinert P. The effect of supplementation with milk fermented by *Lactobacillus casei* (strain DN-114 001) on acute diarrhoea in children attending day care centres. *Int J Clin Pract.* 1999 Apr-May;53(3):179-84.

Pedrosa MC, Golner BB, Goldin AJ, Barakat S, Dallal GE, Russell RM. Survival of yogurt-containing organisms and *Lactobacillus gasseri* (ADH) and their effect on bacterial enzyme activity in the gastrointestinal tract of healthy and hypochlorhydric elderly subjects. *Am J Clin Nutr.* 1995 Feb;61(2):353-9.

Pehowich DJ, Gomes AV, Barnes JA. Fatty acid composition and possible health effects of coconut constituents. *West Indian Med J.* 2000 Jun;49(2):128-33.

Peral MC, Martinez MA, Valdez JC. Bacteriotherapy with *Lactobacillus plantarum* in burns. *Int Wound J.* 2009 Feb;6(1):73-81.

Perez-Galvez A, Martin HD, Sies H, Stahl W. Incorporation of carotenoids from paprika oleoresin into human chylomicrons. *Br J Nutr.* 2003 Jun;89(6):787-93.

Perez-Pena R. Secrets of the Mummy's Medicine Chest. *NY Times.* 2005 Sept 10.

Persson R, Orbaek P, Kecklund G, Akerstedt T. Impact of an 84-hour workweek on biomarkers for stress, metabolic processes and diurnal rhythm. *Scand J Work Environ Health.* 2006 Oct;32(5):349-58.

Pessi T, Sütas Y, Hurme M, Isolauri E. Interleukin-10 generation in atopic children following oral *Lactobacillus rhamnosus* GG. *Clin Exp Allergy.* 2000 Dec;30(12):1804-8.

Peters JI, McKinney JM, Smith B, Wood P, Forkner E, Galbreath AD. Impact of obesity in asthma: evidence from a large prospective disease management study. *Ann Allergy Asthma Immunol.* 2011 Jan;106(1):30-5.

Peterson CG, Hansson T, Skott A, Bengtsson U, Ahlstedt S, Magnussons J. Detection of local mast-cell activity in patients with food hypersensitivity. *J Investig Allergol Clin Immunol.* 2007;17(5):314-20.

Peterson KA, Samuelson WM, Ryujin DT, Young DC, Thomas KL, Hilden K, Fang JC. The role of gastroesophageal reflux in exercise-triggered asthma: a randomized controlled trial. *Dig Dis Sci.* 2009 Mar;54(3):564-71. 2008 Aug 8.

Petlevski R, Hadzija M, Slijepcević M, Juretić D, Petrik J. Glutathione S-transferases and malondialdehyde in the liver of NOD mice on short-term treatment with plant mixture extract P-9801091. *Phytother Res.* 2003 Apr;17(4):311-4.

Petricevic L, Unger FM, Viernstein H, Kiss H. Randomized, double-blind, placebo-controlled study of oral lactobacilli to improve the vaginal flora of postmenopausal women. *Eur J Obstet Gynecol Reprod Biol.* 2008 Nov;141(1):54-7.

Petricevic L, Witt A. The role of *Lactobacillus casei* rhamnosus Lcr35 in restoring the normal vaginal flora after antibiotic treatment of bacterial vaginosis. *BJOG.* 2008 Oct;115(11):1369-74.

Petrunov B, Marinova S, Markova R, Nenkov P, Nikolaeva S, Nikolova M, Taskov H, Cvetanov J. Cellular and humoral systemic and mucosal immune responses stimulated in volunteers by an oral polybacterial immunomodulator "Dentavax". *Int Immunopharmacol.* 2006 Jul;6(7):1181-93.

Petti S, Tarsitani G, D'Arca AS. A randomized clinical trial of the effect of yoghurt on the human salivary microflora. *Arch Oral Biol.* 2001 Aug;46(8):705-12.

Pfefferle PI, Sel S, Ege MJ, Büchele G, Blümer N, Krauss-Etschmann S, Herzum I, Albers CE, Lauener RP, Roponen M, Hirvonen MR, Vuitton DA, Riedler J, Brunekreef B, Dalphin JC, Braun-Fahrländer C, Pekkanen J, von Mutius E, Renz H; PASTURE Study Group. Cord blood allergen-specific IgE is associated with reduced IFN-gamma production by cord blood cells: the Protection against Allergy-Study in Rural Environments (PASTURE) Study. *J Allergy Clin Immunol.* 2008 Oct;122(4):711-6.

Pfundstein B, El Desouky SK, Hull WE, Haubner R, Erben G, Owen RW. Polyphenolic compounds in the fruits of Egyptian medicinal plants (Terminalia bellerica, Terminalia chebula and Terminalia horrida): characterization, quantitation and determination of antioxidant capacities. *Phytochemistry.* 2010 Jul;71(10):1132-48.

Phuapradit P, Varavithya W, Vathanophas K, Sangchai R, Podhipak A, Suthutvoravut U, Nopchinda S, Chantraruksa V, Haschke F. Reduction of rotavirus infection in children receiving bifidobacteria-supplemented formula. *J Med Assoc Thai.* 1999 Nov;82 Suppl 1:S43-8.

Physicians' Desk Reference. Montvale, NJ: Thomson, 2003-2008.

Pierce SK, Klinman NR. Antibody-specific immunoregulation. *J Exp Med.* 1977 Aug 1;146(2):509-19.

Piirainen L, Haahtela S, Helin T, Korpela R, Haahtela T, Vaarala O. Effect of Lactobacillus rhamnosus GG on rBet v1 and rMal d1 specific IgA in the saliva of patients with birch pollen allergy. *Ann Allergy Asthma Immunol.* 2008 Apr;100(4):338-42.

Piirainen L, Haahtela S, Helin T, Korpela R, Haahtela T, Vaarala O. Effect of *Lactobacillus rhamnosus* GG on rBet v1 and rMal d1 specific IgA in the saliva of patients with birch pollen allergy. *Ann Allergy Asthma Immunol.* 2008 Apr;100(4):338-42.

Pike MG, Heddle RJ, Boulton P, Turner MW, Atherton DJ. Increased intestinal permeability in atopic eczema. *J Invest Dermatol.* 1986 Feb;86(2):101-4.

Pines JM, Prabhu A, Hilton JA, Hollander JE, Datner EM. The effect of emergency department crowding on length of stay and medication treatment times in discharged patients with acute asthma. *Acad Emerg Med.* 2010 Aug;17(8):834-9.

Pitkala KH, Strandberg TE, Finne Soveri UH, Ouwehand AC, Poussa T, Salminen S. Fermented cereal with specific bifidobacteria normalizes bowel movements in elderly nursing home residents. A randomized, controlled trial. *J Nutr Health Aging.* 2007 Jul-Aug;11(4):305-11.

Pitten FA, Scholler M, Krüger U, Effendy I, Kramer A. Filamentous fungi and yeasts on mattresses covered with different encasings. Eur J Dermatol. 2001 Nov-Dec;11(6):534-7.

Pitt-Rivers R, Trotter WR. *The Thyroid Gland.* London: Butterworth Publ, 1954.

Plaschke P, Janson C, Norrman E, Björnsson E, Ellbjär S, Järvholm B. Association between atopic sensitization and asthma and bronchial hyperresponsiveness in swedish adults: pets, and not mites, are the most important allergens. *J Allergy Clin Immunol.* 1999 Jul;104(1):58-65.

Plaut M, Valentine MD. Clinical practice. Allergic rhinitis. *N Engl J Med.* 2005 Nov 3;353(18):1934-44.

Plaut TE, Jones TB. *Dr. Tom Plaut's Asthma guide for people of all ages.* Amherst, MA: Pedipress, 1999.

Plaza V, Miguel E, Bellido-Casado J, Lozano MP, Ríos L, Bolíbar I. [Usefulness of the Guidelines of the Spanish Society of Pulmonology and Thoracic Surgery (SEPAR) in identifying the causes of chronic cough]. Arch Bronconeumol. 2006 Feb;42(2):68-73.

Plein K, Hotz J. Therapeutic effects of *Saccharomyces boulardii* on mild residual symptoms in a stable phase of Crohn's disease with special respect to chronic diarrhea—a pilot study. *Z Gastroenterol.* 1993 Feb;31(2):129-34.

Plohmann B, Bader G, Hiller K, Franz G. Immunomodulatory and antitumoral effects of triterpenoid saponins. *Pharmazie.* 1997 Dec;52(12):953-7.

Poblocka-Olech L, Krauze-Baranowska M. SPE-HPTLC of procyanidins from the barks of different species and clones of Salix. *J Pharm Biomed Anal.* 2008 Nov 4;48(3):965-8.

Pohjavuori E, Viljanen M, Korpela R, Kuitunen M, Tiittanen M, Vaarala O, Savilahti E. Lactobacillus GG effect in increasing IFN-gamma production in infants with cow's milk allergy. *J Allergy Clin Immunol.* 2004 Jul;114(1):131-6.

Pohjavuori E, Viljanen M, Korpela R, Kuitunen M, Tiittanen M, Vaarala O, Savilahti E. Lactobacillus GG effect in increasing IFN-gamma production in infants with cow's milk allergy. *J Allergy Clin Immunol.* 2004 Jul;114(1):131-6.

Polito A, Aboab J, Annane D. The hypothalamic pituitary adrenal axis in sepsis. *Novartis Found Symp.* 2007;280:182-203.

Polk S, Sunyer J, Muñoz-Ortiz L, Barnes M, Torrent M, Figueroa C, Harris J, Vall O, Antó JM, Cullinan P. A prospective study of Fel d1 and Der p1 exposure in infancy and childhood wheezing. *Am J Respir Crit Care Med.* 2004 Aug 1;170(3):273-8.

Pollini F, Capristo C, Boner AL. Upper respiratory tract infections and atopy. *Int J Immunopathol Pharmacol.* 2010 Jan-Mar;23(1 Suppl):32-7.

Ponsonby AL, McMichael A, van der Mei I. Ultraviolet radiation and autoimmune disease: insights from epidemiological research. *Toxicology.* 2002 Dec 27;181-182:71-8.

Postlethwait EM. Scavenger receptors clear the air. *J Clin Invest.* 2007 Mar;117(3):601-4.

Postma DS. Gender Differences in Asthma Development and Progression. *Gender Medicine.* 2007;4:S133-146.

Postolache TT, Lapidus M, Sander ER, Langenberg P, Hamilton RG, Soriano JJ, McDonald JS, Furst N, Bai J, Scrandis DA, Cabassa JA, Stiller JW, Balis T, Guzman A, Togias A, Tonelli LH. Changes in allergy symptoms and depression scores are positively correlated in patients with recurrent mood disorders exposed to seasonal peaks in aeroallergens. *ScientificWorldJournal.* 2007 Dec 17;7:1968-77.

Potterton D. (Ed.) *Culpeper's Color Herbal.* New York: Sterling, 1983.

Poulos LM, Waters AM, Correll PK, Loblay RH, Marks GB. Trends in hospitalizations for anaphylaxis, angioedema, and urticaria in Australia, 1993-1994 to 2004-2005. *J Allergy Clin Immunol.* 2007 Oct;120(4):878-84.

Powe DG, Groot Kormelink T, Sisson M, Blokhuis BJ, Kramer MF, Jones NS, Redegeld FA. Evidence for the involvement of free light chain immunoglobulins in allergic and nonallergic rhinitis. *J Allergy Clin Immunol.* 2010 Jan;125(1):139-45.e1-3.

Pregliasco F, Anselmi G, Fonte L, Giussani F, Schieppati S, Soletti L. A new chance of preventing winter diseases by the administration of synbiotic formulations. *J Clin Gastroenterol.* 2008 Sep;42 Suppl 3 Pt 2:S224-33.

Prescott SL, Wickens K, Westcott L, Jung W, Currie H, Black PN, Stanley TV, Mitchell EA, Fitzharris P, Siebers R, Wu L, Crane J; Probiotic Study Group. Supplementation with Lactobacillus rhamnosus or Bifidobacterium lactis probiotics in pregnancy increases cord blood interferon-gamma and breast milk transforming growth factor-beta and immunoglobin A detection. *Clin Exp Allergy.* 2008 Oct;38(10):1606-14.

Prescott SL, Wickens K, Westcott L, Jung W, Currie H, Black PN, Stanley TV, Mitchell EA, Fitzharris P, Siebers R, Wu L, Crane J; Probiotic Study Group. Supplementation with *Lactobacillus rhamnosus* or *Bifidobacterium lactis* probiotics in pregnancy increases cord blood interferon-gamma and breast milk transforming growth factor-beta and immunoglobin A detection. *Clin Exp Allergy.* 2008 Oct;38(10):1606-14.

Priftis KN, Panagiotakos DB, Anthracopoulos MB, Papadimitriou A, Nicolaidou P. Aims, methods and preliminary findings of the Physical Activity, Nutrition and Allergies in Children Examined in Athens (PANACEA) epidemiological study. *BMC Public Health.* 2007 Jul 4;7:140.

Prioult G, Fliss I, Pecquet S. Effect of probiotic bacteria on induction and maintenance of oral tolerance to beta-lactoglobulin in gnotobiotic mice. *Clin Diagn Lab Immunol.* 2003 Sep;10(5):787-92.

Prucksunand C, Indrasukhsri B, Leethochawalit M, Hungspreugs K. Phase II clinical trial on effect of the long turmeric (Curcuma longa Linn) on healing of peptic ulcer. *Southeast Asian J Trop Med Public Health.* 2001 Mar;32(1):208-15.

Pruthi S, Thapa MM. Infectious and inflammatory disorders. *Magn Reson Imaging Clin N Am.* 2009 Aug;17(3):423-38, v.

Qin HL, Zheng JJ, Tong DN, Chen WX, Fan XB, Hang XM, Jiang YQ. Effect of Lactobacillus plantarum enteral feeding on the gut permeability and septic complications in the patients with acute pancreatitis. *Eur J Clin Nutr.* 2008 Jul;62(7):923-30.

Qin HL, Zheng JJ, Tong DN, Chen WX, Fan XB, Hang XM, Jiang YQ. Effect of *Lactobacillus plantarum* enteral feeding on the gut permeability and septic complications in the patients with acute pancreatitis. *Eur J Clin Nutr.* 2008 Jul;62(7):923-30.

Qu C, Srivastava K, Ko J, Zhang TF, Sampson HA, Li XM. Induction of tolerance after establishment of peanut allergy by the food allergy herbal formula-2 is associated with up-regulation of interferon-gamma. *Clin Exp Allergy.* 2007 Jun;37(6):846-55.

Radon K, Danuser B, Iversen M, Jörres R, Monso E, Opravil U, Weber C, Donham KJ, Nowak D. Respiratory symptoms in European animal farmers. *Eur Respir J.* 2001 Apr;17(4):747-54.

Rafter J, Bennett M, Caderni G, Clune Y, Hughes R, Karlsson PC, Klinder A, O'Riordan M, O'Sullivan GC, Pool-Zobel B, Rechkemmer G, Roller M, Rowland I, Salvadori M, Thijs H, Van Loo J, Watzl B, Collins JK. Dietary synbiotics reduce cancer risk factors in polypectomized and colon cancer patients. *Am J Clin Nutr.* 2007 Feb;85(2):488-96.

Raherison C, Pénard-Morand C, Moreau D, Caillaud D, Charpin D, Kopferschmitt C, Lavaud F, Taytard A, Maesano IA. Smoking exposure and allergic sensitization in children according to maternal allergies. *Ann Allergy Asthma Immunol.* 2008 Apr;100(4):351-7.

Rahman MM, Bhattacharya A, Fernandes G. Docosahexaenoic acid is more potent inhibitor of osteoclast differentiation in RAW 264.7 cells than eicosapentaenoic acid. *J Cell Physiol.* 2008 Jan;214(1):201-9.

Raithel M, Weidenhiller M, Abel R, Baenkler HW, Hahn EG. Colorectal mucosal histamine release by mucosa oxygenation in comparison with other established clinical tests in patients with gastrointestinally mediated allergy. *World J Gastroenterol.* 2006 Aug 7;12(29):4699-705.

Raloff J. Ill Winds. *Science News:* 2001;160(14):218.

Rampton DS, Murdoch RD, Sladen GE. Rectal mucosal histamine release in ulcerative colitis. *Clin Sci (Lond).* 1980 Nov;59(5):389-91.

Rancé F, Kanny G, Dutau G, Moneret-Vautrin DA. Food allergens in children. *Arch Pediatr.* 1999;6(Suppl 1):61S-66S.

Randal Bollinger R, Barbas AS, Bush EL, Lin SS, Parker W. Biofilms in the large bowel suggest an apparent function of the human vermiform appendix. *J Theor Biol.* 2007 Dec 21;249(4):826-31.

Randal Bollinger R, Barbas AS, Bush EL, Lin SS, Parker W. Biofilms in the large bowel suggest an apparent function of the human vermiform appendix. *J Theor Biol.* 2007 Dec 21;249(4):826-31.

Rangavajhyala N, Shahani KM, Sridevi G, Srikumaran S. Nonlipopolysaccharide component(s) of Lactobacillus acidophilus stimulate(s) the production of interleukin-1 alpha and tumor necrosis factor-alpha by murine macrophages. *Nutr Cancer.* 1997;28(2):130-4.

Ranjbaran Z, Keefer L, Stepanski E, Farhadi A, Keshavarzian A. The relevance of sleep abnormalities to chronic inflammatory conditions. *Inflamm Res.* 2007 Feb;56(2):51-7.

Rao SK, Rao PS, Rao BN. Preliminary investigation of the radiosensitizing activity of guduchi (Tinospora cordifolia) in tumor-bearing mice. *Phytother Res.* 2008 Nov;22(11):1482-9.

Rapin JR, Wiernsperger N. Possible links between intestinal permeablity and food processing: A potential therapeutic niche for glutamine. *Clinics (Sao Paulo).* 2010 Jun;65(6):635-43.

Rappoport J. Both sides of the pharmaceutical death coin. *Townsend Letter for Doctors and Patients.* 2006 Oct.

Rauha JP, Remes S, Heinonen M, Hopia A, Kähkönen M, Kujala T, Pihlaja K, Vuorela H, Vuorela P. Antimicrobial effects of Finnish plant extracts containing flavonoids and other phenolic compounds. *Int J Food Microbiol.* 2000 May 25;56(1):3-12.

Rauma A. Antioxidant status in vegetarians versus omnivores. *Nutrition.* 2003;16(2): 111-119.

Rautava S, Isolauri E. Cow's milk allergy in infants with atopic eczema is associated with aberrant production of interleukin-4 during oral cow's milk challenge. *J Pediatr Gastroenterol Nutr.* 2004 Nov;39(5):529-35.

Rautava S, Salminen S, Isolauri E. Specific probiotics in reducing the risk of acute infections in infancy—a randomised, double-blind, placebo-controlled study. *Br J Nutr.* 2009 Jun;101(11):1722-6.

Rayes N, Seehofer D, Hansen S, Boucsein K, Müller AR, Serke S, Bengmark S, Neuhaus P. Early enteral supply of lactobacillus and fiber versus selective bowel decontamination: a controlled trial in liver transplant recipients. *Transplantation.* 2002 Jul 15;74(1):123-7.

Rayes N, Seehofer D, Müller AR, Hansen S, Bengmark S, Neuhaus P. Influence of probiotics and fibre on the incidence of bacterial infections following major abdominal surgery - results of a prospective trial. *Z Gastroenterol.* 2002 Oct;40(10):869-76.

Raza S, Graham SM, Allen SJ, Sultana S, Cuevas L, Hart CA, Kaila M, Isolauri E, Saxelin M, Arvilommi H, *et al.* Lactobacillus GG in acute diarrhea. *Indian Pediatr.* 1995 Oct;32(10):1140-2.

Raza S, Graham SM, Allen SJ, Sultana S, Cuevas L, Hart CA. Lactobacillus GG promotes recovery from acute nonbloody diarrhea in Pakistan. Pediatr Infect Dis J. 1995 Feb;14(2):107-11.

Rebhun J. Coexisting immune complex diseases in atopy. *Ann Allergy.* 1980 Dec;45(6):368-71.

Reddy KP, Shahani KM, Kulkarni SM. B-complex vitamins in cultured and acidified yogurt. *J Dairy Sci.* 1976 Feb;59(2):191-5.

Reger D, Goode S, Mercer E. *Chemistry: Principles & Practice.* Fort Worth, TX: Harcourt Brace, 1993.

Reger D, Goode S, Mercer E. *Chemistry: Principles & Practice.* Fort Worth, TX: Harcourt Brace, 1993.

REFERENCES AND BIBLIOGRAPHY

Regis E. *Virus Ground Zero.* New York: Pocket, 1996.

Reha CM, Ebru A. Specific immunotherapy is effective in the prevention of new sensitivities. *Allergol Immunopathol (Madr).* 2007 Mar-Apr;35(2):44-51.

Rehm J, Taylor B, Mohapatra S, Irving H, Baliunas D, Patra J, Roerecke M. Alcohol as a risk factor for liver cirrhosis: a systematic review and meta-analysis. Drug Alcohol Rev. 2010 Jul;29(4):437-45.

Reid G, Beuerman D, Heinemann C, Bruce AW. Probiotic Lactobacillus dose required to restore and maintain a normal vaginal flora. *FEMS Immunol Med Microbiol.* 2001 Dec;32(1):37-41.

Reid G, Burton J, Hammond JA, Bruce AW. Nucleic acid-based diagnosis of bacterial vaginosis and improved management using probiotic lactobacilli. *J Med Food.* 2004 Summer;7(2):223-8.

Reid G, Charbonneau D, Erb J, Kochanowski B, Beuerman D, Poehner R, Bruce AW. Oral use of *Lactobacillus rhamnosus* GR-1 and L. fermentum RC-14 significantly alters vaginal flora: randomized, placebo-controlled trial in 64 healthy women. *FEMS Immunol Med Microbiol.* 2003 Mar 20;35(2):131-4.

Renkonen R, Renkonen J, Joenväärä S, Mattila P, Parviainen V, Toppila-Salmi S. Allergens are transported through the respiratory epithelium. *Expert Rev Clin Immunol.* 2010 Jan;6(1):55-9.

Renvert S, Lindahl C, Renvert H, Persson GR. Clinical and microbiological analysis of subjects treated with Brånemark or AstraTech implants: a 7-year follow-up study. *Clin Oral Implants Res.* 2008 Apr;19(4):342-7.

Reuter A, Lidholm J, Andersson K, Ostling J, Lundberg M, Scheurer S, Enrique E, Cistero-Bahima A, San Miguel-Moncin M, Ballmer-Weber BK, Vieths S. A critical assessment of allergen component-based in vitro diagnosis in cherry allergy across Europe. *Clin Exp Allergy.* 2006 Jun;36(6):815-23.

Reznik M, Sharif I, Ozuah PO. Rubbing ointments and asthma morbidity in adolescents. *J Altern Complement Med.* 2004 Dec;10(6):1097-9. Uu

Riccia DN, Bizzini F, Perilli MG, Polimeni A, Trinchieri V, Amicosante G, Cifone MG. Anti-inflammatory effects of *Lactobacillus brevis* (CD2) on periodontal disease. *Oral Dis.* 2007 Jul;13(4):376-85.

Riccia DN, Bizzini F, Perilli MG, Polimeni A, Trinchieri V, Amicosante G, Cifone MG. Anti-inflammatory effects of *Lactobacillus brevis* (CD2) on periodontal disease. *Oral Dis.* 2007 Jul;13(4):376-85.

Riccioni G, Barbara M, Bucciarelli T, di Ilio C, D'Orazio N. Antioxidant vitamin supplementation in asthma. *Ann Clin Lab Sci.* 2007 Winter;37(1):96-101.

Riccioni G, Bucciarelli T, Mancini B, Di Ilio C, Della Vecchia R, D'Orazio N. Plasma lycopene and antioxidant vitamins in asthma: the PLAVA study. *J Asthma.* 2007 Jul-Aug;44(6):429-32.

Riccioni G, D'Orazio N. The role of selenium, zinc and antioxidant vitamin supplementation in the treatment of bronchial asthma: adjuvant therapy or not? *Expert Opin Investig Drugs.* 2005 Sep;14(9):1145-55.

Riccioni G, Di Stefano F, De Benedictis M, Verna N, Cavallucci E, Paolini F, Di Sciascio MB, Della Vecchia R, Schiavone C, Boscolo P, Conti P, Di Gioacchino M. Seasonal variability of non-specific bronchial responsiveness in asthmatic patients with allergy to house dust mites. *Allergy Asthma Proc.* 2001 Jan-Feb;22(1):5-9.

Riedler J, Braun-Fahrländer C, Eder W, Schreuer M, Waser M, Maisch S, Carr D, Schierl R, Nowak D, von Mutius E; ALEX Study Team. Exposure to farming in early life and development of asthma and allergy: a cross-sectional survey. *Lancet.* 2001 Oct 6;358(9288):1129-33.

Rimkiene S, Ragazinskiene O, Savickiene N. The cumulation of Wild pansy (Viola tricolor L.) accessions: the possibility of species preservation and usage in medicine. *Medicina (Kaunas).* 2003;39(4):411-6.

Rinne M, Kalliomaki M, Arvilommi H, Salminen S, Isolauri E. Effect of probiotics and breastfeeding on the bifidobacterium and lactobacillus/enterococcus microbiota and humoral immune responses. *J Pediatr.* 2005 Aug;147(2):186-91.

Rinne M, Kalliomaki M, Arvilommi H, Salminen S, Isolauri E. Effect of probiotics and breastfeeding on the bifidobacterium and lactobacillus/enterococcus microbiota and humoral immune responses. *J Pediatr.* 2005 Aug;147(2):186-91.

Rinne M, Kalliomäki M, Salminen S, Isolauri E. Probiotic intervention in the first months of life: short-term effects on gastrointestinal symptoms and long-term effects on gut microbiota. *J Pediatr Gastroenterol Nutr.* 2006 Aug;43(2):200-5.

Río ME, Zago Beatriz L, Garcia H, Winter L. The nutritional status change the effectiveness of a dietary supplement of lactic bacteria on the emerging of respiratory tract diseases in children. *Arch Latinoam Nutr.* 2002 Mar;52(1):29-34.

Río ME, Zago Beatriz L, Garcia H, Winter L. The nutritional status change the effectiveness of a dietary supplement of lactic bacteria on the emerging of respiratory tract diseases in children. *Arch Latinoam Nutr.* 2002 Mar;52(1):29-34.

Río ME, Zago LB, Garcia H, Winter L. Influence of nutritional status on the effectiveness of a dietary supplement of live lactobacillus to prevent and cure diarrhoea in children. *Arch Latinoam Nutr.* 2004 Sep;54(3):287-92.

Robert AM, Groult N, Six C, Robert L. The effect of procyanidolic oligomers on mesenchymal cells in culture II—Attachment of elastic fibers to the cells. *Pathol Biol.* 1990 Jun;38(6):601-7.

Robert AM, Groult N, Six C, Robert L. The effect of procyanidolic oligomers on mesenchymal cells in culture II—Attachment of elastic fibers to the cells. *Pathol Biol.* 1990 Jun;38(6):601-7.

Robert AM, Robert L, Renard G. Protection of cornea against proteolytic damage. Experimental study of procyanidolic oligomers (PCO) on bovine cornea. *J Fr Ophtalmol.* 2002 Apr;25(4):351-5.

Robert AM, Tixier JM, Robert L, Legeais JM, Renard G. Effect of procyanidolic oligomers on the permeability of the blood-brain barrier. *Pathol Biol.* 2001 May;49(4):298-304.

Roberts G, Lack G. Diagnosing peanut allergy with skin prick and specific IgE testing. *J Allergy Clin Immunol.* 2005 Jun;115(6):1291-6.

Robinson L, Cherewatenko VS, Reeves S. *Epicor: The Key to a Balanced Immune System.* Sherman Oaks, CA: Health Point, 2009.

Rodriguez E, Valbuena MC, Rey M, Porras de Quintana L. Causal agents of photoallergic contact dermatitis diagnosed in the national institute of dermatology of Colombia. *Photodermatol Photoimmunol Photomed.* 2006 Aug;22(4):189-92.

Rodriguez J, Crespo JF, Burks W, Rivas-Plata C, Fernandez-Anaya S, Vives R, Daroca P. Randomized, double-blind, crossover challenge study in 53 subjects reporting adverse reactions to melon (Cucumis melo). *J Allergy Clin Immunol.* 2000 Nov;106(5):968-72.

Rodriguez-Fragoso L, Reyes-Esparza J, Burchiel SW, Herrera-Ruiz D, Torres E. Risks and benefits of commonly used herbal medicines in Mexico. *Toxicol Appl Pharmacol.* 2008 Feb 15;227(1):125-35.

Rodríguez-Ortiz PG, Muñoz-Mendoza D, Arias-Cruz A, González-Díaz SN, Herrera-Castro D, Vidaurri-Ojeda AC. Epidemiological characteristics of patients with food allergy assisted at Regional Center of Allergies and Clinical Immunology of Monterrey. *Rev Alerg Mex.* 2009 Nov-Dec;56(6):185-91.

Roduit C, Scholtens S, de Jongste JC, Wijga AH, Gerritsen J, Postma DS, Brunekreef B, Hoekstra MO, Aalberse R, Smit HA. Asthma at 8 years of age in children born by caesarean section. *Thorax.* 2009 Feb;64(2):107-13.

Roessler A, Friedrich U, Vogelsang H, Bauer A, Kaatz M, Hipler UC, Schmidt I, Jahreis G. The immune system in healthy adults and patients with atopic dermatitis seems to be affected differently by a probiotic intervention. *Clin Exp Allergy.* 2008 Jan;38(1):93-102.

Roessler A, Friedrich U, Vogelsang H, Bauer A, Kaatz M, Hipler UC, Schmidt I, Jahreis G. The immune system in healthy adults and patients with atopic dermatitis seems to be affected differently by a probiotic intervention. *Clin Exp Allergy.* 2008 Jan;38(1):93-102.

Roger A, Justicia JL, Navarro LÁ, Eseverri JL, Ferrès J, Malet A, Alvà V. Observational study of the safety of an ultra-rush sublingual immunotherapy regimen to treat rhinitis due to house dust mites. *Int Arch Allergy Immunol.* 2011;154(1):69-75. 2010 Jul 27.

Roller M, Clune Y, Collins K, Rechkemmer G, Watzl B. Consumption of prebiotic inulin enriched with oligofructose in combination with the probiotics *Lactobacillus rhamnosus* and *Bifidobacterium lactis* has minor effects on selected immune parameters in polypectomised and colon cancer patients. *Br J Nutr.* 2007 Apr;97(4):676-84.

Romeo J, Wärnberg J, Nova E, Díaz LE, González-Gross M, Marcos A. Changes in the immune system after moderate beer consumption. *Ann Nutr Metab.* 2007;51(4):359-66.

Romieu I, Barraza-Villarreal A, Escamilla-Núñez C, Texcalac-Sangrador JL, Hernandez-Cadena L, Díaz-Sánchez D, De Batlle J, Del Rio-Navarro BE. Dietary intake, lung function and airway inflammation in Mexico City school children exposed to air pollutants. *Respir Res.* 2009 Dec 10;10:122.

Ronteltap A, van Schaik J, Wensing M, Rynja FJ, Knulst AC, de Vries JH. Sensory testing of recipes masking peanut or hazelnut for double-blind placebo-controlled food challenges. Allergy. 2004 Apr;59(4):457-60. Clark S, Bock SA, Gaeta TJ, Brenner BE, Cydulka RK, Camargo CA; Multicenter Airway Research Collaboration-8 Investigators. Multicenter study of emergency department visits for food allergies. *J Allergy Clin Immunol.* 2004 Feb;113(2):347-52.

Rook GA, Hernandez-Pando R. Pathogenetic role, in human and murine tuberculosis, of changes in the peripheral metabolism of glucocorticoids and antiglucocorticoids. *Psychoneuroendocrinology.* 1997;22 Suppl 1:S109-13.

Ros E, Mataix J. Fatty acid composition of nuts—implications for cardiovascular health. *Br J Nutr.* 2006 Nov;96 Suppl 2:S29-35.

Rosander A, Connolly E, Roos S. Removal of antibiotic resistance gene-carrying plasmids from *Lactobacillus reuteri* ATCC 55730 and characterization of the resulting daughter strain, *L. reuteri* DSM 17938. *Appl Environ Microbiol.* 2008 Oct;74(19):6032-40.

Rosenfeldt V, Benfeldt E, Nielsen SD, Michaelsen KF, Jeppesen DL, Valerius NH, Paerregaard A. Effect of probiotic Lactobacillus strains in children with atopic dermatitis. *J Allergy Clin Immunol.* 2003 Feb;111(2):389-95.

Rosenfeldt V, Benfeldt E, Valerius NH, Paerregaard A, Michaelsen KF. Effect of probiotics on gastrointestinal symptoms and small intestinal permeability in children with atopic dermatitis. *J Pediatr.* 2004 Nov;145(5):612-6.

REFERENCES AND BIBLIOGRAPHY

Rosenfeldt V, Michaelsen KF, Jakobsen M, Larsen CN, Møller PL, Pedersen P, Tvede M, Weyrehter H, Valerius NH, Paerregaard A. Effect of probiotic Lactobacillus strains in young children hospitalized with acute diarrhea. *Pediatr Infect Dis J.* 2002 May;21(5):411-6.

Rosenkranz SK, Swain KE, Rosenkranz RR, Beckman B, Harms CA. Modifiable lifestyle factors impact airway health in non-asthmatic prepubescent boys but not girls. *Pediatr Pulmonol.* 2010 Dec 30.

Rosenlund H, Bergström A, Alm JS, Swartz J, Scheynius A, van Hage M, Johansen K, Brunekreef B, von Mutius E, Ege MJ, Riedler J, Braun-Fahrländer C, Waser M, Pershagen G; PARSIFAL Study Group. Allergic disease and atopic sensitization in children in relation to measles vaccination and measles infection. *Pediatrics.* 2009 Mar;123(3):771-8.

Rousseaux C, Thuru X, Gelot A, Barnich N, Neut C, Dubuquoy L, Dubuquoy C, Merour E, Geboes K, Chamaillard M, Ouwehand A, Leyer G, Carcano D, Colombel JF, Ardid D, Desreumaux P. Lactobacillus acidophilus modulates intestinal pain and induces opioid and cannabinoid receptors. *Nat Med.* 2007 Jan;13(1):35-7

Royer RJ, Schmidt CL. Evaluation of venotropic drugs by venous gas plethysmography. A study of procyanidolic oligomers *Sem Hop.* 1981 Dec 18-25;57(47-48):2009-13.

Rozycki VR, Baigorria CM, Freyre MR, Bernard CM, Zannier MS, Charpentier M. Nutrient content in vegetable species from the Argentine Chaco. *Arch Latinoam Nutr.* 1997 Sep;47(3):265-70.

Rubin E., Farber JL. *Pathology.* 3rd Ed. Philadelphia: Lippincott-Raven, 1999.

Rudders SA, Espinola JA, Camargo CA Jr. North-south differences in US emergency department visits for acute allergic reactions. *Ann Allergy Asthma Immunol.* 2010 May;104(5):413-6.

Rynard PB, Palij B, Galloway CA, Roughley FR. Resperin inhalation treatment for chronic respiratory diseases. *Can Fam Physician.* 1968 Oct;14(10):70-1.

Saarinen KM, Juntunen-Backman K, Järvenpää AL, Klemetti P, Kuitunen P, Lope L, Renlund M, Siivola M, Vaarala O, Savilahti E. Breast-feeding and the development of cows' milk protein allergy. *Adv Exp Med Biol.* 2000;478:121-30.

Saavedra JM, Abi-Hanna A, Moore N, Yolken RH. Long-term consumption of infant formulas containing live probiotic bacteria: tolerance and safety. *Am J Clin Nutr.* 2004 Feb;79(2):261-7.

Saavedra JM, Bauman NA, Oung I, Perman JA, Yolken RH. Feeding of *Bifidobacterium bifidum* and *Streptococcus thermophilus* to infants in hospital for prevention of diarrhoea and shedding of rotavirus. *Lancet.* 1994 Oct 15;344(8929):1046-9.

Saggioro A. Probiotics in the treatment of irritable bowel syndrome. *J Clin Gastroenterol.* 2004 Jul;38(6 Suppl):S104-6.

Sahagún-Flores JE, López-Peña LS, de la Cruz-Ramírez Jaimes J, García-Bravo MS, Peregrina-Gómez R, de Alba-García JE. Eradication of Helicobacter pylori: triple treatment scheme plus Lactobacillus vs. triple treatment alone. *Cir Cir.* 2007 Sep-Oct;75(5):333-6.

Sahagún-Flores JE, López-Peña LS, de la Cruz-Ramírez Jaimes J, García-Bravo MS, Peregrina-Gómez R, de Alba-García JE. Eradication of *Helicobacter pylori*: triple treatment scheme plus Lactobacillus vs. triple treatment alone. *Cir Cir.* 2007 Sep-Oct;75(5):333-6.

Sahakian NM, White SK, Park JH, Cox-Ganser JM, Kreiss K. Identification of mold and dampness-associated respiratory morbidity in 2 schools: comparison of questionnaire survey responses to national data. *J Sch Health.* 2008 Jan;78(1):32-7.

Sahin-Yilmaz A, Nocon CC, Corey JP. Immunoglobulin E-mediated food allergies among adults with allergic rhinitis. *Otolaryngol Head Neck Surg.* 2010 Sep;143(3):379-85.

Salazar-Lindo E, Figueroa-Quintanilla D, Caciano MI, Reto-Valiente V, Chauviere G, Colin P; Lacteol Study Group. Effectiveness and safety of Lactobacillus LB in the treatment of mild acute diarrhea in children. *J Pediatr Gastroenterol Nutr.* 2007 May;44(5):571-6.

Salazar-Lindo E, Miranda-Langschwager P, Campos-Sanchez M, Chea-Woo E, Sack RB. *Lactobacillus casei* strain GG in the treatment of infants with acute watery diarrhea: a randomized, double-blind, placebo controlled clinical trial [ISRCTN67363048]. *BMC Pediatr.* 2004 Sep 2;4:18.

Salem N, Wegher B, Mena P, Uauy R. Arachidonic and docosahexaenoic acids are biosynthesized from their 18-carbon precursors in human infants. *Proc Natl Acad Sci.* 1996;93:49-54.

Salib RJ, Howarth PH. Remodelling of the upper airways in allergic rhinitis: is it a feature of the disease? *Clin Exp Allergy.* 2003 Dec;33(12):1629-33.

Salim AS. Sulfhydryl-containing agents in the treatment of gastric bleeding induced by nonsteroidal anti-inflammatory drugs. *Can J Surg.* 1993 Feb;36(1):53-8.

Salmi H, Kuitunen M, Viljanen M, Lapatto R. Cow's milk allergy is associated with changes in urinary organic acid concentrations. *Pediatr Allergy Immunol.* 2010 Mar;21(2 Pt 2):e401-6.

Salminen E, Elomaa I, Minkkinen J, Vapaatalo H, Salminen S. Preservation of intestinal integrity during radiotherapy using live *Lactobacillus acidophilus* cultures. *Clin Radiol.* 1988 Jul;39(4):435-7.

Salminen S, Isolauri E, Salminen E. Clinical uses of probiotics for stabilizing the gut mucosal barrier: successful strains and future challenges. *Antonie Van Leeuwenhoek.* 1996 Oct;70(2-4):347-58.

Salom IL, Silvis SE, Doscherholmen A. Effect of cimetidine on the absorption of vitamin B12. *Scand J Gastroenterol.* 1982;17:129-31.

Salome CM, Marks GB. Sex, asthma and obesity: an intimate relationship? *Clin Exp Allergy.* 2011 Jan;41(1):6-8.

Salpietro CD, Gangemi S, Briuglia S, Meo A, Merlino MV, Muscolino G, Bisignano G, Trombetta D, Saija A. The almond milk: a new approach to the management of cow-milk allergy/intolerance in infants. *Minerva Pediatr.* 2005 Aug;57(4):173-80.

Salvi SS, Barnes PJ. Chronic obstructive pulmonary disease in non-smokers. *Lancet.* 2009 Aug 29;374(9691):733-43.

Samanta M, Sarkar M, Ghosh P, Ghosh J, Sinha M, Chatterjee S. Prophylactic probiotics for prevention of necrotizing enterocolitis in very low birth weight newborns. *J Trop Pediatr.* 2009 Apr;55(2):128-31.

Sancho AI, Hoffmann-Sommergruber K, Alessandri S, Conti A, Giuffrida MG, Shewry P, Jensen BM, Skov P, Vieths S. Authentication of food allergen quality by physicochemical and immunological methods. *Clin Exp Allergy.* 2010 Jul;40(7):973-86.

Santos A, Dias A, Pinheiro JA. Predictive factors for the persistence of cow's milk allergy. *Pediatr Allergy Immunol.* 2010 Apr 27.

Sanz Ortega J, Martorell Aragonés A, Michavila Gómez A, Nieto García A; Grupo de Trabajo para el Estudio de la Alergia Alimentaria. Incidence of IgE-mediated allergy to cow's milk proteins in the first year of life. *An Esp Pediatr.* 2001 Jun;54(6):536-9.

Saran S, Gopalan S, Krishna TP. Use of fermented foods to combat stunting and failure to thrive. *Nutrition.* 2002 May;18(5):393-6.

Sato Y, Akiyama H, Matsuoka H, Sakata K, Nakamura R, Ishikawa S, Inakuma T, Totsuka M, Sugita-Konishi Y, Ebisawa M, Teshima R. Dietary carotenoids inhibit oral sensitization and the development of food allergy. *J Agric Food Chem.* 2010 Jun 23;58(12):7180-6.

Satyanarayana S, Sushruta K, Sarma GS, Srinivas N, Subba Raju GV. Antioxidant activity of the aqueous extracts of spicy food additives—evaluation and comparison with ascorbic acid in in-vitro systems. *J Herb Pharmacother.* 2004;4(2):1-10.

Savage JH, Kaeding AJ, Matsui EC, Wood RA. The natural history of soy allergy. *J Allergy Clin Immunol.* 2010 Mar;125(3):683-6.

Savilahti EM, Karinen S, Salo HM, Klemetti P, Saarinen KM, Klemola T, Kuitunen M, Hautaniemi S, Savilahti E, Vaarala O. Combined T regulatory cell and Th2 expression profile identifies children with cow's milk allergy. *Clin Immunol.* 2010 Jul;136(1):16-20.

Savilahti EM, Rantanen V, Lin JS, Karinen S, Saarinen KM, Goldis M, Mäkelä MJ, Hautaniemi S, Savilahti E, Sampson HA. Early recovery from cow's milk allergy is associated with decreasing IgE and increasing IgG4 binding to cow's milk epitopes. *J Allergy Clin Immunol.* 2010 Jun;125(6):1315-1321.e9.

Savino F, Pelle E, Palumeri E, Oggero R, Miniero R. *Lactobacillus reuteri* (American Type Culture Collection Strain 55730) versus simethicone in the treatment of infantile colic: a prospective randomized study. Pediatrics. 2007 Jan;119(1):e124-30.

Sazanova NE, Varnacheva LN, Novikova AV, Pletneva NB. Immunological aspects of food intolerance in children during first years of life. *Pediatriia.* 1992;(3):14-8.

Scadding G, Bjarnason I, Brostoff J, Levi AJ, Peters TJ. Intestinal permeability to 51Cr-labelled ethylenediaminetetraacetate in food-intolerant subjects. *Digestion.* 1989;42(2):104-9.

Scalabrin DM, Johnston WH, Hoffman DR, P'Pool VL, Harris CL, Mitmesser SH. Growth and tolerance of healthy term infants receiving hydrolyzed infant formulas supplemented with Lactobacillus rhamnosus GG: randomized, double-blind, controlled trial. *Clin Pediatr (Phila).* 2009 Sep;48(7):734-44.

Schaafsma G, Meuling WJ, van Dokkum W, Bouley C. Effects of a milk product, fermented by *Lactobacillus acidophilus* and with fructo-oligosaccharides added, on blood lipids in male volunteers. *Eur J Clin Nutr.* 1998 Jun;52(6):436-40.

Schauenberg P, Paris F. *Guide to Medicinal Plants.* New Canaan, CT: Keats Publ, 1977.

Schauss AG, Wu X, Prior RL, Ou B, Huang D, Owens J, Agarwal A, Jensen GS, Hart AN, Shanbrom E. Antioxidant capacity and other bioactivities of the freeze-dried Amazonian palm berry, Euterpe oleraceae mart. (acai). *J Agric Food Chem.* 2006 Nov 1;54(22):8604-10.

Schempp H, Weiser D, Elstner EF. Biochemical model reactions indicative of inflammatory processes. Activities of extracts from Fraxinus excelsior and Populus tremula. *Arzneimittelforschung.* 2000 Apr;50(4):362-72.

Schiffrin EJ, Brassart D, Servin AL, Rochat F, Donnet-Hughes A. Immune modulation of blood leukocytes in humans by lactic acid bacteria: criteria for strain selection. *Am J Clin Nutr.* 1997 Aug;66(2):515S-520S.

Schillaci D, Arizza V, Dayton T, Camarda L, Di Stefano V. In vitro anti-biofilm activity of Boswellia spp. oleogum resin essential oils. *Lett Appl Microbiol.* 2008 Nov;47(5):433-8.

Schlumpf M, Cotton B, Conscience M, Haller V, Steinmann B, Lichtensteiger W. In vitro and in vivo estrogenicity of UV screens. *Environ Health Perspect.* 2001 Mar;109(3):239-44.

Schmid B, Kötter I, Heide L. Pharmacokinetics of salicin after oral administration of a standardised willow bark extract. *Eur J Clin Pharmacol.* 2001 Aug;57(5):387-91.

Schmitt DA, Maleki SJ (2004) Comparing the effects of boiling, frying and roasting on the allergenicity of peanuts. *J Allergy Clin Immunol.* 113: S155.

Schnappinger M, Sausenthaler S, Linseisen J, Hauner H, Heinrich J. Fish consumption, allergic sensitisation and allergic diseases in adults. *Ann Nutr Metab.* 2009;54(1):67-74.

Schnappinger M, Sausenthaler S, Linseisen J, Hauner H, Heinrich J. Fish consumption, allergic sensitisation and allergic diseases in adults. *Ann Nutr Metab.* 2009;54(1):67-74.

Scholz-Ahrens KE, Ade P, Marten B, Weber P, Timm W, Açil Y, Glüer CC, Schrezenmeir J. Prebiotics, probiotics, and synbiotics affect mineral absorption, bone mineral content, and bone structure. *J Nutr.* 2007 Mar;137(3 Suppl 2):838S-46S.

Schönfeld P. Phytanic Acid toxicity: implications for the permeability of the inner mitochondrial membrane to ions. *Toxicol Mech Methods.* 2004;14(1-2):47-52.

Schottner M, Gansser D, Spiteller G. Lignans from the roots of Urtica dioica and their metabolites bind to human sex hormone binding globulin (SHBG). *Planta Med.* 1997;65:529-532.

Schouten B, van Esch BC, Hofman GA, Boon L, Knippels LM, Willemsen LE, Garssen J. Oligosaccharide-induced whey-specific CD25(+) regulatory T-cells are involved in the suppression of cow milk allergy in mice. *J Nutr.* 2010 Apr;140(4):835-41.

Schroecksnadel S, Jenny M, Fuchs D. Sensitivity to sulphite additives. *Clin Exp Allergy.* 2010 Apr;40(4):688-9.

Schulick P. *Ginger: Common Spice & Wonder Drug.* Brattleboro, VT: Herbal Free Perss, 1996.

Schulman G. A nexus of progression of chronic kidney disease: charcoal, tryptophan and profibrotic cytokines. *Blood Purif.* 2006;24(1):143-8.

Schulz V, Hansel R, Tyler VE. *Rational Phytotherapy.* Berlin: Springer-Verlag; 1998.

Schumacher P. *Biophysical Therapy Of Allergies.* Stuttgart: Thieme, 2005.

Schütz K, Carle R, Schieber A. Taraxacum—a review on its phytochemical and pharmacological profile. *J Ethnopharmacol.* 2006 Oct 11;107(3):313-23.

Schwab D, Hahn EG, Raithel M. Enhanced histamine metabolism: a comparative analysis of collagenous colitis and food allergy with respect to the role of diet and NSAID use. *Inflamm Res.* 2003 Apr;52(4):142-7.

Schwab D, Müller S, Aigner T, Neureiter D, Kirchner T, Hahn EG, Raithel M. Functional and morphologic characterization of eosinophils in the lower intestinal mucosa of patients with food allergy. *Am J Gastroenterol.* 2003 Jul;98(7):1525-34.

Schwelberger HG. Histamine intolerance: a metabolic disease? *Inflamm Res.* 2010 Mar;59 Suppl 2:S219-21.

Schwellenbach LJ, Olson KL. McConnell KJ, Stolepart RS, Nash JD, Merenich JA. The triglyceride-lowering effects of a modest dose of docosahexaenoic acid alone versus in combination with low dose eicosapentaenoic acid in patients with coronary artery disease and elevated triglycerides. *J Am Coll Nutr.* 2006;25(6):480-485.

Scott-Taylor TH, O'B Hourihane J, Strobel S. Correlation of allergen-specific IgG subclass antibodies and T lymphocyte cytokine responses in children with multiple food allergies. *Pediatr Allergy Immunol.* 2010 Sep;21(6):935-44.

Scurlock AM, Jones SM. An update on immunotherapy for food allergy. *Curr Opin Allergy Clin Immunol.* 2010 Dec;10(6):587-93.

Sealey-Voyksner JA, Khosla C, Voyksner RD, Jorgenson JW. Novel aspects of quantitation of immunogenic wheat gluten peptides by liquid chromatography-mass spectrometry. *J Chromatogr A.* 2010 Jun 18;1217(25):4167-83.

Searing DA, Leung DY. Vitamin D in atopic dermatitis, asthma and allergic diseases. *Immunol Allergy Clin North Am.* 2010 Aug;30(3):397-409.

Sekine K, Toida T, Saito M, Kuboyama M, Kawashima T, Hashimoto Y. A new morphologically characterized cell wall preparation (whole peptidoglycan) from Bifidobacterium infantis with a higher efficacy on the regression of an established tumor in mice. *Cancer Res.* 1985 Mar;45(3):1300-7.

Senior F. Fallout. *New York Magazine.* Fall: 2003.

Senna G, Gani F, Leo G, Schiappoli M. Alternative tests in the diagnosis of food allergies. *Recenti Prog Med.* 2002 May;93(5):327-34.

Seo K, Jung S, Park M, Song Y, Choung S. Effects of leucocyanidines on activities of metabolizing enzymes and antioxidant enzymes. *Biol Pharm Bull.* 2001 May;24(5):592-3.

Seo K, Jung S, Park M, Song Y, Choung S. Effects of leucocyanidines on activities of metabolizing enzymes and antioxidant enzymes. *Biol Pharm Bull.* 2001 May;24(5):592-3.

Seo SW, Koo HN, An HJ, Kwon KB, Lim BC, Seo EA, Ryu DG, Moon G, Kim HY, Kim HM, Hong SH. Taraxacum officinale protects against cholecystokinin-induced acute pancreatitis in rats. *World J Gastroenterol.* 2005 Jan 28;11(4):597-9.

Seppo L, Jauhiainen T, Poussa T, Korpela R. A fermented milk high in bioactive peptides has a blood pressure-lowering effect in hypertensive subjects. *Am J Clin Nutr.* 2003 Feb;77(2):326-30.

Seppo L, Korpela R, Lönnerdal B, Metsäniitty L, Juntunen-Backman K, Klemola T, Paganus A, Vanto T. A follow-up study of nutrient intake, nutritional status, and growth in infants with cow milk allergy fed either a soy formula or an extensively hydrolyzed whey formula. *Am J Clin Nutr.* 2005 Jul;82(1):140-5.

Serra A, Cocuzza S, Poli G, La Mantia I, Messina A, Pavone P. Otologic findings in children with gastroesophageal reflux. *Int J Pediatr Otorhinolaryngol.* 2007 Nov;71(11):1693-7. 2007 Aug 22.

Sevar R. Audit of outcome in 455 consecutive patients treated with homeopathic medicines. *Homeopathy.* 2005 Oct;94(4):215-21.

Shahani KM, Ayebo AD. Role of dietary lactobacilli in gastrointestinal microecology. *Am J Clin Nutr.* 1980 Nov;33(11 Suppl):2448-57.

Shahani KM, Chandan RC. Nutritional and healthful aspects of cultured and culture-containing dairy foods. *J Dairy Sci.* 1979 Oct;62(10):1685-94.

Shahani KM, Friend BA. Properties of and prospects for cultured dairy foods. *Soc Appl Bacteriol Symp Ser.* 1983;11:257-69.

Shahani KM, Herper WJ, Jensen RG, Parry RM Jr, Zittle CA. Enzymes in bovine milk: a review. *J Dairy Sci.* 1973 May;56(5):531-43.

Shahani KM, Kwan AJ, Friend BA. Role and significance of enzymes in human milk. *Am J Clin Nutr.* 1980 Aug;33(8):1861-8.

Shahani KM, Meshbesher BF, Mangalampalli V. *Cultivate Health From Within.* Danbury, CT: Vital Health Publ, 2005.

Shaheen S, Potts J, Gnatiuc L, Makowska J, Kowalski ML, Joos G, van Zele T, van Durme Y, De Rudder I, Wöhrl S, Godnic-Cvar J, Skadhauge L, Thomsen G, Zuberbier T, Bergmann KC, Heinzerling L, Gjomarkaj M, Bruno A, Pace E, Bonini S, Fokkens W, Weersink EJ, Loureiro C, Todo-Bom A, Villanueva CM, Sanjuas C, Zock JP, Janson C, Burney P; Selenium and Asthma Research Integration project; GA2LEN. The relation between paracetamol use and asthma: a GA2LEN European case-control study. *Eur Respir J.* 2008 Nov;32(5):1231-6.

Shaheen SO, Newson RB, Rayman MP, Wong AP, Tumilty MK, Phillips JM, Potts JF, Kelly FJ, White PT, Burney PG. Randomised, double blind, placebo-controlled trial of selenium supplementation in adult asthma. *Thorax.* 2007 Jun;62(6):483-90.

Shakib F, Brown HM, Phelps A, Redhead R. Study of IgG sub-class antibodies in patients with milk intolerance. *Clin Allergy.* 1986 Sep;16(5):451-8.

Shalev E, Battino S, Weiner E, Colodner R, Keness Y. Ingestion of yogurt containing *Lactobacillus acidophilus* compared with pasteurized yogurt as prophylaxis for recurrent *Candidal* vaginitis and bacterial vaginosis. *Arch Fam Med.* 1996 Nov-Dec;5(10):593-6.

Shamir R, Makhoul IR, Etzioni A, Shehadeh N. Evaluation of a diet containing probiotics and zinc for the treatment of mild diarrheal illness in children younger than one year of age. *J Am Coll Nutr.* 2005 Oct;24(5):370-5.

Sharma P, Sharma BC, Puri V, Sarin SK. An open-label randomized controlled trial of lactulose and probiotics in the treatment of minimal hepatic encephalopathy. *Eur J Gastroent Hepatol.* 2008 Jun;20(6):506-11.

Sharma SC, Sharma S, Gulati OP. Pycnogenol inhibits the release of histamine from mast cells. *Phytother Res.* 2003 Jan;17(1):66-9.

Sharnan J, Kumar L, Singh S. Comparison of results of skin prick tests, enzyme-linked immunosorbent assays and food challenges in children with respiratory allergy. *J Trop Pediatr.* 2001 Dec;47(6):367-8.

Shawcross DL, Wright G, Olde Damink SW, Jalan R. Role of ammonia and inflammation in minimal hepatic encephalopathy. *Metab Brain Dis.* 2007 Mar;22(1):125-38.

Shea KM, Trucker RT, Weber RW, Peden DB. Climate change and allergic disease. *Clin Rev Allergy Immunol.* 2008;6:443-453.

Shea-Donohue T, Stiltz J, Zhao A, Notari L. Mast Cells. *Curr Gastroenterol Rep.* 2010 Aug 14.

Sheih YH, Chiang BL, Wang LH, Liao CK, Gill HS. Systemic immunity-enhancing effects in healthy subjects following dietary consumption of the lactic acid bacterium *Lactobacillus rhamnosus* HN001. *J Am Coll Nutr.* 2001 Apr;20(2 Suppl):149-56.

Shen FY, Lee MS, Jung SK. Effectiveness of pharmacopuncture for asthma: a systematic review and meta-analysis. *Evid Based Complement Alternat Med.* 2011;2011. pii: 678176.

Sheth SS, Waserman S, Kagan R, Alizadehfar R, Primeau MN, Elliot S, St Pierre Y, Wickett R, Joseph L, Harada L, Dufresne C, Allen M, Allen M, Godefroy SB, Clarke AE. Role of food labels in accidental exposures in food-allergic individuals in Canada. *Ann Allergy Asthma Immunol.* 2010 Jan;104(1):60-5.

Shi S, Zhao Y, Zhou H, Zhang Y, Jiang X, Huang K. Identification of antioxidants from Taraxacum mongolicum by high-performance liquid chromatography-diode array detection-radical-scavenging detection-electrospray ionization mass spectrometry and nuclear magnetic resonance experiments. *J Chromatogr A.* 2008 Oct 31;1209(1-2):145-52

Shi S, Zhou H, Zhang Y, Huang K, Liu S. Chemical constituents from Neo-Taraxacum siphonathum. *Zhongguo Zhong Yao Za Zhi.* 2009 Apr;34(8):1002-4.

REFERENCES AND BIBLIOGRAPHY

Shi SY, Zhou CX, Xu Y, Tao QF, Bai H, Lu FS, Lin WY, Chen HY, Zheng W, Wang LW, Wu YH, Zeng S, Huang KX, Zhao Y, Li XK, Qu J. Studies on chemical constituents from herbs of Taraxacum mongolicum. *Zhongguo Zhong Yao Za Zhi*. 2008 May;33(10):1147-57.

Shibata H, Nabe T, Yamamura H, Kohno S. l-Ephedrine is a major constituent of Mao-Bushi-Saishin-To, one of the formulas of Chinese medicine, which shows immediate inhibition after oral administration of passive cutaneous anaphylaxis in rats. *Inflamm Res*. 2000 Aug;49(8):398-403.

Shichinohe K, Shimizu M, Kurokawa K. Effect of M-711 on experimental asthma in rats. *J Vet Med Sci*. 1996 Jan;58(1):55-9.

Shimauchi H, Mayanagi G, Nakaya S, Minamibuchi M, Ito Y, Yamaki K, Hirata H. Improvement of periodontal condition by probiotics with *Lactobacillus salivarius* WB21: a randomized, double-blind, placebo-controlled study. *J Clin Periodontol*. 2008 Oct;35(10):897-905.

Shimizu K, Ogura H, Goto M, Asahara T, Nomoto K, Morotomi M, Matsushima A, Tasaki O, Fujita K, Hosotsubo H, Kuwagata Y, Tanaka H, Shimazu T, Sugimoto H. Synbiotics decrease the incidence of septic complications in patients with severe SIRS: a preliminary report. *Dig Dis Sci*. 2009 May;54(5):1071-8.

Shimoi T, Ushiyama H, Kan K, Saito K, Kamata K, Hirokado M. Survey of glycoalkaloids content in the various potatoes. *Shokuhin Eiseigaku Zasshi*. 2007 Jun;48(3):77-82.

Shishehbor F, Behroo L, Ghafouriyan Broujerdnia M, Namjoyan F, Latifi SM. Quercetin effectively quells peanut-induced anaphylactic reactions in the peanut sensitized rats. *Iran J Allergy Asthma Immunol*. 2010 Mar;9(1):27-34.

Shishodia S, Harikumar KB, Dass S, Ramawat KG, Aggarwal BB. The guggul for chronic diseases: ancient medicine, modern targets. *Anticancer Res*. 2008 Nov-Dec;28(6A):3647-64.

Shivpuri DN, Menon MP, Parkash D. Preliminary studies in Tylophora indica in the treatment of asthma and allergic rhinitis. *J Assoc Physicians India*. 1968 Jan;16(1):9-15.

Shivpuri DN, Menon MP, Prakash D. A crossover double-blind study on Tylophora indica in the treatment of asthma and allergic rhinitis. *J Allergy*. 1969 Mar;43(3):145-50.

Shivpuri DN, Singhal SC, Parkash D. Treatment of asthma with an alcoholic extract of Tylophora indica: a cross-over, double-blind study. *Ann Allergy*. 1972; 30:407-12.

Shoaf K, Mulvey GL, Armstrong GD, Hutkins RW. Prebiotic galactooligosaccharides reduce adherence of enteropathogenic *Escherichia coli* to tissue culture cells. Infect Immun. 2006 Dec;74(12):6920-8.

Shoaf, K., Muvey, G.L., Armstrong, G.D., Hutkins, R.W. (2006) Prebiotic galactooligosaccharides reduce adherence of enteropathogenic Escherichia coli to tissue culture cells. *Infect Immun*. Dec;74(12):6920-8.

Shornikova AV, Casas IA, Isolauri E, Mykkänen H, Vesikari T. *Lactobacillus reuteri* as a therapeutic agent in acute diarrhea in young children. *J Pediatr Gastroenterol Nutr*. 1997 Apr;24(4):399-404.

Shornikova AV, Casas IA, Mykkänen H, Salo E, Vesikari T. Bacteriotherapy with *Lactobacillus reuteri* in rotavirus gastroenteritis. *Pediatr Infect Dis J*. 1997 Dec;16(12):1103-7.

Sicherer SH, Muñoz-Furlong A, Godbold JH, Sampson HA. US prevalence of self-reported peanut, tree nut, and sesame allergy: 11-year follow-up. *J Allergy Clin Immunol*. 2010 Jun;125(6):1322-6.

Sicherer SH, Noone SA, Koerner CB, Christie L, Burks AW, Sampson HA. Hypoallergenicity and efficacy of an amino acid-based formula in children with cow's milk and multiple food hypersensitivities. *J Pediatr*. 2001 May;138(5):688-93.

Sicherer SH, Sampson HA. Food allergy. *J Allergy Clin Immunol*. 2010 Feb;125(2 Suppl 2):S116-25.

Sidoroff V, Hyvärinen M, Piippo-Savolainen E, Korppi M. Lung function and overweight in school aged children after early childhood wheezing. *Pediatr Pulmonol*. 2010 Dec 30.

Sigstedt SC, Hooten CJ, Callewaert MC, Jenkins AR, Romero AE, Pullin MJ, Kornienko A, Lowrey TK, Slambrouck SV, Steelant WF. Evaluation of aqueous extracts of Taraxacum officinale on growth and invasion of breast and prostate cancer cells. *Int J Oncol*. 2008 May;32(5):1085-90.

Silman AJ, MacGregor AJ, Thomson W, Holligan S, Carthy D, Farhan A, Ollier WE. Twin concordance rates for rheumatoid arthritis: results from a nationwide study. *Br J Rheumatol*. 1993 Oct;32(10):903-7.

Silva MF, Kamphorst AO, Hayashi EA, Bellio M, Carvalho CR, Faria AM, Sabino KC, Coelho MG, Nobrega A, Tavares D, Silva AC. Innate profiles of cytokines implicated on oral tolerance correlate with low- or high-suppression of humoral response. *Immunology*. 2010 Jul;130(3):447-57.

Silva MR, Dias G, Ferreira CL, Franceschini SC, Costa NM. Growth of preschool children was improved when fed an iron-fortified fermented milk beverage supplemented with *Lactobacillus acidophilus*. *Nutr Res*. 2008 Apr;28(4):226-32.

Simakachorn N, Pichaipat V, Rithipornpaisarn P, Kongkaew C, Tongpradit P, Varavithya W. Clinical evaluation of the addition of lyophilized, heat-killed *Lactobacillus acidophilus* LB to oral rehydration therapy in the treatment of acute diarrhea in children. *J Pediatr Gastroenterol Nutr*. 2000 Jan;30(1):68-72.

Simenhoff ML, Dunn SR, Zollner GP, Fitzpatrick ME, Emery SM, Sandine WE, Ayres JW. Biomodulation of the toxic and nutritional effects of small bowel bacterial overgrowth in end-stage kidney disease using freeze-dried *Lactobacillus acidophilus*. *Miner Electrolyte Metab*. 1996;22(1-3):92-6.

Simeone D, Miele E, Boccia G, Marino A, Troncone R, Staiano A. Prevalence of atopy in children with chronic constipation. *Arch Dis Child.* 2008 Dec;93(12):1044-7.

Simões EA, Carbonell-Estrany X, Rieger CH, Mitchell I, Fredrick L, Groothuis JR; Palivizumab Long-Term Respiratory Outcomes Study Group. The effect of respiratory syncytial virus on subsequent recurrent wheezing in atopic and nonatopic children. *J Allergy Clin Immunol.* 2010 Aug;126(2):256-62. 2010 Jul 10.

Simons FER. What's in a name? The allergic rhinitis-asthma connection. *Clin Exp All Rev.* 2003;3:9-17.

Simonte SJ, Ma S, Mofidi S, Sicherer SH. Relevance of casual contact with peanut butter in children with peanut allergy. *J Allergy Clin Immunol.* 2003 Jul;112(1):180-2.

Simopoulos AP. Essential fatty acids in health and chronic disease. *Am J Clin Nutr.* 1999 Sep;70(3 Suppl):560S-569S.

Simpson A, Tan VY, Winn J, Svensén M, Bishop CM, Heckerman DE, Buchan I, Custovic A. Beyond atopy: multiple patterns of sensitization in relation to asthma in a birth cohort study. *Am J Respir Crit Care Med.* 2010 Jun 1;181(11):1200-6.

Simpson AB, Yousef E, Hossain J. Association between peanut allergy and asthma morbidity. *J Pediatr.* 2010 May;156(5):777-81.

Sin A, Terzioğlu E, Kokuludağ A, Sebik F, Kabakçi T. Serum eosinophil cationic protein (ECP) levels in patients with seasonal allergic rhinitis and allergic asthma. *Allergy Asthma Proc.* 1998 Mar-Apr;19(2):69-73.

Singer P, Shapiro H, Theilla M, Anbar R, Singer J, Cohen J. Anti-inflammatory properties of omega-3 fatty acids in critical illness: novel mechanisms and an integrative perspective. *Intensive Care Med.* 2008 Sep;34(9):1580-92.

Singh BB, Khorsan R, Vinjamury SP, Der-Martirosian C, Kizhakkeveettil A, Anderson TM. Herbal treatments of asthma: a systematic review. *J Asthma.* 2007 Nov;44(9):685-98.

Singh S, Khajuria A, Taneja SC, Johri RK, Singh J, Qazi GN. Boswellic acids: A leukotriene inhibitor also effective through topical application in inflammatory disorders. *Phytomedicine.* 2008 Jun;15(6-7):400-7.

Singh V, Jain NK. Asthma as a cause for, rather than a result of, gastroesophageal reflux. *J Asthma.* 1983;20(4):241-3. 3.

Sinn DH, Song JH, Kim HJ, Lee JH, Son HJ, Chang DK, Kim YH, Kim JJ, Rhee JC, Rhee PL. Therapeutic effect of *Lactobacillus acidophilus*-SDC 2012, 2013 in patients with irritable bowel syndrome. *Dig Dis Sci.* 2008 Oct;53(10):2714-8.

Sirvent S, Palomares O, Vereda A, Villalba M, Cuesta-Herranz J, Rodríguez R. nsLTP and profilin are allergens in mustard seeds: cloning, sequencing and recombinant production of Sin a 3 and Sin a 4. *Clin Exp Allergy.* 2009 Dec;39(12):1929-36.

Sistek D, Kelly R, Wickens K, Stanley T, Fitzharris P, Crane J. Is the effect of probiotics on atopic dermatitis confined to food sensitized children? *Clin Exp Allergy.* 2006 May;36(5):629-33.

Skamstrup Hansen K, Vieths S, Vestergaard H, Skov PS, Bindslev-Jensen C, Poulsen LK. Seasonal variation in food allergy to apple. *J Chromatogr B Biomed Sci Appl.* 2001 May 25;756(1-2):19-32.

Skovbjerg S, Roos K, Holm SE, Grahn Håkansson E, Nowrouzian F, Ivarsson M, Adlerberth I, Wold AE. Spray bacteriotherapy decreases middle ear fluid in children with secretory otitis media. *Arch Dis Child.* 2009 Feb;94(2):92-8.

Skripak JM, Nash SD, Rowley H, Brereton NH, Oh S, Hamilton RG, Matsui EC, Burks AW, Wood RA. A randomized, double-blind, placebo-controlled study of milk oral immunotherapy for cow's milk allergy. *J Allergy Clin Immunol.* 2008 Dec;122(6):1154-60.

Sletten GB, Halvorsen R, Egaas E, Halstensen TS. Changes in humoral responses to beta-lactoglobulin in tolerant patients suggest a particular role for IgG4 in delayed, non-IgE-mediated cow's milk allergy. *Pediatr Allergy Immunol.* 2006 Sep;17(6):435-43.

Smith J. *Genetic Roulette: The Documented Health Risks of Genetically Engineered Foods.* White River Jct, Vermont: Chelsea Green, 2007.

Smith K, Warholak T, Armstrong E, Leib M, Rehfeld R, Malone D. Evaluation of risk factors and health outcomes among persons with asthma. *J Asthma.* 2009 Apr;46(3):234-7.

Smith LJ, Holbrook JT, Wise R, Blumenthal M, Dozor AJ, Mastronarde J, Williams L; American Lung Association Asthma Clinical Research Centers. Dietary intake of soy genistein is associated with lung function in patients with asthma. *J Asthma.* 2004;41(8):833-43.

Smith S, Sullivan K. Examining the influence of biological and psychological factors on cognitive performance in chronic fatigue syndrome: a randomized, double-blind, placebo-controlled, crossover study. *Int J Behav Med.* 2003;10(2):162-73.

Sofic E, Denisova N, Youdim K, Vatrenjak-Velagic V, De Filippo C, Mehmedagic A, Causevic A, Cao G, Joseph JA, Prior RL. Antioxidant and pro-oxidant capacity of catecholamines and related compounds. Effects of hydrogen peroxide on glutathione and sphingomyelinase activity in pheochromocytoma PC12 cells: potential relevance to age-related diseases. *J Neural Transm.* 2001;108(5):541-57.

Soleo L, Colosio C, Alinovi R, Guarneri D, Russo A, Lovreglio P, Vimercati L, Birindelli S, Cortesi I, Flore C, Carta P, Colombi A, Parrinello G, Ambrosi L. Immunologic effects of exposure to low levels of inorganic mercury. *Med Lav.* 2002 May-Jun;93(3):225-32.

Solomons NW, Guerrero AM, Torun B. Effective in vivo hydrolysis of milk lactose by beta-galactosidases in the presence of solid foods. *Am J Clin Nutr.* 1985 Feb;41(2):222-7.

Sompamit K, Kukongviriyapan U, Nakmareong S, Pannangpetch P, Kukongviriyapan V. Curcumin improves vascular function and alleviates oxidative stress in non-lethal lipopolysaccharide-induced endotoxaemia in mice. *Eur J Pharmacol.* 2009 Aug 15;616(1-3):192-9.

Sonibare MA, Gbile ZO. Ethnobotanical survey of anti-asthmatic plants in South Western Nigeria. *Afr J Tradit Complement Altern Med.* 2008 Jun 18;5(4):340-5.

Sontag SJ, O'Connell S, Khandelwal S, Greenlee H, Schnell T, Nemchausky B, Chejfec G, Miller T, Seidel J, Sonnenberg A. Asthmatics with gastroesophageal reflux: long term results of a randomized trial of medical and surgical antireflux therapies. *Am J Gastroenterol.* 2003 May;98(5):987-99.

Sosa M, Saavedra P, Valero C, Guañabens N, Nogués X, del Pino-Montes J, Mosquera J, Alegre J, Gómez-Alonso C, Muñoz-Torres M, Quesada M, Pérez-Cano R, Jódar E, Torrijos A, Lozano-Tonkin C, Díaz-Curiel M; GIUMO Study Group. Inhaled steroids do not decrease bone mineral density but increase risk of fractures: data from the GIUMO Study Group. *J Clin Densitom.* 2006 Apr-Jun;9(2):154-8.

Soyka F, Edmonds A. *The Ion Effect: How Air Electricity Rules your Life and Health.* Bantam, New York: Bantam, 1978.

Spence A. *Basic Human Anatomy.* Menlo Park, CA: Benjamin/Commings, 1986.

Spiller G. *The Super Pyramid.* New York: HRS Press, 1993.

Sporik R, Squillace SP, Ingram JM, Rakes G, Honsinger RW, Platts-Mills TA. Mite, cat, and cockroach exposure, allergen sensitisation, and asthma in children: a case-control study of three schools. *Thorax.* 1999 Aug;54(8):675-80.

Srivastava K, Zou ZM, Sampson HA, Dansky H, Li XM. Direct Modulation of Airway Reactivity by the Chinese Anti-Asthma Herbal Formula ASHMI. *J Allergy Clin Immunol.* 2005;115:S7.

Srivastava KD, Qu C, Zhang T, Goldfarb J, Sampson HA, Li XM. Food Allergy Herbal Formula-2 silences peanut-induced anaphylaxis for a prolonged posttreatment period via IFN-gamma-producing CD8+ T cells. *J Allergy Clin Immunol.* 2009 Feb;123(2):443-51.

Srivastava KD, Zhang TF, Qu C, Sampson HA, Li XM. Silencing Peanut Allergy: A Chinese Herbal Formula, FAHF-2, Completely Blocks Peanut-induced Anaphylaxis for up to 6 Months Following Therapy in a Murine Model Of Peanut Allergy. *J Allergy Clin Immunol.* 2006;117:S328.

Stach A, Emberlin J, Smith M, Adams-Groom B, Myszkowska D. Factors that determine the severity of Betula spp. pollen seasons in Poland (Poznań and Krakow) and the United Kingdom (Worcester and London). *Int J Biometeorol.* 2008 Mar;52(4):311-21.

Stachowska E, Dolegowska B, Chlubek D, Wesolowska T, Ciechanowski K, Gutowski P, Szumilowicz H, Turowski R. Dietary trans fatty acids and composition of human atheromatous plaques. *Eur J Nutr.* 2004 Oct;43(5):313-8.

Staden U, Rolinck-Werninghaus C, Brewe F, Wahn U, Niggemann B, Beyer K. Specific oral tolerance induction in food allergy in children: efficacy and clinical patterns of reaction. *Allergy.* 2007 Nov;62(11):1261-9.

Stadlbauer V, Mookerjee RP, Hodges S, Wright GA, Davies NA, Jalan R. Effect of probiotic treatment on deranged neutrophil function and cytokine responses in patients with compensated alcoholic cirrhosis. *J Hepatol.* 2008 Jun;48(6):945-51.

Stahl SM. Selective histamine H1 antagonism: novel hypnotic and pharmacologic actions challenge classical notions of antihistamines. *CNS Spectr.* 2008 Dec;13(12):1027-38.

State Pharmacopoeia Commission of The People's Republic of China. *Pharmacopoeia of the People's Republic of China.* Beijing: Chemical Industry Press; 2005.

Steinman HA, Le Roux M, Potter PC. Sulphur dioxide sensitivity in South African asthmatic children. *S Afr Med J.* 1993 Jun;83(6):387-90.

Stenberg JA, Hambäck PA, Ericson L. Herbivore-induced "rent rise" in the host plant may drive a diet breadth enlargement in the tenant. *Ecology.* 2008 Jan;89(1):126-33.

Stengler M. *The Natural Physician's Healing Therapies.* Stamford, CT: Bottom Line Books, 2008.

Stensrud T, Carlsen KH. Can one single test protocol for provoking exercise-induced bronchoconstriction also be used for assessing aerobic capacity? *Clin Respir J.* 2008 Jan;2(1):47-53.

Steurer-Stey C, Russi EW, Steurer J: Complementary and alternative medicine in asthma: do they work? *Swiss Med Wkly.* 2002, 132:338-344.

Stillerman A, Nachtsheim C, Li W, Albrecht M, Waldman J. Efficacy of a novel air filtration pillow for avoidance of perennial allergens in symptomatic adults. *Ann Allergy Asthma Immunol.* 2010 May;104(5):440-9.

Stirapongsasuti P, Tanglertsampan C, Aunhachoke K, Sangasapaviliya A. Anaphylactic reaction to phukwaan-ban in a patient with latex allergy. *J Med Assoc Thai.* 2010 May;93(5):616-9.

Størdal K, Johannesdottir GB, Bentsen BS, Knudsen PK, Carlsen KC, Closs O, Handeland M, Holm HK, Sandvik L. Acid suppression does not change respiratory symptoms in children with asthma and gastro-oesophageal reflux disease. *Arch Dis Child.* 2005 Sep;90(9):956-60.

Stratiki Z, Costalos C, Sevastiadou S, Kastanidou O, Skouroliakou M, Giakoumatou A, Petrohilou V. The effect of a bifidobacter supplemented bovine milk on intestinal permeability of preterm infants. *Early Hum Dev.* 2007 Sep;83(9):575-9.

Stratiki Z, Costalos C, Sevastiadou S, Kastanidou O, Skouroliakou M, Giakoumatou A, Petrohilou V. The effect of a bifidobacter supplemented bovine milk on intestinal permeability of preterm infants. *Early Hum Dev.* 2007 Sep;83(9):575-9.

Strinnholm A, Brulin C, Lindh V. Experiences of double-blind, placebo-controlled food challenges (DBPCFC): a qualitative analysis of mothers' experiences. *J Child Health Care.* 2010 Jun;14(2):179-88.

Strozzi GP, Mogna L. Quantification of folic acid in human feces after administration of *Bifidobacterium* probiotic strains. *J Clin Gastroenterol.* 2008 Sep;42 Suppl 3 Pt 2:S179-84.

Stuck BA, Czajkowski J, Hagner AE, Klimek L, Verse T, Hörmann K, Maurer JT. Changes in daytime sleepiness, quality of life, and objective sleep patterns in seasonal allergic rhinitis: a controlled clinical trial. *J Allergy Clin Immunol.* 2004 Apr;113(4):663-8.

Stull DE, Schaefer M, Crespi S, Sandor DW. Relative strength of relationships of nasal congestion and ocular symptoms with sleep, mood and productivity. *Curr Med Res Opin.* 2009 Jul;25(7):1785-92.

Sturtzel B, Mikulits C, Gisinger C, Elmadfa I. Use of fiber instead of laxative treatment in a geriatric hospital to improve the wellbeing of seniors. *J Nutr Health Aging.* 2009 Feb;13(2):136-9.

Stutius LM, Sheehan WJ, Rangsithienchai P, Bharmanee A, Scott JE, Young MC, Dioun AF, Schneider LC, Phipatanakul W. Characterizing the relationship between sesame, coconut, and nut allergy in children. *Pediatr Allergy Immunol.* 2010 Dec;21(8):1114-8.

Su P, Henriksson A, Tandianus JE, Park JH, Foong F, Dunn NW. Detection and quantification of *Bifidobacterium lactis* LAFTI B94 in human faecal samples from a consumption trial. *FEMS Microbiol Lett.* 2005 Mar 1;244(1):99-103.

Sugawara G, Nagino M, Nishio H, Ebata T, Takagi K, Asahara T, Nomoto K, Nimura Y. Perioperative synbiotic treatment to prevent postoperative infectious complications in biliary cancer surgery: a randomized controlled trial. *Ann Surg.* 2006 Nov;244(5):706-14.

Sugnanam KK, Collins JT, Smith PK, Connor F, Lewindon P, Cleghorn G, Withers G. Dichotomy of food and inhalant allergen sensitization in eosinophilic esophagitis. *Allergy.* 2007 Nov;62(11):1257-60.

Sullivan A, Barkholt L, Nord CE. *Lactobacillus acidophilus, Bifidobacterium lactis* and *Lactobacillus* F19 prevent antibiotic-associated ecological disturbances of Bacteroides fragilis in the intestine. *J Antimicrob Chemother.* 2003 Aug;52(2):308-11.

Sulman FG, Levy D, Lunkan L, Pfeifer Y, Tal E. New methods in the treatment of weather sensitivity. *Fortschr Med.* 1977 Mar 17;95(11):746-52.

Sulman FG. Migraine and headache due to weather and allied causes and its specific treatment. *Ups J Med Sci Suppl.* 1980;31:41-4.

Sumantran VN, Kulkarni AA, Harsulkar A, Wele A, Koppikar SJ, Chandwaskar R, Gaire V, Dalvi M, Wagh UV. Hyaluronidase and collagenase inhibitory activities of the herbal formulation Triphala guggulu. *J Biosci.* 2007 Jun;32(4):755-61.

Sumiyoshi M, Sakanaka M, Kimura Y. Effects of Red Ginseng extract on allergic reactions to food in Balb/c mice. *J Ethnopharmacol.* 2010 Aug 14.

Sung JH, Lee JO, Son JK, Park NS, Kim MR, Kim JG, Moon DC. Cytotoxic constituents from Solidago virga-aurea var. gigantea MIQ. *Arch Pharm Res.* 1999 Dec;22(6):633-7.

Suomalainen H, Isolauri E. New concepts of allergy to cow's milk. *Ann Med.* 1994 Aug;26(4):289-96.

Sur S, Camara M, Buchmeier A, Morgan S, Nelson HS. Double-blind trial of pyridoxine (vitamin B6) in the treatment of steroid-dependent asthma. *Ann Allergy.* 1993 Feb;70(2):147-52.

Sütas Y, Kekki OM, Isolauri E. Late onset reactions to oral food challenge are linked to low serum interleukin-10 concentrations in patients with atopic dermatitis and food allergy. *Clin Exp Allergy.* 2000 Aug;30(8):1121-8.

Suzuki Y, Kondo K, Ichise H, Tsukamoto Y, Urano T, Umemura K. Dietary supplementation with fermented soybeans suppresses intimal thickening. *Nutrition.* 2003 Mar;19(3):261-4.

Svanes C, Heinrich J, Jarvis D, Chinn S, Omenaas E, Gulsvik A, Künzli N, Burney P. Pet-keeping in childhood and adult asthma and hay fever: European community respiratory health survey. *J Allergy Clin Immunol.* 2003 Aug;112(2):289-300.

Svendsen AJ, Holm NV, Kyvik K, *et al.* Relative importance of genetic effects in rheumatoid arthritis: historical cohort study of Danish nationwide twin population. *BMJ* 2002;324(7332): 264-266.

Sweeney B, Vora M, Ulbricht C, Basch E. Evidence-based systematic review of dandelion (Taraxacum officinale) by natural standard research collaboration. *J Herb Pharmacother.* 2005;5(1):79-93.

Swett. JA. *A Treatise on Disease of the Chest.* New York, 1852.

REFERENCES AND BIBLIOGRAPHY

Swiderska-Kiełbik S, Krakowiak A, Wiszniewska M, Dudek W, Walusiak-Skorupa J, Krawczyk-Szulc P, Michowicz A, Pałczyński C. Health hazards associated with occupational exposure to birds. *Med Pr.* 2010;61(2):213-22.

Szyf M, McGowan P, Meaney MJ. The social environment and the epigenome. *Environ Mol Mutagen.* 2008 Jan;49(1):46-60.

Szymański H, Chmielarczyk A, Strus M, Pejcz J, Jawień M, Kochan P, Heczko PB. Colonisation of the gastrointestinal tract by probiotic *L. rhamnosus* strains in acute diarrhoea in children. *Dig Liver Dis.* 2006 Dec;38 Suppl 2:S274-6.

Szymański H, Pejcz J, Jawień M, Chmielarczyk A, Strus M, Heczko PB. Treatment of acute infectious diarrhoea in infants and children with a mixture of three *Lactobacillus rhamnosus* strains—a randomized, double-blind, placebo-controlled trial. *Aliment Pharmacol Ther.* 2006 Jan 15;23(2):247-53.

Takada Y, Ichikawa H, Badmaev V, Aggarwal BB. Acetyl-11-keto-beta-boswellic acid potentiates apoptosis, inhibits invasion, and abolishes osteoclastogenesis by suppressing NF-kappa B and NF-kappa B-regulated gene expression. *J Immunol.* 2006 Mar 1;176(5):3127-40.

Takagi A, Ikemura H, Matsuzaki T, Sato M, Nomoto K, Morotomi M, Yokokura T. Relationship between the in vitro response of dendritic cells to *Lactobacillus* and prevention of tumorigenesis in the mouse. *J Gastroenterol.* 2008;43(9):661-9.

Takahashi N, Eisenhuth G, Lee I, Schachtele C, Laible N, Binion S. Nonspecific antibacterial factors in milk from cows immunized with human oral bacterial pathogens. *J Dairy Sci.* 1992 Jul;75(7):1810-20.

Takasaki M, Konoshima T, Tokuda H, Masuda K, Arai Y, Shiojima K, Ageta H. Anti-carcinogenic activity of Taraxacum plant. I. *Biol Pharm Bull.* 1999 Jun;22(6):602-5.

Takeda K, Okumura K. Effects of a fermented milk drink containing *Lactobacillus casei* strain Shirota on the human NK-cell activity. *J Nutr.* 2007 Mar;137(3 Suppl 2):791S-3S.

Takeda K, Suzuki T, Shimada SI, Shida K, Nanno M, Okumura K. Interleukin-12 is involved in the enhancement of human natural killer cell activity by *Lactobacillus casei* Shirota. *Clin Exp Immunol.* 2006 Oct;146(1):109-15.

Tamaoki J, Chiyotani A, Sakai A, Takemura H, Konno K. Effect of menthol vapour on airway hyperresponsiveness in patients with mild asthma. *Respir Med.* 1995 Aug;89(7):503-4.

Tamura M, Shikina T, Morihana T, Hayama M, Kajimoto O, Sakamoto A, Kajimoto Y, Watanabe O, Nonaka C, Shida K, Nanno M. Effects of probiotics on allergic rhinitis induced by Japanese cedar pollen: randomized double-blind, placebo-controlled clinical trial. *Int Arch Allergy Imml.* 2007;143(1):75-82.

Taniguchi C, Homma M, Takano O, Hirano T, Oka K, Aoyagi Y, Niitsuma T, Hayashi T. Pharmacological effects of urinary products obtained after treatment with saiboku-to, a herbal medicine for bronchial asthma, on type IV allergic reaction. *Planta Med.* 2000 Oct;66(7):607-11.

Tapiero H, Ba GN, Couvreur P, Tew KD. Polyunsaturated fatty acids (PUFA) and eicosanoids in human health and pathologies. *Biomed Pharmacother.* 2002 Jul;56(5):215-22.

Tapsell LC, Hemphill I, Cobiac L, Patch CS, Sullivan DR, Fenech M, Roodenrys S, Keogh JB, Clifton PM, Williams PG, Fazio VA, Inge KE. Health benefits of herbs and spices: the past, the present, the future. *Med J Aust.* 2006 Aug 21;185(4 Suppl):S4-24.

Tasli L, Mat C, De Simone C, Yazici H. Lactobacilli lozenges in the management of oral ulcers of Behçet's syndrome. *Clin Exp Rheumatol.* 2006 Sep-Oct;24(5 Suppl 42):S83-6.

Tasli L, Mat C, De Simone C, Yazici H. Lactobacilli lozenges in the management of oral ulcers of Behçet's syndrome. *Clin Exp Rheumatol.* 2006 Sep-Oct;24(5 Suppl 42):S83-6.

Taussig SJ, Batkin S. Bromelain, the enzyme complex of pineapple (Ananas comosus) and its clinical application. An update. *J Ethnopharmacol.* 1988 Feb-Mar;22(2):191-203.

Taylor AL, Dunstan JA, Prescott SL. Probiotic supplementation for the first 6 months of life fails to reduce the risk of atopic dermatitis and increases the risk of allergen sensitization in high-risk children: a randomized controlled trial. *J Allergy Clin Immunol.* 2007 Jan;119(1):184-91.

Taylor AL, Hale J, Wiltschut J, Lehmann H, Dunstan JA, Prescott SL. Effects of probiotic supplementation for the first 6 months of life on allergen- and vaccine-specific immune responses. *Clin Exp Allergy.* 2006 Oct;36(10):1227-35.

Taylor RB, Lindquist N, Kubanek J, Hay ME. Intraspecific variation in palatability and defensive chemistry of brown seaweeds: effects on herbivore fitness. *Oecologia.* 2003 Aug;136(3):412-23.

Teitelbaum J. *From Fatigue to Fantastic.* New York: Avery, 2001.

Terheggen-Lagro SW, Khouw IM, Schaafsma A, Wauters EA. Safety of a new extensively hydrolysed formula in children with cow's milk protein allergy: a double blind crossover study. *BMC Pediatr.* 2002 Oct 14;2:10.

Terracciano L, Bouygue GR, Sarratud T, Veglia F, Martelli A, Fiocchi A. Impact of dietary regimen on the duration of cow's milk allergy: a random allocation study. *Clin Exp Allergy.* 2010 Apr;40(4):637-42.

Tesse R, Schieck M, Kabesch M. Asthma and endocrine disorders: Shared mechanisms and genetic pleiotropy. *Mol Cell Endocrinol.* 2010 Dec 4. [ahead of print] .

Tevini M, ed. *UV-B Radiation and Ozone Depletion: Effects on humans, animals, plants, microorganisms and materials.* Boca Raton: Lewis Pub, 1993.

Thakkar K, Boatright RO, Gilger MA, El-Serag HB. Gastroesophageal reflux and asthma in children: a systematic review. *Pediatrics.* 2010 Apr;125(4):e925-30. 2010 Mar 29.

Tham KW, Zuraimi MS, Koh D, Chew FT, Ooi PL. Associations between home dampness and presence of molds with asthma and allergic symptoms among young children in the tropics. *Pediatr Allergy Immunol.* 2007 Aug;18(5):418-24.

Thampithak A, Jaisin Y, Meesarapee B, Chongthammakun S, Piyachaturawat P, Govitrapong P, Supavilai P, Sanvarinda Y. Transcriptional regulation of iNOS and COX-2 by a novel compound from Curcuma comosa in lipopolysaccharide-induced microglial activation. *Neurosci Lett.* 2009 Sep 22;462(2):171-5.

Theler B, Brockow K, Ballmer-Weber BK. Clinical presentation and diagnosis of meat allergy in Switzerland and Southern Germany. *Swiss Med Wkly.* 2009 May 2;139(17-18):264-70.

Theofilopoulos AN, Kono DH: The genes of systemic autoimmunity. *Proc Assoc Am Physicians.* 1999;111(3): 228-240.

Thibault H, Aubert-Jacquin C, Goulet O. Effects of long-term consumption of a fermented infant formula (with *Bifidobacterium breve* c50 and *Streptococcus thermophilus* 065) on acute diarrhea in healthy infants. *J Pediatr Gastroenterol Nutr.* 2004 Aug;39(2):147-52.

Thiruvengadam KV, Haranath K, Sudarsan S, Sekar TS, Rajagopal KR, Zacharian MG, Devarajan TV. Tylophora indica in bronchial asthma (a controlled comparison with a standard anti-asthmatic drug). *J Indian Med Assoc.* 1978 Oct 1;71(7):172-6.

Thomas M. Are breathing exercises an effective strategy for people with asthma? *Nurs Times.* 2009 Mar 17-23;105(10):22-7.

Thomas Y, Schiff M, Belkadi L, Jurgens P, Kahhak L, Benveniste J. Activation of human neutrophils by electronically transmitted phorbol-myristate acetate. *Med Hypoth.* 2000;54: 33-39.

Thomas, R.G., Gebhardt, S.E. 2008. Nutritive value of pomegranate fruit and juice. *Maryland Dietetic Association Annual Meeting, USDA-ARS.* 2008 April 11.

Thompson D. *On Growth and Form.* Cambridge: Cambridge University Press, 1992.

Thompson T, Lee AR, Grace T. Gluten contamination of grains, seeds, and flours in the United States: a pilot study. *J Am Diet Assoc.* 2010 Jun;110(6):937-40.

Tierra L. *The Herbs of Life.* Freedom, CA: Crossing Press, 1992.

Tierra M. *The Way of Herbs.* New York: Pocket Books, 1990.

Tietze H. *Kombucha: The Miracle Fungus.* Gateway Books: Bath, UK, 1995.

Tisserand R. *The Art of Aromatherapy.* New York: Inner Traditions, 1979.

Tiwari M. *Ayurveda: A Life of Balance.* Rochester, VT: Healing Arts, 1995.

Tlaskalová-Hogenová H, Stepánková R, Hudcovic T, Tucková L, Cukrowska B, Lodinová-Zádníková R, Kozáková H, Rossmann P, Bártová J, Sokol D, Funda DP, Borovská D, Reháková Z, Sinkora J, Hofman J, Drastich P, Kokesová A. Commensal bacteria (normal microflora), mucosal immunity and chronic inflammatory and autoimmune diseases. *Immunol Lett.* 2004 May 15;93(2-3):97-108.

Todd GR, Acerini CL, Ross-Russell R, Zahra S, Warner JT, McCance D. Survey of adrenal crisis associated with inhaled corticosteroids in the United Kingdom. *Arch Dis Child.* 2002 Dec;87(6):457-61.

Tonkal AM, Morsy TA. An update review on Commiphora molmol and related species. *J Egypt Soc Parasitol.* 2008 Dec;38(3):763-96.

Topçu G, Erenler R, Cakmak O, Johansson CB, Celik C, Chai HB, Pezzuto JM. Diterpenes from the berries of Juniperus excelsa. *Phytochemistry.* 1999 Apr;50(7):1195-9.

Toppila-Salmi S, Renkonen J, Joenväärä S, Mattila P, Renkonen R. Allergen interactions with epithelium. *Curr Opin Allergy Clin Immunol.* 2011 Feb;11(1):29-32.

Tordesillas L, Pacios LF, Palacín A, Cuesta-Herranz J, Madero M, Díaz-Perales A. Characterization of IgE epitopes of Cuc m 2, the major melon allergen, and their role in cross-reactivity with pollen profilins. *Clin Exp Allergy.* 2010 Jan;40(1):174-81.

Tormo Carnicer R, Infante Piña D, Roselló Mayans E, Bartolomé Comas R. Intake of fermented milk containing *Lactobacillus casei* DN-114 001 and its effect on gut flora. *An Pediatr.* 2006 Nov;65(5):448-53.

Torrent M, Sunyer J, Muñoz L, Cullinan P, Iturriaga MV, Figueroa C, Vall O, Taylor AN, Anto JM. Early-life domestic aeroallergen exposure and IgE sensitization at age 4 years. *J Allergy Clin Immunol.* 2006 Sep;118(3):742-8.

Touhami M, Boudraa G, Mary JY, Soltana R, Desjeux JF. Clinical consequences of replacing milk with yogurt in persistent infantile diarrhea. *Ann Pediatr.* 1992 Feb;39(2):79-86.

Towers GH. FAHF-1 purporting to block peanut-induced anaphylaxis. *J Allergy Clin Immunol.* 2003 May;111(5):1140; author reply 1140-1.

Towle A. *Modern Biology.* Austin: Harcourt Brace, 1993.

Trenev N. *Probiotics: Nature's Internal Healers.* New York: Avery, 1998.

Tripkovic L, Lambert H, Hart K, Smith CP, Bucca G, Penson S, Chope G, Hyppönen E, Berry J, Vieth R, Lanham-New S. Comparison of vitamin D2 and vitamin D3 supplementation in raising serum 25-

hydroxyvitamin D status: a systematic review and meta-analysis. Am J Clin Nutr. 2012 Jun;95(6):1357-64.

Trois L, Cardoso EM, Miura E. Use of probiotics in HIV-infected children: a randomized double-blind controlled study. J Trop Pediatr. 2008 Feb;54(1):19-24.

Trojanová I, Rada V, Kokoska L, Vlková E. The bifidogenic effect of Taraxacum officinale root. Fitoterapia. 2004 Dec;75(7-8):760-3.

Troncone R, Caputo N, Florio G, Finelli E. Increased intestinal sugar permeability after challenge in children with cow's milk allergy or intolerance. Allergy. 1994 Mar;49(3):142-6.

Trout L, King M, Feng W, Inglis SK, Ballard ST. Inhibition of airway liquid secretion and its effect on the physical properties of airway mucus. Am J Physiol. 1998 Feb;274(2 Pt 1):L258-63.

Tsai JC, Tsai S, Chang WC. Comparison of two Chinese medical herbs, Huangbai and Qianniuzi, on influence of short circuit current across the rat intestinal epithelia. J Ethnopharmacol. 2004 Jul;93(1):21-5.

Tsong T. Deciphering the language of cells. Trends in Biochem Sci. 1989;14:89-92.

Tsuchiya J, Barreto R, Okura R, Kawakita S, Fesce E, Marotta F. Single-blind follow-up study on the effectiveness of a symbiotic preparation in irritable bowel syndrome. Chin J Dig Dis. 2004;5(4):169-74.

Tubelius P, Stan V, Zachrisson A. Increasing work-place healthiness with the probiotic Lactobacillus reuteri: a randomised, double-blind placebo-controlled study. Environ Health. 2005 Nov 7;4:25.

Tucker KL, Olson B, Bakun P, Dallal GE, Selhub J, Rosenberg IH. Breakfast cereal fortified with folic acid, vitamin B-6, and vitamin B-12 increases vitamin concentrations and reduces homocysteine concentrations: a randomized trial. Am J Clin Nutr. 2004 May;79(5):805-11.

Tulk HM, Robinson LE. Modifying the n-6/n-3 polyunsaturated fatty acid ratio of a high-saturated fat challenge does not acutely attenuate postprandial changes in inflammatory markers in men with metabolic syndrome. Metabolism. 2009 Jul 20.

Tunnicliffe WS, Burge PS, Ayres JG. Effect of domestic concentrations of nitrogen dioxide on airway responses to inhaled allergen in asthmatic patients. Lancet. 1994 Dec 24-31;344(8939-8940):1733-6.

Tunnicliffe WS, Fletcher TJ, Hammond K, Roberts K, Custovic A, Simpson A, Woodcock A, Ayres JG. Sensitivity and exposure to indoor allergens in adults with differing asthma severity. Eur Respir J. 1999 Mar;13(3):654-9.

Tuomilehto J, Lindström J, Hyyrynen J, Korpela R, Karhunen ML, Mikkola L, Jauhiainen T, Seppo L, Nissinen A. Effect of ingesting sour milk fermented using Lactobacillus helveticus bacteria producing tripeptides on blood pressure in subjects with mild hypertension. J Hum Hypertens. 2004 Nov;18(11):795-802.

Turchet P, Laurenzano M, Auboiron S, Antoine JM. Effect of fermented milk containing the probiotic Lactobacillus casei DN-114001 on winter infections in free-living elderly subjects: a randomised, controlled pilot study. J Nutr Health Aging. 2003;7(2):75-7.

Tursi A, Brandimarte G, Giorgetti GM, Elisei W. Mesalazine and/or Lactobacillus casei in maintaining long-term remission of symptomatic uncomplicated diverticular disease of the colon. Hepatogastroenterology. 2008 May-Jun;55(84):916-20.

Twetman S, Derawi B, Keller M, Ekstrand K, Yucel-Lindberg T, Stecksen-Blicks C. Short-term effect of chewing gums containing probiotic Lactobacillus reuteri on the levels of inflammatory mediators in gingival crevicular fluid. Acta Odontol Scand. 2009 Feb;67(1):19-24.

U.S. Food and Drug Administration Guidance for Industry Botanical Drug Products. CfDEaR. 2000

Uddenfeldt M, Janson C, Lampa E, Leander M, Norbäck D, Larsson L, Rask-Andersen A. High BMI is related to higher incidence of asthma, while a fish and fruit diet is related to a lower- Results from a long-term follow-up study of three age groups in Sweden. Respir Med. 2010 Jul;104(7):972-80.

Udupa AL, Udupa SL, Guruswamy MN. The possible site of anti-asthmatic action of Tylophora asthmatica on pituitary-adrenal axis in albino rats. Planta Med. 1991 Oct;57(5):409-13.

Ueno H, Yoshioka K, Matsumoto T. Usefulness of the skin index in predicting the outcome of oral challenges in children. J Investig Allergol Clin Immunol. 2007;17(4):207-10.

Ueno M, Adachi A, Fukumoto T, Nishitani N, Fujiwara N, Matsuo H, Kohno K, Morita E. Analysis of causative allergen of the patient with baker's asthma and wheat-dependent exercise-induced anaphylaxis (WDEIA). Arerugi. 2010 May;59(5):552-7.

Ukabam SO, Mann RJ, Cooper BT. Small intestinal permeability to sugars in patients with atopic eczema. Br J Dermatol. 1984 Jun;110(6):649-52.

Ulrich RS, Simons RF, Losito BD, Fiorito E, Miles MA, Zelson M. Stress recovery during exposure to natural and urban environments. J Envir Psychol. 1991;11:201-30.

Unknown. Proteolytic activity of various lactic acid bacteria. Japan Jnl Dairy Food Sci. 1990;39(4).

Unsel M, Sin AZ, Ardeniz O, Erdem N, Ersoy R, Gulbahar O, Mete N, Kokuludağ A. New onset egg allergy in an adult. J Investig Allergol Clin Immunol. 2007;17(1):55-8.

Upadhyay AK, Kumar K, Kumar A, Mishra HS. Tinospora cordifolia (Willd.) Hook. f. and Thoms. (Guduchi) - validation of the Ayurvedic pharmacology through experimental and clinical studies. Int J Ayurveda Res. 2010 Apr;1(2):112-21.

Urata Y, Yoshida S, Irie Y, Tanigawa T, Amayasu H, Nakabayashi M, Akahori K. Treatment of asthma patients with herbal medicine TJ-96: a randomized controlled trial. *Respir Med.* 2002 Jun;96(6):469-74.

Vakil JR, Shahani KM. Carbohydrate metabolism of lactic acid cultures. V. Lactobionate and gluconate metabolism of *Streptococcus lactis* UN. *J Dairy Sci.* 1969 Dec;52(12):1928-34.

Valeur N, Engel P, Carbajal N, Connolly E, Ladefoged K. Colonization and immunomodulation by *Lactobacillus reuteri* ATCC 55730 in the human gastrointestinal tract. *Appl Environ Microbiol.* 2004 Feb;70(2):1176-81.

Vally H, Thompson PJ, Misso NL. Changes in bronchial hyperresponsiveness following high- and low-sulphite wine challenges in wine-sensitive asthmatic patients. *Clin Exp Allergy.* 2007 Jul;37(7):1062-6.

van Baarlen P, Troost FJ, van Hemert S, van der Meer C, de Vos WM, de Groot PJ, Hooiveld GJ, Brummer RJ, Kleerebezem M. Differential NF-kappaB pathways induction by *Lactobacillus plantarum* in the duodenum of healthy humans correlating with immune tolerance. *Proc Natl Acad Sci U S A.* 2009 Feb 17;106(7):2371-6

van Beelen VA, Roeleveld J, Mooibroek H, Sijtsma L, Bino RJ, Bosch D, Rietjens IM, Alink GM. A comparative study on the effect of algal and fish oil on viability and cell proliferation of Caco-2 cells. *Food Chem Toxicol.* 2007 May;45(5):716-24.

van den Heuvel EG, Schoterman MH, Muijs T. Transgalactooligosaccharides stimulate calcium absorption in postmenopausal women. *J Nutr.* 2000 Dec;130(12):2938-42.

van Elburg RM, Uil JJ, de Monchy JG, Heymans HS. Intestinal permeability in pediatric gastroenterology. *Scand J Gastroenterol Suppl.* 1992;194:19-24.

van Huisstede A, Braunstahl GJ. Obesity and asthma: co-morbidity or causal relationship? *Monaldi Arch Chest Dis.* 2010 Sep;73(3):116-23.

van Kampen V, Merget R, Rabstein S, Sander I, Bruening T, Broding HC, Keller C, Muesken H, Overlack A, Schultze-Werninghaus G, Walusiak J, Raulf-Heimsoth M. Comparison of wheat and rye flour solutions for skin prick testing: a multi-centre study (Stad 1). *Clin Exp Allergy.* 2009 Dec;39(12):1896-902.

van Odijk J, Peterson CG, Ahlstedt S, Bengtsson U, Borres MP, Hulthén L, Magnusson J, Hansson T. Measurements of eosinophil activation before and after food challenges in adults with food hypersensitivity. *Int Arch Allergy Immunol.* 2006;140(4):334-41.

van Zwol A, Moll HA, Fetter WP, van Elburg RM. Glutamine-enriched enteral nutrition in very low birthweight infants and allergic and infectious diseases at 6 years of age. *Paediatr Perinat Epidemiol.* 2011 Jan;25(1):60-6.

Vanderhoof JA. Probiotics in allergy management. *J Pediatr Gastroenterol Nutr.* 2008 Nov;47 Suppl 2:S38-40.

VanHaitsma TA, Mickleborough T, Stager JM, Koceja DM, Lindley MR, Chapman R. Comparative effects of caffeine and albuterol on the bronchoconstrictor response to exercise in asthmatic athletes. *Int J Sports Med.* 2010 Apr;31(4):231-6.

Vanto T, Helppilä S, Juntunen-Backman K, Kalimo K, Klemola T, Korpela R, Koskinen P. Prediction of the development of tolerance to milk in children with cow's milk hypersensitivity. *J Pediatr.* 2004 Feb;144(2):218-22.

Vargas C, Bustos P, Diaz PV, Amigo H, Rona RJ. Childhood environment and atopic conditions, with emphasis on asthma in a Chilean agricultural area. *J Asthma.* 2008 Jan-Feb;45(1):73-8.

Varonier HS, de Haller J, Schopfer C. Prevalence of allergies in children and adolescents. *Helv Paediatr Acta.* 1984;39:129-136.

Varraso R, Fung TT, Barr RG, Hu FB, Willett W, Camargo CA Jr. Prospective study of dietary patterns and chronic obstructive pulmonary disease among US women. *Am J Clin Nutr.* 2007 Aug;86(2):488-95.

Varraso R, Fung TT, Hu FB, Willett W, Camargo CA. Prospective study of dietary patterns and chronic obstructive pulmonary disease among US men. *Thorax.* 2007 Sep;62(9):786-91. 2007 May 15.

Varraso R, Jiang R, Barr RG, Willett WC, Camargo CA Jr. Prospective study of cured meats consumption and risk of chronic obstructive pulmonary disease in men. *Am J Epidemiol.* 2007 Dec 15;166(12):1438-45. 2007 Sep 4. 17785711; .

Vassallo MF, Banerji A, Rudders SA, Clark S, Mullins RJ, Camargo CA Jr. Season of birth and food allergy in children. *Ann Allergy Asthma Immunol.* 2010 Apr;104(4):307-13.

Vauthier JM, Lluch A, Lecomte E, Artur Y, Herbeth B. Family resemblance in energy and macronutrient intakes: the Stanislas Family Study. *Int J Epidemiol.*1996 Oct;25(5):1030-7.

Vempati R, Bijlani RL, Deepak KK. The efficacy of a comprehensive lifestyle modification programme based on yoga in the management of bronchial asthma: a randomized controlled trial. *BMC Pulm Med.* 2009 Jul 30;9:37.

Vendt N, Grünberg H, Tuure T, Malminiemi O, Wuolijoki E, Tillmann V, Sepp E, Korpela R. Growth during the first 6 months of life in infants using formula enriched with Lactobacillus rhamnosus GG: double-blind, randomized trial. *J Hum Nutr Diet.* 2006 Feb;19(1):51-8.

Vendt N, Grünberg H, Tuure T, Malminiemi O, Wuolijoki E, Tillmann V, Sepp E, Korpela R. Growth during the first 6 months of life in infants using formula enriched with *Lactobacillus rhamnosus* GG: double-blind, randomized trial. *J Hum Nutr Diet.* 2006 Feb;19(1):51-8.

Venkatachalam KV. Human 3'-phosphoadenosine 5'-phosphosulfate (PAPS) synthase: biochemistry, molecular biology and genetic deficiency. *IUBMB Life.* 2003 Jan;55(1):1-11.

Venkatesan N, Punithavathi D, Babu M. Protection from acute and chronic lung diseases by curcumin. *Adv Exp Med Biol.* 2007;595:379-405.

Venter C, Hasan Arshad S, Grundy J, Pereira B, Bernie Clayton C, Voigt K, Higgins B, Dean T. Time trends in the prevalence of peanut allergy: three cohorts of children from the same geographical location in the UK. *Allergy.* 2010 Jan;65(1):103-8.

Venter C, Meyer R. Session 1: Allergic disease: The challenges of managing food hypersensitivity. *Proc Nutr Soc.* 2010 Feb;69(1):11-24.

Ventura MT, Polimeno L, Amoruso AC, Gatti F, Annoscia E, Marinaro M, Di Leo E, Matino MG, Buquicchio R, Bonini S, Tursi A, Francavilla A. Intestinal permeability in patients with adverse reactions to food. *Dig Liver Dis.* 2006 Oct;38(10):732-6.

Venturi A, Gionchetti P, Rizzello F, Johansson R, Zucconi E, Brigidi P, Matteuzzi D, Campieri M. Impact on the composition of the faecal flora by a new probiotic preparation: preliminary data on maintenance treatment of patients with ulcerative colitis. *Aliment Pharmacol Ther.* 1999 Aug;13(8):1103-8.

Venturi A, Gionchetti P, Rizzello F, Johansson R, Zucconi E, Brigidi P, Matteuzzi D, Campieri M. Impact on the composition of the faecal flora by a new probiotic preparation: preliminary data on maintenance treatment of patients with ulcerative colitis. *Aliment Pharmacol Ther.* 1999 Aug;13(8):1103-8.

Verhasselt V. Oral tolerance in neonates: from basics to potential prevention of allergic disease. *Mucosal Immunol.* 2010 Jul;3(4):326-33.

Verstege A, Mehl A, Rolinck-Werninghaus C, Staden U, Nocon M, Beyer K, Niggemann B. The predictive value of the skin prick test weal size for the outcome of oral food challenges. Clin Exp Allergy. 2005 Sep;35(9):1220-6. Rolinck-Werninghaus C, Staden U, Mehl A, Hamelmann E, Beyer K, Niggemann B. Specific oral tolerance induction with food in children: transient or persistent effect on food allergy? *Allergy.* 2005 Oct;60(10):1320-2.

Vidgren HM, Agren JJ, Schwab U, Rissanen T, Hanninen O, Uusitupa MI. Incorporation of n-3 fatty acids into plasma lipid fractions, and erythrocyte membranes and platelets during dietary supplementation with fish, fish oil, and docosahexaenoic acid-rich oil among healthy young men. *Lipids.* 1997 Jul;32(7):697-705.

Vidgren HM, Agren JJ, Schwab U, Rissanen T, Hanninen O, Uusitupa MI. Incorporation of n-3 fatty acids into plasma lipid fractions, and erythrocyte membranes and platelets during dietary supplementation with fish, fish oil, and docosahexaenoic acid-rich oil among healthy young men. *Lipids.* 1997 Jul;32(7):697-705.

Viinanen A, Munhbayarlah S, Zevgee T, Narantsetseg L, Naidansuren Ts, Koskenvuo M, Helenius H, Terho EO. Prevalence of asthma, allergic rhinoconjuctivitis and allergic sensitization in Mongolia. *Allergy.* 2005;60:1370-1377.

Vila R, Mundina M, Tomi F, Furlán R, Zacchino S, Casanova J, Cañigueral S. Composition and antifungal activity of the essential oil of Solidago chilensis. *Planta Med.* 2002 Feb;68(2):164-7.

Viljanen M, Kuitunen M, Haahtela T, Juntunen-Backman K, Korpela R, Savilahti E. Probiotic effects on faecal inflammatory markers and on faecal IgA in food allergic atopic eczema/dermatitis syndrome infants. *Pediatr Allergy Immunol.* 2005 Feb;16(1):65-71.

Viljanen M, Savilahti E, Haahtela T, Juntunen-Backman K, Korpela R, Poussa T, Tuure T, Kuitunen M. Probiotics in the treatment of atopic eczema/dermatitis syndrome in infants: a double-blind placebo-controlled trial. *Allergy.* 2005 Apr;60(4):494-500.

Villarruel G, Rubio DM, Lopez F, Cintioni J, Gurevech R, Romero G, Vandenplas Y. *Saccharomyces boulardii* in acute childhood diarrhoea: a randomized, placebo-controlled study. *Acta Paediatr.* 2007 Apr;96(4):538-41.

Vinson JA, Proch J, Bose P. MegaNatural((R)) Gold Grapeseed Extract: In Vitro Antioxidant and In Vivo Human Supplementation Studies. *J Med Food.* 2001 Spring;4(1):17-26.

Vinson JA, Proch J, Bose P. MegaNatural((R)) Gold Grapeseed Extract: In Vitro Antioxidant and In Vivo Human Supplementation Studies. *J Med Food.* 2001 Spring;4(1):17-26.

Visitsunthorn N, Pacharn P, Jirapongsananuruk O, Weeravejsukit S, Sripramong C, Sookrung N, Bunnag C. Comparison between Siriraj mite allergen vaccine and standardized commercial mite vaccine by skin prick testing in normal Thai adults. *Asian Pac J Allergy Immunol.* 2010 Mar;28(1):41-5.

Visness CM, London SJ, Daniels JL, Kaufman JS, Yeatts KB, Siega-Riz AM, Liu AH, Calatroni A, Zeldin DC. Association of obesity with IgE levels and allergy symptoms in children and adolescents: results from the National Health and Nutrition Examination Survey 2005-2006. *J Allergy Clin Immunol.* 2009 May;123(5):1163-9, 1169.e1-4.

Visness CM, London SJ, Daniels JL, Kaufman JS, Yeatts KB, Siega-Riz AM, Calatroni A, Zeldin DC. Association of childhood obesity with atopic and nonatopic asthma: results from the National Health and Nutrition Examination Survey 1999-2006. *J Asthma.* 2010 Sep;47(7):822-9.

Vivatvakin B, Kowitdamrong E. Randomized control trial of live *Lactobacillus acidophilus* plus *Bifidobacterium infantis* in treatment of infantile acute watery diarrhea. *J Med Assoc Thai.* 2006 Sep;89 Suppl 3:S126-33.

Vlieg-Boerstra BJ, Dubois AE, van der Heide S, Bijleveld CM, Wolt-Plompen SA, Oude Elberink JN, Kukler J, Jansen DF, Venter C, Duiverman EJ. Ready-to-use introduction schedules for first exposure to allergenic foods in children at home. *Allergy.* 2008 Jul;63(7):903-9.

Vlieg-Boerstra BJ, van der Heide S, Bijleveld CM, Kukler J, Duiverman EJ, Wolt-Plompen SA, Dubois AE. Dietary assessment in children adhering to a food allergen avoidance diet for allergy prevention. *Eur J Clin Nutr.* 2006 Dec;60(12):1384-90.

Voicekovska JG, Orlikov GA, Karpov IuG, Teibe U, Ivanov AD, Baidekalne I, Voicehovskis NV, Maulins E. External respiration function and quality of life in patients with bronchial asthma in correction of selenium deficiency. *Ter Arkh.* 2007;79(8):38-41.

Voïtsekhovskaia IuG, Skesters A, Orlikov GA, Silova AA, Rusakova NE, Larmane LT, Karpov IuG, Ivanov AD, Maulins E. Assessment of some oxidative stress parameters in bronchial asthma patients beyond add-on selenium supplementation. *Biomed Khim.* 2007 Sep-Oct;53(5):577-84.

Vojdani A. Antibodies as predictors of complex autoimmune diseases. *Int J Immunopathol Pharmacol.* 2008 Apr-Jun;21(2):267-78.

von Berg A, Filipiak-Pittroff B, Krämer U, Link E, Bollrath C, Brockow I, Koletzko S, Grübl A, Heinrich J, Wichmann HE, Bauer CP, Reinhardt D, Berdel D; GINIplus study group. Preventive effect of hydrolyzed infant formulas persists until age 6 years: long-term results from the German Infant Nutritional Intervention Study (GINI). *J Allergy Clin Immunol.* 2008 Jun;121(6):1442-7.

von Berg A, Koletzko S, Grübl A, Filipiak-Pittroff B, Wichmann HE, Bauer CP, Reinhardt D, Berdel D; German Infant Nutritional Intervention Study Group. The effect of hydrolyzed cow's milk formula for allergy prevention in the first year of life: the German Infant Nutritional Intervention Study, a randomized double-blind trial. *J Allergy Clin Immunol.* 2003 Mar;111(3):533-40.

von Kruedener S, Schneider W, Elstner EF. A combination of Populus tremula, Solidago virgaurea and Fraxinus excelsior as an anti-inflammatory and antirheumatic drug. A short review. *Arzneimittelforschung.* 1995 Feb;45(2):169-71.

von Mutius E, Vercelli D. Farm living: effects on childhood asthma and allergy. *Nat Rev Immunol.* 2010 Dec;10(12):861-8. 2010 Nov 9.

Vuksan V, Whitham D, Sievenpiper JL, Jenkins AL, Rogovik AL, Bazinet RP, Vidgen E, Hanna A. Supplementation of conventional therapy with the novel grain Salba (Salvia hispanica L.) improves major and emerging cardiovascular risk factors in type 2 diabetes: results of a randomized controlled trial. *Diabetes Care.* 2007 Nov;30(11):2804-10.

Vulevic J, Drakoularakou A, Yaqoob P, Tzortzis G and Gibson GR; Modulation of the fecal microflora profile and immune function by a novel trans-galactooligosaccharide mixture (B-GOS) in healthy elderly volunteers. *Am J Clin Nutr.* 1988 88;1438-1446.

Waddell L. Food allergies in children: the difference between cow's milk protein allergy and food intolerance. *J Fam Health Care.* 2010;20(3):104.

Wahler D, Gronover CS, Richter C, Foucu F, Twyman RM, Moerschbacher BM, Fischer R, Muth J, Prufer D. Polyphenoloxidase silencing affects latex coagulation in Taraxacum spp. *Plant Physiol.* 2009 Jul 15.

Waite DA, Eyles EF, Tonkin SL, O'Donnell TV. Asthma prevalence in Tokelauan children in two environments. *Clin Allergy.* 1980;10:71-75.

Waked M, Salameh P. Risk factors for asthma and allergic diseases in school children across Lebanon. *J Asthma Allergy.* 2008 Nov 11;2:1-7.

Walders-Abramson N, Wamboldt FS, Curran-Everett D, Zhang L. Encouraging physical activity in pediatric asthma: a case-control study of the wonders of walking (WOW) program. *Pediatr Pulmonol.* 2009 Sep;44(9):909-16.

Walker S, Wing A. Allergies in children. *J Fam Health Care.* 2010;20(1):24-6.

Walker WA. Antigen absorption from the small intestine and gastrointestinal disease. *Pediatr Clin North Am.* 1975 Nov;22(4):731-46.

Walker WA. Antigen handling by the small intestine. *Clin Gastroenterol.* 1986 Jan;15(1):1-20.

Walle UK, Walle T. Transport of the cooked-food mutagen 2-amino-1-methyl-6-phenylimidazo- 4,5-b pyridine (PhIP) across the human intestinal Caco-2 cell monolayer: role of efflux pumps. *Carcinogenesis.* 1999 Nov;20(11):2153-7.

Walsh MG. Toxocara infection and diminished lung function in a nationally representative sample from the United States population. *Int J Parasitol.* 2010 Nov 8.

Walsh SJ, Rau LM: Autoimmune diseases: a leading cause of death among young and middle-aged women in the United States. *Am J Public Health* 2000, 90(9): 1463-1466.

Wang G, Liu CT, Wang ZL, Yan CL, Luo FM, Wang L, Li TQ. Effects of Astragalus membranaceus in promoting T-helper cell type 1 polarization and interferon-gamma production by up-regulating T-bet expression in patients with asthma. *Chin J Integr Med.* 2006 Dec;12(4):262-7.

REFERENCES AND BIBLIOGRAPHY

Wang H, Chang B, Wang B. The effect of herbal medicine including astragalus membranaceus (fisch) bge, codonpsis pilosula and glycyrrhiza uralensis fisch on airway responsiveness. *Zhonghua Jie He He Hu Xi Za Zhi.* 1998 May;21(5):287-8.

Wang J, Lin J, Bardina L, Goldis M, Nowak-Wegrzyn A, Shreffler WG, Sampson HA. Correlation of IgE/IgG4 milk epitopes and affinity of milk-specific IgE antibodies with different phenotypes of clinical milk allergy. *J Allergy Clin Immunol.* 2010 Mar;125(3):695-702, 702.e1-702.e6.

Wang J, Patil SP, Yang N, Ko J, Lee J, Noone S, Sampson HA, Li XM. Safety, tolerability, and immunologic effects of a food allergy herbal formula in food allergic individuals: a randomized, double-blinded, placebo-controlled, dose escalation, phase 1 study. *Ann Allergy Asthma Immunol.* 2010 Jul;105(1):75-84.

Wang J. Management of the patient with multiple food allergies. *Curr Allergy Asthma Rep.* 2010 Jul;10(4):271-7.

Wang JL, Shaw NS, Kao MD. Magnesium deficiency and its lack of association with asthma in Taiwanese elementary school children. *Asia Pac J Clin Nutr.* 2007;16 Suppl 2:579-84.

Wang JS, Hung WP. The effects of a swimming intervention for children with asthma. *Respirology.* 2009 Aug;14(6):838-42.

Wang KY, Li SN, Liu CS, Perng DS, Su YC, Wu DC, Jan CM, Lai CH, Wang TN, Wang WM. Effects of ingesting Lactobacillus- and Bifidobacterium-containing yogurt in subjects with colonized Helicobacter pylori. *Am J Clin Nutr.* 2004 Sep;80(3):737-41.

Wang KY, Li SN, Liu CS, Perng DS, Su YC, Wu DC, Jan CM, Lai CH, Wang TN, Wang WM. Effects of ingesting *Lactobacillus-* and *Bifidobacterium-*containing yogurt in subjects with colonized *Helicobacter pylori. Am J Clin Nutr.* 2004 Sep;80(3):737-41.

Wang YH, Yang CP, Ku MS, Sun HL, Lue KH. Efficacy of nasal irrigation in the treatment of acute sinusitis in children. *Int J Pediatr Otorhinolaryngol.* 2009 Dec;73(12):1696-701. 2009 Sep 27.

Wang YM, Huan GX. *Utilization of Classical Formulas.* Beijing, China: Chinese Medicine and Pharmacology Publishing Co, 1998.

Waring G, Levy D. Challenging adverse reactions in children with food allergies. *Paediatr Nurs.* 2010 Jul;22(6):16-22.

Waser M, Michels KB, Bieli C, Flöistrup H, Pershagen G, von Mutius E, Ege M, Riedler J, Schram-Bijkerk D, Brunekreef B, van Hage M, Lauener R, Braun-Fahrländer C; PARSIFAL Study team. Inverse association of farm milk consumption with asthma and allergy in rural and suburban populations across Europe. *Clin Exp Allergy.* 2007 May;37(5):661-70.

Watkins BA, Hannon K, Ferruzzi M, Li Y. Dietary PUFA and flavonoids as deterrents for environmental pollutants. *J Nutr Biochem.* 2007 Mar;18(3):196-205.

Watson L. *Supernature.* New York: Bantam, 1973.

Watson R. Preedy VR. Botanical Medicine in Clinical Practice. Oxfordshire: CABI, 2008.

Watve MG, Tickoo R, Jog MM, Bhole BD. How many antibiotics are produced by the genus Streptomyces? *Arch Microbiol.* 2001 Nov;176(5):386-90.

Watzl B, Bub A, Blockhaus M, Herbert BM, Lührmann PM, Neuhäuser-Berthold M, Rechkemmer G. Prolonged tomato juice consumption has no effect on cell-mediated immunity of well-nourished elderly men and women. *J Nutr.* 2000 Jul;130(7):1719-23.

Webber CM, England RW. Oral allergy syndrome: a clinical, diagnostic, and therapeutic challenge. *Ann Allergy Asthma Immunol.* 2010 Feb;104(2):101-8; quiz 109-10, 117.

Webster D, Taschereau P, Belland RJ, Sand C, Rennie RP. Antifungal activity of medicinal plant extracts; preliminary screening studies. *J Ethnopharmacol.* 2008 Jan 4;115(1):140-6.

Weekes DJ. Management of Herpes Simplex with Virostatic Bacterial Agent. *EENT Dig.* 1963;25(12).

Weekes DJ. The treatment of aphthous stomatitis with Lactobacillus tablets. *NY State J Med.* 1958 Aug 15;58(16):2672-3.

Wegrowski J, Robert AM, Moczar M. The effect of procyanidolic oligomers on the composition of normal and hypercholesterolemic rabbit aortas. *Biochem Pharmacol.* 1984 Nov 1;33(21):3491-7.

Wei A, Shibamoto T. Antioxidant activities and volatile constituents of various essential oils. *J Agric Food Chem.* 2007 Mar 7;55(5):1737-42.

Weiler JM, Layton T, Hunt M. Asthma in United States Olympic athletes who participated in the 1996 Summer Games. J Allergy Clin Immunol. 1998 Nov;102(5):722-6. 7.

Weiner MA. *Secrets of Fijian Medicine.* Berkeley, CA: Univ. of Calif., 1969.

Weisgerber M, Webber K, Meurer J, Danduran M, Berger S, Flores G. Moderate and vigorous exercise programs in children with asthma: safety, parental satisfaction, and asthma outcomes. Pediatr Pulmonol. 2008 Dec;43(12):1175-82.

Weiss RF. *Herbal Medicine.* Gothenburg, Sweden: Beaconsfield, 1988.

Weizman Z, Asli G, Alsheikh A. Effect of a probiotic infant formula on infections in child care centers: comparison of two probiotic agents. *Pediatrics.* 2005 Jan;115(1):5-9.

Wen MC, Huang CK, Srivastava KD, Zhang TF, Schofield B, Sampson HA, Li XM. Ku-Shen (Sophora flavescens Ait), a single Chinese herb, abrogates airway hyperreactivity in a murine model of asthma. *J Allergy Clin Immunol.* 2004;113:218.

Wen MC, Taper A, Srivastava KD, Huang CK, Schofield B, Li XM. Immunology of T cells by the Chinese Herbal Medicine Ling Zhi (Ganoderma lucidum) *J Allergy Clin Immunol.* 2003;111:S320.

Wen MC, Wei CH, Hu ZQ, Srivastava K, Ko J, Xi ST, Mu DZ, Du JB, Li GH, Wallenstein S, Sampson H, Kattan M, Li XM. Efficacy and tolerability of anti-asthma herbal medicine intervention in adult patients with moderate-severe allergic asthma. *J Allergy Clin Immunol.* 2005;116:517-24.

Wenus C, Goll R, Loken EB, Biong AS, Halvorsen DS, Florholmen J. Prevention of antibiotic-associated diarrhoea by a fermented probiotic milk drink. *Eur J Clin Nutr.* 2008 Feb;62(2):299-301.

Werbach M. *Nutritional Influences on Illness.* Tarzana, CA: Third Line Press, 1996.

West CE, Hammarström ML, Hernell O. Probiotics during weaning reduce the incidence of eczema. *Pediatr Allergy Immunol.* 2009 Aug;20(5):430-7.

West R. Risk of death in meat and non-meat eaters. *BMJ.* 1994 Oct 8;309(6959):955.

Westerholm-Ormio M, Vaarala O, Tiittanen M, Savilahti E. Infiltration of Foxp3- and Toll-like receptor-4-positive cells in the intestines of children with food allergy. *J Pediatr Gastroenterol Nutr.* 2010 Apr;50(4):367-76.

Wheeler JG, Bogle ML, Shema SJ, Shirrell MA, Stine KC, Pittler AJ, Burks AW, Helm RM. Impact of dietary yogurt on immune function. *Am J Med Sci.* 1997 Feb;313(2):120-3.

Wheeler JG, Shema SJ, Bogle ML, Shirrell MA, Burks AW, Pittler A, Helm RM. Immune and clinical impact of *Lactobacillus acidophilus* on asthma. *Ann Allergy Asthma Immunol.* 1997 Sep;79(3):229-33.

Wheeler JG, Shema SJ, Bogle ML, Shirrell MA, Burks AW, Pittler A, Helm RM. Immune and clinical impact of *Lactobacillus acidophilus* on asthma. *Ann Allergy Asthma Immunol.* 1997 Sep;79(3):229-33.

White LB, Foster S. The Herbal Drugstore. Emmaus, PA: Rodale, 2000.

Whitfield KE, Wiggins SA, Belue R, Brandon DT. Genetic and environmental influences on forced expiratory volume in African Americans: the Carolina African-American Twin Study of Aging. *Ethn Dis.* 2004 Spring;14(2):206-11.

WHO. *Guidelines for Drinking-water Quality.* 2nd ed, vol. 2. Geneva: World Health Organization, 1996.

WHO. How trace elements in water contribute to health. *WHO Chronicle.* 1978;32:382-385.

WHO. *INFOSAN Food Allergies. Information Note No. 3.* Geneva, Switzerland: World Health Organization, 2006.

Whorwell PJ, Altringer L, Morel J, Bond Y, Charbonneau D, O'Mahony L, Kiely B, Shanahan F, Quigley EM. Efficacy of an encapsulated probiotic *Bifidobacterium infantis* 35624 in women with irritable bowel syndrome. *Am J Gastroenterol.* 2006 Jul;101(7):1581-90.

Wickens K, Black PN, Stanley TV, Mitchell E, Fitzharris P, Tannock GW, Purdie G, Crane J; Probiotic Study Group. A differential effect of 2 probiotics in the prevention of eczema and atopy: a double-blind, randomized, placebo-controlled trial. *J Allergy Clin Immunol.* 2008 Oct;122(4):788-94.

Widdicombe JG, Ernst E. Clinical cough V: complementary and alternative medicine: therapy of cough. *Handb Exp Pharmacol.* 2009;(187):321-42.

Wildt S, Munck LK, Vinter-Jensen L, Hanse BF, Nordgaard-Lassen I, Christensen S, Avnstroem S, Rasmussen SN, Rumessen JJ. Probiotic treatment of collagenous colitis: a randomized, double-blind, placebo-controlled trial with *Lactobacillus acidophilus* and *Bifidobacterium animalis* subsp. *Lactis. Inflamm Bowel Dis.* 2006 May;12(5):395-401.

Wilkens H, Wilkens JH, Uffmann J, Bövers J, Fröhlich JC, Fabel H. Effect of the platelet-activating factor antagonist BN 52063 on exertional asthma. *Pneumologie.* 1990 Feb;44 Suppl 1:347-8.

Willard T, Jones K. *Reishi Mushroom: Herb of Spiritual Potency and Medical Wonder.* Issaquah, Washington: Sylvan Press, 1990.

Willard T. *Edible and Medicinal Plants of the Rocky Mountains and Neighbouring Territories.* Calgary: 1992.

Willemsen LE, Koetsier MA, Balvers M, Beermann C, Stahl B, van Tol EA. Polyunsaturated fatty acids support epithelial barrier integrity and reduce IL-4 mediated permeability in vitro. *Eur J Nutr.* 2008 Jun;47(4):183-91.

Williams AB, Yu C, Tashima K, Burgess J, Danvers K. Evaluation of two self-care treatments for prevention of vaginal candidiasis in women with HIV. *J Assoc Nurses AIDS Care.* 2001 Jul-Aug;12(4):51-7.

Williams DM. Considerations in the long-term management of asthma in ambulatory patients. *AM J Health Sits Pham.* 2006;63:S14-21.

Wilson D, Evans M, Guthrie N, Sharma P, Baisley J, Schonlau F, Burki C. A randomized, double-blind, placebo-controlled exploratory study to evaluate the potential of pycnogenol for improving allergic rhinitis symptoms. *Phytother Res.* 2010 Aug;24(8):1115-9.

Wilson K, McDowall L, Hodge D, Chetcuti P, Cartledge P. Cow's milk protein allergy. *Community Pract.* 2010 May;83(5):40-1.

Wilson L. *Nutritional Balancing and Hair Mineral Analysis.* Prescott, AZ: LD Wilson, 1998.

REFERENCES AND BIBLIOGRAPHY

Wilson NM, Charette L, Thomson AH, Silverman M. Gastro-oesophageal reflux and childhood asthma: the acid test. *Thorax.* 1985 Aug;40(8):592-7.

Winchester AM. *Biology and its Relation to Mankind.* New York: Van Nostrand Reinhold, 1969.

Wiseman H. Vitamin D is a membrane antioxidant. Ability to inhibit iron-dependent lipid peroxidation in liposomes compared to cholesterol, ergosterol and tamoxifen and relevance to anticancer action. FEBS Lett. 1993 Jul 12;326(1-3):285-8.

Witsell DL, Garrett CG, Yarbrough WG, Dorrestein SP, Drake AF, Weissler MC. Effect of *Lactobacillus acidophilus* on antibiotic-associated gastrointestinal morbidity: a prospective randomized trial. *J Otolaryngol.* 1995 Aug;24(4):230-3.

Wittenberg JS. *The Rebellious Body.* New York: Insight, 1996.

Woessner KM, Simon RA, Stevenson DD. Monosodium glutamate sensitivity in asthma. *J Allergy Clin Immunol.* 1999 Aug;104(2 Pt 1):305-10.

Wöhrl S, Hemmer W, Focke M, Rappersberger K, Jarisch R. Histamine intolerance-like symptoms in healthy volunteers after oral provocation with liquid histamine. *Allergy Asthma Proc.* 2004 Sep-Oct;25(5):305-11.

Wolvers DA, van Herpen-Broekmans WM, Logman MH, van der Wielen RP, Albers R. Effect of a mixture of micronutrients, but not of bovine colostrum concentrate, on immune function parameters in healthy volunteers: a randomized placebo-controlled study. *Nutr J.* 2006 Nov 21;5:28.

Wolverton BC. *How to grow fresh air: 50 houseplants that purify your home or office.* New York: Penguin, 1997.

Wong GWK, Hui DSC, Chan HH, Fox TF, Leung R, Zhong NS, Chen YZ, Lai CKW. Prevalence of respiratory and atopic disorders in Chinese schoolchildren. *Clinical and Experimental Allergy.* 2001;31:1125-1231.

Wong WM, Lai KC, Lam KF, Hui WM, Hu WH, Lam CL, Xia HH, Huang JQ, Chan CK, Lam SK, Wong BC. Prevalence, clinical spectrum and health care utilization of gastro-oesophageal reflux disease in a Chinese population: a population-based study. *Aliment Pharmacol Ther.* 2003 Sep 15;18(6):595-604.

Wood M. *The Book of Herbal Wisdom.* Berkeley, CA: North Atlantic, 1997.

Wood RA, Kraynak J. *Food Allergies for Dummies.* Hoboken, NJ: Wiley Publ, 2007.

Woods RK, Abramson M, Bailey M, Walters EH. International prevalences of reported food allergies and intolerances. Comparisons arising from the European Community Respiratory Health Survey (ECRHS) 1991-1994. *Eur J Clin Nutr* 2001;55:298-304.

Woods RK, Abramson M, Raven JM, Bailey M, Weiner JM, Walters EH. Reported food intolerance and respiratory symptoms in young adults. *Eur Respir J.* 1998;11: 151-155.

Wouters EF, Reynaert NL, Dentener MA, Vernooy JH. Systemic and local inflammation in asthma and chronic obstructive pulmonary disease: is there a connection? *Proc Am Thorac Soc.* 2009 Dec;6(8):638-47.

Wright GR, Howieson S, McSharry C, McMahon AD, Chaudhuri R, Thompson J, Donnelly I, Brooks RG, Lawson A, Jolly L, McAlpine L, King EM, Chapman MD, Wood S, Thomson NC. Effect of improved home ventilation on asthma control and house dust mite allergen levels. *Allergy.* 2009 Nov;64(11):1671-80.

Wright RJ. Epidemiology of stress and asthma: from constricting communities and fragile families to epigenetics. *Immunol Allergy Clin North Am.* 2011 Feb;31(1):19-39.

Wu B, Yu J, Wang Y. Effect of Chinese herbs for tonifying Shen on balance of Th1 /Th2 in children with asthma in remission stage. *Zhongguo Zhong Xi Yi Jie He Za Zhi.* 2007 Feb;27(2):120-2.

Wu Q, Wu K, Ye Y, Dong X, Zhang J. Quorum sensing and its roles in pathogenesis among animal-associated pathogens—a review. *Wei Sheng Wu Xue Bao.* 2009 Jul 4;49(7):853-8.

Xi L, Han DM, Lü XF, Zhang L. Psychological characteristics in patients with allergic rhinitis and its associated factors analysis.. *Zhonghua Er Bi Yan Hou Tou Jing Wai Ke Za Zhi.* 2009 Dec;44(12):982-5.

Xiao JZ, Kondo S, Takahashi N, Miyaji K, Oshida K, Hiramatsu A, Iwatsuki K, Kokubo S, Hosono A. Effects of milk products fermented by *Bifidobacterium longum* on blood lipids in rats and healthy adult male volunteers. *J Dairy Sci.* 2003 Jul;86(7):2452-61.

Xiao JZ, Kondo S, Yanagisawa N, Miyaji K, Enomoto K, Sakoda T, Iwatsuki K, Enomoto T. Clinical efficacy of probiotic *Bifidobacterium longum* for the treatment of symptoms of Japanese cedar pollen allergy in subjects evaluated in an environmental exposure unit. *Allergol Int.* 2007 Mar;56(1):67-75.

Xiao JZ, Kondo S, Yanagisawa N, Takahashi N, Odamaki T, Iwabuchi N, Miyaji K, Iwatsuki K, Togashi H, Enomoto K, Enomoto T. Probiotics in the treatment of Japanese cedar pollinosis: a double-blind placebo-controlled trial. *Clin Exp Allergy.* 2006 Nov;36(11):1425-35.

Xiao JZ, Kondo S, Yanagisawa N, Takahashi N, Odamaki T, Iwabuchi N, Iwatsuki K, Kokubo S, Togashi H, Enomoto K, Enomoto T. Effect of probiotic *Bifidobacterium longum* BB536 in relieving clinical symptoms and modulating plasma cytokine levels of Japanese cedar pollinosis during the pollen season. A randomized double-blind, placebo-controlled trial. *J Investig Allergol Clin Immunol.* 2006;16(2):86-93.

Xiao P, Kubo H, Ohsawa M, Higashiyama K, Nagase H, Yan YN, Li JS, Kamei J, Ohmiya S. kappa-Opioid receptor-mediated antinociceptive effects of stereoisomers and derivatives of (+)-matrine in mice. *Planta Med.* 1999 Apr;65(3):230-3.

Xiao SD, Zhang DZ, Lu H, Jiang SH, Liu HY, Wang GS, Xu GM, Zhang ZB, Lin GJ, Wang GL. Multicenter, randomized, controlled trial of heat-killed *Lactobacillus acidophilus* LB in patients with chronic diarrhea. *Adv Ther.* 2003 Sep-Oct;20(5):253-60.

Xie JY, Dong JC, Gong ZH. Effects on herba epimedii and radix Astragali on tumor necrosis factor-alpha and nuclear factor-kappa B in asthmatic rats. *Zhongguo Zhong Xi Yi Jie He Za Zhi.* 2006 Aug;26(8):723-7.

Xu X, Zhang D, Zhang H, Wolters PJ, Killeen NP, Sullivan BM, Locksley RM, Lowell CA, Caughey GH. Neutrophil histamine contributes to inflammation in mycoplasma pneumonia. *J Exp Med.* 2006 Dec 25;203(13):2907-17.

Yadav H, Jain S, Sinha PR. Antidiabetic effect of probiotic dahl containing *Lactobacillus acidophilus* and *Lactobacillus casei* in high fructose fed rats. *Nutrition.* 2007 Jan;23(1):62-8.

Yadav RK, Ray RB, Vempati R, Bijlani RL. Effect of a comprehensive yoga-based lifestyle modification program on lipid peroxidation. *Indian J Physiol Pharmacol.* 2005 Jul-Sep;49(3):358-62.

Yadav VS, Mishra KP, Singh DP, Mehrotra S, Singh VK. Immunomodulatory effects of curcumin. *Immunopharmacol Immunotoxicol.* 2005;27(3):485-97.

Yadzir ZH, Misnan R, Abdullah N, Bakhtiar F, Arip M, Murad S. Identification of Ige-binding proteins of raw and cooked extracts of Loligo edulis (white squid). *Southeast Asian J Trop Med Public Health.* 2010 May;41(3):653-9.

Yamamura S, Morishima H, Kumano-go T, Suganuma N, Matsumoto H, Adachi H, Sigedo Y, Mikami A, Kai T, Masuyama A, Takano T, Sugita Y, Takeda M. The effect of *Lactobacillus helveticus* fermented milk on sleep and health perception in elderly subjects. *Eur J Clin Nutr.* 2009 Jan;63(1):100-5.

Yang Z. Are peanut allergies a concern for using peanut-based formulated foods in developing countries? *Food Nutr Bull.* 2010 Jun;31(2 Suppl):S147-53.

Yasuda T, Takeyama Y, Ueda T, Shinzeki M, Sawa H, Nakajima T, Kuroda Y. Breakdown of Intestinal Mucosa Via Accelerated Apoptosis Increases Intestinal Permeability in Experimental Severe Acute Pancreatitis. *J Surg Res.* 2006 Apr 4.

Yeager S. *The Doctor's Book of Food Remedies.* Emmaus, PA: Rodale Press, 1998.

Yeager S. The Doctor's Book of Food Remedies. Emmaus, PA: Rodale Press, 1998.

Yeh CC, Lin CC, Wang SD, Chen YS, Su BH, Kao ST. Protective and anti-inflammatory effect of a traditional Chinese medicine, Xia-Bai-San, by modulating lung local cytokine in a murine model of acute lung injury. *Int Immunopharmacol.* 2006 Sep;6(9):1506-14.

Yonekura S, Okamoto Y, Okawa T, Hisamitsu M, Chazono H, Kobayashi K, Sakurai D, Horiguchi S, Hanazawa T. Effects of daily intake of Lactobacillus paracasei strain KW3110 on Japanese cedar pollinosis. *Allergy Asthma Proc.* 2009 Jul-Aug;30(4):397-405.

Yu L, Zhang Y, Chen C, Cui HF, Yan XK. Meta-analysis on randomized controlled clinical trials of acupuncture for asthma. *Zhongguo Zhen Jiu.* 2010 Sep;30(9):787-92.

Yu LC. The epithelial gatekeeper against food allergy. *Pediatr Neonatol.* 2009 Dec;50(6):247-54.

Yusoff NA, Hampton SM, Dickerson JW, Morgan JB. The effects of exclusion of dietary egg and milk in the management of asthmatic children: a pilot study. *J R Soc Promot Health.* 2004 Mar;124(2):74-80.

Zanjanian MH. The intestine in allergic diseases. *Ann Allergy.* 1976 Sep;37(3):208-18.

Zarate G, Gonzalez S, Chaia AP. *Assessing survival of dairy propionibacteria in gastrointestinal conditions and adherence to intestinal epithelia. Centro de Referencia para Lactobacilos-CONICET.* Tucuman, Argentina: Humana Press. 2004.

Zarkadas M, Scott FW, Salminen J, Ham Pong A. Common Allergenic Foods and Their Labelling in Canada. *Can J Allergy Clin Immun.* 1999; 4:118-141.

Zeiger RS, Heller S. The development and prediction of atopy in high-risk children: follow-up at age seven years in a prospective randomized study of combined maternal and infant food allergen avoidance. *J Allergy Clin Immunol.* 1995 Jun;95(6):1179-90.

Zeng J, Li YQ, Zuo XL, Zhen YB, Yang J, Liu CH. Clinical trial: effect of active lactic acid bacteria on mucosal barrier function in patients with diarrhoea-predominant irritable bowel syndrome. *Aliment Pharmacol Ther.* 2008 Oct 15;28(8):994-1002.

Zhang CS, Yang AW, Zhang AL, Fu WB, Thien FU, Lewith G, Xue CC. Ear-acupressure for allergic rhinitis: a systematic review. *Clin Otolaryngol.* 2010 Feb;35(1):6-12.

Zhang T, Srivastava K, Wen MC, Yang N, Cao J, Busse P, Birmingham N, Goldfarb J, Li XM. Pharmacology and immunological actions of a herbal medicine ASHMI on allergic asthma. *Phytother Res.* 2010 Jul;24(7):1047-55.

Zhang Z, Lai HJ, Roberg KA, Gangnon RE, Evans MD, Anderson EL, Pappas TE, Dasilva DF, Tisler CJ, Salazar LP, Gern JE, Lemanske RF Jr. Early childhood weight status in relation to asthma development in high-risk children. *J Allergy Clin Immunol.* 2010 Dec;126(6):1157-62. 2010 Nov 4.

REFERENCES AND BIBLIOGRAPHY

Zhao FD, Dong JC, Xie JY. Effects of Chinese herbs for replenishing shen and strengthening qi on some indexes of neuro-endocrino-immune network in asthmatic rats. *Zhongguo Zhong Xi Yi Jie He Za Zhi.* 2007 Aug;27(8):715-9.

Zhao HY, Wang HJ, Lu Z, Xu SZ. Intestinal microflora in patients with liver cirrhosis. *Chin J Dig Dis.* 2004;5(2):64-7.

Zhao J, Bai J, Shen K, Xiang L, Huang S, Chen A, Huang Y, Wang J, Ye R. Self-reported prevalence of childhood allergic diseases in three cities of China: a multicenter study. *BMC Public Health.* 2010 Sep 13;10:551.

Zheng M. Experimental study of 472 herbs with antiviral action against the herpes simplex virus. *Zhong Xi Yi Jie He Za Zhi.* 1990 Jan;10(1):39-41, 6.

Zhou Q, Zhang B, Verne GN. Intestinal membrane permeability and hypersensitivity in the irritable bowel syndrome. *Pain.* 2009 Nov;146(1-2):41-6.

Zhu DD, Zhu XW, Jiang XD, Dong Z. Thymic stromal lymphopoietin expression is increased in nasal epithelial cells of patients with mugwort pollen sensitive-seasonal allergic rhinitis. *Chin Med J (Engl).* 2009 Oct 5;122(19):2303-7.

Zhu HH, Chen YP, Yu JE, Wu M, Li Z. Therapeutic effect of Xincang Decoction on chronic airway inflammation in children with bronchial asthma in remission stage. *Zhong Xi Yi Jie He Xue Bao.* 2005 Jan;3(1):23-7.

Ziaei Kajbaf T, Asar S, Alipoor MR. Relationship between obesity and asthma symptoms among children in Ahvaz, Iran:A cross sectional study. *Ital J Pediatr.* 2011 Jan 6;37(1):1.

Zielen S, Kardos P, Madonini E. Steroid-sparing effects with allergen-specific immunotherapy in children with asthma: a randomized controlled trial. *J Allergy Clin Immunol.* 2010 Nov;126(5):942-9. 2010 Jul 10.

Ziemniak W. Efficacy of *Helicobacter pylori* eradication taking into account its resistance to antibiotics. *J Physiol Pharmacol.* 2006 Sep;57 Suppl 3:123-41.

Ziment I, Tashkin DP. Alternative medicine for allergy and asthma. *J Allergy Clin Immunol.* 2000 Oct;106(4):603-14.

Ziment I. Alternative therapies for asthma. *Curr Opin Pulm Med.* 1997 Jan;3(1):61-71.

Zizza, C. The nutrient content of the Italian food supply 1961-1992. *Euro J Clin Nutr.* 1997;51: 259-265.

Zoccatelli G, Pokoj S, Foetisch K, Bartra J, Valero A, Del Mar San Miguel-Moncin M, Vieths S, Scheurer S. Identification and characterization of the major allergen of green bean (Phaseolus vulgaris) as a nonspecific lipid transfer protein (Pha v 3). *Mol Immunol.* 2010 Apr;47(7-8):1561-8.

Zwolińska-Wcisło M, Brzozowski T, Mach T, Budak A, Trojanowska D, Konturek PC, Pajdo R, Drozdowicz D, Kwiecień S. Are probiotics effective in the treatment of fungal colonization of the gastrointestinal tract? Experimental and clinical studies. *J Physiol Pharmacol.* 2006 Nov;57 Suppl 9:35-49.

Index

(Herbs, foods and other natural solutions are too numerous to index)

* 9 7 8 1 9 3 6 2 5 1 4 7 6 *